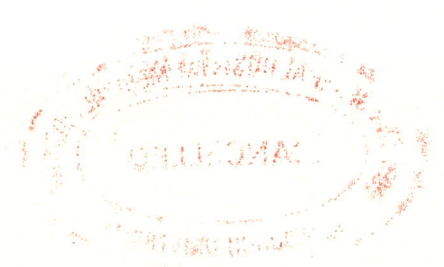

Carcinoma-in-situ and Cancer of the Testis
BIOLOGY AND TREATMENT

Proceedings of a workshop held in Copenhagen, Denmark August 1986

EDITED BY
M. RØRTH
G. DAUGAARD
N. E. SKAKKEBÆK
K. M. GRIGOR
A. GIWERCMAN

BLACKWELL SCIENTIFIC PUBLICATIONS
OXFORD LONDON EDINBURGH
BOSTON PALO ALTO MELBOURNE

© 1987 by
Blackwell Scientific Publications
Editorial offices:
Osney Mead, Oxford OX2 0EL
8 John Street, London WC1N 2ES
23 Ainslie Place, Edinburgh EH3 6AJ
52 Beacon Street, Boston
   Massachusetts 02108, USA
667 Lytton Avenue, Palo Alto
   California 94301, USA
107 Barry Street, Carlton
   Victoria 3053, Australia

All rights reserved. No part of this publication may be reproduced, stored in a retrieval system, or transmitted, in any form or by any means, electronic, mechanical, photocopying, recording or otherwise without the prior permission of the copyright owner

First published 1987
Reprinted 1988

Printed in Great Britain at the Alden Press, Oxford

DISTRIBUTORS

USA
   Year Book Medical Publishers
   35 East Wacker Drive
   Chicago, Illinois 60601

Canada
   The C. V. Mosby Company
   5240 Finch Avenue East,
   Scarborough, Ontario

Australia
   Blackwell Scientific Publications
   (Australia) Pty Ltd
   107 Barry Street
   Carlton, Victoria 3053

British Library
Cataloguing in Publication Data

Carcinoma-in-situ and cancer of the testis :
   biology and treatment : proceedings of a
   workshop held in Copenhagen, Denmark,
   August 1986.
   1. Testis—Cancer
   I. Rørth, Mikael   II. International Journal
   of Andrology
   616.99'463   RC280.T4

ISBN 0-632-01706-6

INTERNATIONAL JOURNAL OF ANDROLOGY
Volume 10, Number 1, 1987, Special Issue

Contents

Foreword ix

Session 1: Normal and malignant germ cell, comparative aspects
    Chairman: K. M. Grigor

A. F. Holstein, B. Schütte, H. Becker and M. Hartmann:
Morphology of normal and malignant germ cells 1
    Discussion: Grigor, Holstein, Jacobsen, Niemi, Jacobsen, Skakkebæk, Müller

N. E. Skakkebæk, J. Berthelsen, A. Giwercman and J. Müller:
Carcinoma-in-situ of the testis: possible origin from gonocytes and precursor of all types of germ cell tumours, except spermatocytoma 19
    Discussion: Holstein, Skakkebæk, Grigor, Jacobsen

J. Hustin, J. Collette and P. Franchimont:
Immunohistochemical demonstration of placental alkaline phosphatase in various states of testicular development and in germ cell tumours 29
    Discussion: Grigor, Hustin, Jacobsen

P. Pöllänen and M. Niemi:
Immunohistochemical identification of macrophages, lymphoid cells and HLA antigens in the human testis 37
    Discussion: Hargreave, Pöllänen, Müller, Skakkebæk

N. B. Friedman:
The function of the primordial germ cell in extragonadal tissues 43
    Discussion: Grigor, Friedman

W. F. J. Feitz, F. M. J. Debruyne and F. C. S. Ramaekers:
Intermediate filament proteins as tissue specific markers in normal and neoplastic testicular tissue 51
    Discussion: Skakkebæk, Debruyne, Oliver, Jacobsen, Holstein, Niemi

Session 2: Oncogenes and germ cell cancer
    Chairman: K. M. Grigor

K. Sikora, G. Evan and J. Watson:
Oncogenes and germ cell tumours 57
    Discussion: Engström, Sikora, Niemi, Oosterhuis

Celia D. De Lozier-Blanchet, H. Walt, E. Engel and P. Vaugnat:
Cytogenetic studies of human testicular germ cell tumours 69

W. Engström, B. Hopkins and P. Schofield:
Expression of growth regulatory genes in primary human testicular neoplasms 79
  Discussion: Sikora, Engström, Walt, Niemi

R. T. D. Oliver:
HLA phenotype and clinicopathological behaviour of germ cell tumours: possible evidence for clonal evolution from seminomas to nonseminomas 85
  Discussion: Dieckmann, Oliver, Bannwart, Skakkebæk, Oosterhuis, Grigor, Rørth, Müller

Session 3: Biochemical, histochemical and ultrastructural markers of malignant germ cells. Culture systems
  Chairman: M. Niemi

P. W. Andrews, B. Fenderson and Sen-itiroh Hakamori:
Human embryonal carcinoma cells and their differentiation in culture 95
  Discussion: Holstein, Andrews, Safirstein, Oosterhuis, Walt, Niemi, Vogelzang

J. Casper, H.-J. Schmoll, U. Schnaid and C. Fonatsch:
Cell lines of human germinal cancer 105
  Discussion: Niemi, Casper, Jacobsen, Walt, Oosterhuis, Vogelzang, Oliver

G. W. Sledge, Jr, J. N. Eble, B. J. Roth, B. P. Wuhrman and L. H. Einhorn:
Flow cytometry derived DNA content of the primary lesions of advanced germ cell tumours 115
  Discussion: Oosterhuis, Sledge, Niemi, Rustin

M. Sehested and Grete K. Jacobsen:
Ultrastructure of syncytiotrophoblast-like cells in seminomas of the testis 121
  Discussion: Holstein, Sehested, Niemi, Grigor, Walt

H. M. Rabes:
Proliferation of human testicular tumours 127
  Discussion: Niemi, Rabes, Oliver, Skakkebæk, Safirstein, Ikinger

A. Harstrick, J. Casper and H.-J. Schmoll:
Comparative antitumour activity of cisplatin and two new cisplatin-analogues JM8 and JM9 in human testicular carcinoma xenografts 139
  Discussion: Niemi, Harstrick, Vogelzang, Safirstein, Andrews, Schmoll, Oliver

J. Müller, N. E. Skakkebæk and M. Constance Parkinson:
The spermatocytic seminoma: views on pathogenesis 147
  Discussion: Holstein, Müller, Niemi, Friedman, Jacobsen, Grigor, Skakkebæk

Raija Malmi and K.-O. Söderström
Lectin binding sites in human seminiferous epithelium, in CIS cells and in seminomas 157
  Discussion: Niemi, Malmi

D. Lehmann and Hj. Müller:
Analysis of the autoimmune response in an '*in-situ*' carcinoma of the testis   163
    Discussion: Oliver, Lehmann, Niemi, Walt

M. Niemi (Chairman):
General discussion on the biology of malignant germ cells   169
    Discussion: Hargreave, Holstein, Niemi, Jacobsen, Grigor, Walt, Skakkebæk, Engström

Session 4: Clinical aspects of carcinoma-in-situ
    Chairman: T. B. Hargreave

A. Giwercman, J. G. Berthelsen, J. Müller, H. von der Maase and N. E. Skakkebæk:
Screening for carcinoma-in-situ of the testis   173
    Discussion: Hargreave, Giwercman, Skakkebæk, Bannwart, Rankin, Dieckmann, Vogelzang, Oliver, Jackson, Ikinger

K. V. Pedersen, P. Boiesen and C. G. Zetterlund:
Experience of screening for carcinoma-in-situ of the testis among young men with surgically corrected maldescended testes   181
    Discussion: Hargreave, Pedersen, Skakkebæk, Giwercman, Wahlqvist

Suzan Lenz, A. Giwercman, N. E. Skakkebæk, E. Bruun and C. Frimodt-Møller:
Ultrasound in detection of early neoplasia of the testis   187

C. Thomsen, K. E. Jensen, A. Giwercman, L. Kjær, O. Henriksen and N. E. Skakkebæk:
Magnetic resonance: *in vivo* tissue characterization of the testes in patients with carcinoma-in-situ of the testis and healthy subjects   191

E. Bruun, C. Frimodt-Møller, A. Giwercman, Suzan Lenz and N. E. Skakkebæk:
Testicular biopsy as an outpatient procedure in screening for carcinoma-in-situ: complications and the patients' acceptance   199
    Discussion: Hargreave, Bruun, Schraffordt Koops, Skakkebæk

Anne Østerlind, J. G. Berthelsen, N. Abildgaard, S. O. Hansen and others: (Poster)
Incidence of bilateral testicular germ cell cancer in Denmark 1960–1984: preliminary findings   203

H. von der Maase, A. Giwercman, J. Müller and N. E. Skakkebæk:
Management of carcinoma-in-situ of the testis   209
    Discussion: Hargreave, von der Maase, Skakkebæk, Oliver, Berthelsen, Einhorn, Holstein, Bannwart

T. B. Hargreave (Chairman):
General discussion on carcinoma-in-situ   221
    Discussion: Willis, Pedersen, Müller, Hargreave, Skakkebæk, Jackson, Bannwart, Berthelsen, Grigor, Hartlapp, Bruun, Jacobsen, Dieckmann, Weidner, von der Maase, Friedman

Session 5: Prognostic factors of testicular cancer

Chairman: T. B. Hargreave

N. J. Vogelzang:
Prognostic factors in metastatic testicular cancer 225
Discussion: Hargreave, Oliver, Vogelzang, Hansen, Bosl

G. Stoter, R. Sylvester, D. Th. Sleijfer, W. W. ten Bokkel Huinink and others:
Multivariate analysis of prognostic variables in patients with disseminated non-seminomatous testicular cancer: results from an EORTC multi-institutional phase III study 239
Discussion: Hargreave, Rustin, Stoter, Dieckmann, Levi, Oliver

Session 6: Treatment of testicular tumour patients with good prognosis

Chairman: L. H. Einhorn

M. J. Peckham and M. Brada:
Surveillance following orchidectomy for stage I testicular cancer 247
Discussion: Pizzocaro, Brada, Vogelzang, Debruyne, Oliver, Scardino, Skakkebæk

M. Rørth, H. von der Maase, E. S. Nielsen, M. Pedersen and H. Schultz:
Orchidectomy alone versus orchidectomy plus radiotherapy in stage I nonseminomatous testicular cancer: a randomized study by the Danish Testicular Carcinoma Study Group 255
Discussion: Pizzocaro, Rørth, Einhorn, Oliver, Bannwart, Brada, Skakkebæk, Debruyne

R. T. D. Oliver:
Limitations to the use of surveillance as an option in the management of stage I seminoma 263
Discussion: von der Maase, Oliver

G. Pizzocaro:
Retroperitoneal lymph node dissection in clinical stage IIA and IIB non-seminomatous germ cell tumours of the testis 269
Discussion: Ozols, Pizzocaro, Vogelzang, Einhorn, Debruyne

J. H. Hartlapp, L. Weissbach and R. Bussar-Maatz:
Adjuvant chemotherapy in nonseminomatous testicular tumour stage II 277
Discussion: Rankin, Hartlapp, Oliver, Einhorn, Brada, Pizzocaro

Session 7: Treatment of testicular tumour patients with poor prognosis

Chairman: L. H. Einhorn

G. J. Bosl, D. Bajorin and N. L. Geller:
An analysis of poor risk assignment in patients with germ cell tumours 285
Discussion: Hansen, Bosl, Levi, Oliver

R. F. Ozols:
Treatment of poor prognosis germ cell tumours with high dose cisplatin regimens   291
   Discussion: Safirstein, Ozols, Rørth, Pizzocaro, Levi, Vogelzang

E. S. Newlands, K. D. Bagshawe, R. H. J. Begent, G. J. S. Rustin, S. M. Crawford and L. Holden:
Treatment of patients with poor prognosis anaplastic germ cell tumours (AGCT) of the testis and other sites   301
   Discussion: Schraffordt Koops, Newlands, Grigor, Rørth, Bosl, Safirstein

H. J. Schmoll, I. Schubert, H. Arnold, G. Dölken and others:
Disseminated testicular cancer with bulky disease: results of a phase-II study with cisplatin ultra high dose/VP-16/bleomycin   311
   Discussion: Ozols, Schmoll

Gedske Daugaard, H. H. Hansen and M. Rørth:
Management of advanced metastatic germ cell tumours   319
   Discussion: Pizzocaro, Daugaard, Ozols, Einhorn, Safirstein, Schmoll, Rørth

Session 8: Treatment toxicity
   Chairman: H.-J. Schmoll

R. Safirstein, J. Winston, D. Moel, S. Dikman and J. Guttenplan:
Cisplatin nephrotoxicity: insight into mechanism   325
   Discussion: Levi, Safirstein, Oosterhuis, Friedman, Grigor, Schmoll

Gedske Daugaard, U. Abildgaard, N. H. Holstein-Rathlou, O. Amtorp and P. P. Leyssac:
Effect of cisplatin on renal haemodynamics and tubular function in the dog kidney   347
   Discussion: Vogelzang, Daugaard

G. J. Bosl, S. P. Leitner, S. A. Atlas, J. E. Sealey, J. J. Preibisz and E. Scheiner:
Altered renin and aldosterone excretion in patients treated for metastatic germ cell tumours   353
   Discussion: Rustin, Bosl, Rankin, Einhorn, Safirstein

G. Laurell, B. Engström, A. Hirsch and D. Bagger-Sjöbäck:
Ototoxicity of cisplatin   359
   Discussion: Salomon, Laurell, Safirstein, Schmoll

B. L. Samuels, N. J. Vogelzang and B. J. Kennedy:
Vascular toxicity following vinblastine, bleomycin and cisplatin therapy for germ cell tumours   363
   Discussion: Schmoll, Vogelzang, Oliver, Einhorn

Session 9: Fertility problems

    Chairman: T. B. Hargreave

J. G. Berthelsen:
Testicular cancer and fertility   371

G. J. Bosl and D. Bajorunas:
Pituitary and testicular hormonal function after treatment for germ cell tumours   381

P. Fried, R. Steinfeld, B. Casileth and A. Steinfeld:
Incidence of developmental handicaps among the offspring of men treated for testicular seminoma   385

G. J. S. Rustin, D. Pektasides, K. D. Bagshawe, E. S. Newlands and R. H. J. Begent:
Fertility after chemotherapy for male and female germ cell tumours   389

T. B. Hargreave (Chairman):
General discussion on fertility and testicular cancer   393
    Discussion: Hargreave, Skakkebæk, Bosl, Berthelsen, Rustin, Safirstein, Vogelzang, Friedman, Fried, Grigor, Schmoll, Brada, Delozier-Blanchet

Session 10: Overall treatment planning

    Chairman: H.-J. Schmoll

L. H. Einhorn:
Treatment strategies of testicular cancer in the United States   399
    Discussion: Grigor, Einhorn, Pizzocaro, Schmoll, Oliver, Rørth

G. Stoter:
Treatment strategies of testicular cancer in Europe   407
    Discussion: Rørth, Stoter

Session 11: Concluding remarks

M. Niemi:
Biology of germ cell tumours: Concluding remarks   417

T. B. Hargreave:
Clinical aspects of carcinoma-in-situ (CIS): Concluding remarks   421

N. J. Vogelzang:
Treatment of germ cell tumours: Concluding remarks   423

Author index   425

Subject index   427

Foreword

In November 1980 a workshop entitled 'Early Detection of Testicular Cancer' was held in Copenhagen (Skakkebæk et al., 1981). Since this event remarkable progress has taken place both in the areas of early detection and in the treatment of testicular cancer.

Carcinoma-in-situ has now been widely accepted as the early stage of testicular cancer. The diagnosis of this condition in risk groups has therefore become a major issue.

Concerning patients with testicular cancer, 95% of these can now be completely cured by the combined use of treatment modalities. Efforts are therefore directed towards decreasing overall toxicity of treatment without loss of efficacy in the vast majority of patients and towards the development of more effective drug regimens in the group of patients with poor prognosis.

Despite progress in these areas of research, the aetiology of testicular cancer is still poorly understood, as are the very early stages of neoplastic development. Techniques of modern biology including the use of monoclonal antibodies and cultured cell lines, and the investigation of oncogenes, will conceivably be of great help in increasing our knowledge of aetiology and pathogenesis.

It was with this background that a workshop on testicular cancer was held in Copenhagen in August 1986. This book contains the proceedings of the workshop and includes a full account of the discussions which followed each paper given by experts in their field.

The workshop was supported by the Danish Cancer Society, the Danish Medical Research Council, the Daell Foundation, the Tuborg Foundation, and the Lundbeck Foundation.

The organizing committee is grateful to Ms Birgitte Bruun, Ms Elin Dahms, and Mrs Margo Boyle for their invaluable and very professional help.

Mikael Rørth *Kenneth M. Grigor*
Gedske Daugaard *Aleksander Giwercman*
Niels Erik Skakkebæk

Reference
Skakkebæk, N. E., Berthelsen, J. G., Grigor, K. M. & Visfeldt, J. (Eds) (1981) *Early Detection of Testicular Cancer*. Scriptor, Copenhagen.

The views expressed in these proceedings are the responsibility of the authors of the individual papers and are not necessarily those of the organisers and editors

Carcinoma-in-situ
and Cancer of the Testis
BIOLOGY AND TREATMENT

Morphology of normal and malignant germ cells*

A. F. HOLSTEIN,[1] B. SCHÜTTE,[2] H. BECKER[3] and M. HARTMANN[4]   [1]Department of Microscopical Anatomy, [2]Department of Andrology, [3]Clinic of Urology, University of Hamburg, and [4]Armed Forces Hospital Hamburg-Wandsbek, Federal Republic of Germany

Summary

By means of semithin section histology and electron microscopy the following male germ cells are described: gonocytes and prospermatogonia in the embryonic and fetal testes; spermatogonia and primary spermatocytes in the testis of the adult; abnormal spermatogonia and spermatocytes, which are not tumour cells. In contrast to these cells, four main tumour cell types which on the basis of morphological criteria can be said to be derived from germ cells, are classified and designated as Tc 1 to Tc 4. The various tissues accompanying the tumour cells are briefly described.

Key words. Testis tumour, malignant germ cells, ultrastructure.

Introduction

In the histopathological assessment of testicular tumours, paraffin sections of representative samples of the tissue are normally examined and the diagnosis is based on the overall appearance of the entire surgically excised specimen. A single, supposedly comprehensive, diagnostic term is used to summarize the tumour components and the different types of tissue present.

An alternative approach is to make detailed investigations of the material using semithin sections and finally electron microscopy thereby concentrating on the cellular aspects of testicular tumours. Such studies indicate that uniformity of cellular morphology is only encountered in solid areas of seminoma, and in the cells of carcinoma-in-situ. All other testicular tumours show a combination of diverse tumour cell types with different appearances interspersed with accompanying non-tumour elements so that a single summarizing term does not describe the component parts at the cellular level and may be confusing. The identification of cell types and their variants, and their relationship to germ cells poses the greatest problems.

It may be argued that tumour cells are no longer germ cells, and, if so, the term 'malignant germ cells' is surely inappropriate and misleading. In spite of this reservation, we accept the invitation of the organizing committee of this symposium and we shall describe the cellular elements of testicular tumours.

---

* Parts of Tc4 description will be published separately in cooperation with K. Dressler and H. Lauke in *Andrologia*, 1987.

Correspondence: Prof. Dr. med. A. F. Holstein, Abteilung fur Mikroskopische Anatomie, Martinistr. 52, 2000 Hamburg 20, F.R.G.

Germ cells during embryonic and fetal life

In order to recognize malignant cells and to be able to differentiate them from normal germ cells, a review of the morphology of normal germ cells in the embryo, fetus and adult will be given in the first instance.

The investigation of human germ cells during embryonic and fetal life is incomplete and the results are still fragmentary (Wartenberg, 1981). The names of the different types of germ cell are not strictly defined, and therefore there is uncertainty in the nomenclature used by different research groups.

After primordial germ cells have invaded the gonadal anlage and once they have entered the testicular cords, primitive germ cells can be distinguished from gonocytes (Gondos, 1977). The subsequent developmental stages of germ cells are designated 'prospermatogonia' which turn into type A spermatogonia by the beginning of puberty at the latest. From this developmental sequence of the early germ cells, the stages of the 8th, 10th, 13th and 22nd week of pregnancy have been chosen to describe the characteristic features of the germ cells.

In an 8-week male embryo, the germ cells are located in the testicular cords and are already readily recognized by light microscopy because of their abundance of glycogen (Fig. 1). The cells have a relatively large nucleus with a large nucleolus. The cytoplasm contains round mitochondria whose internal tubular structures appear slightly dilated. The Golgi apparatus is not very prominent. Much glycogen is found equally distributed in the cytoplasm except for a marginal space beneath the plasmalemma. This peripheral margin is filled with microfilaments which lie directly adjacent to the plasmalemma and also the microfilaments extend within cytoplasmic processes in various directions out from the cell. In many cells there are numerous vacuoles and flat cisterns of endoplasmic reticulum (ER).

This very characteristic cellular pattern of germ cells in the 8-week embryo is also seen in 10-week embryos and in some of the cells of fetuses in the 13th week, and these cells may be considered as being 'gonocytes'. Further distinctive types of germ cells can be identified from these gonocytes particularly in older fetuses and these other cells begin to exhibit some of the features of spermatogonia. Their nuclei and nucleoli are a little larger and glycogen deposits are no longer visible (Fig. 2). Furthermore, there are some cell types which are considered as fetal spermatogonia (Wartenberg, Holstein & Vossmeyer, 1971). Their mitochondria are also round but possess internal cristate structures and are connected to each other by intermitochondrial cement, the typical feature of adult spermatozoa.

Spermatogonia and primary spermatocytes in the adult

In the adult, the germ cells comprise all the cell types of complete spermatogenesis. For the estimation of the relationship of germ cells to testicular tumour cells, only the various types of spermatogonia and primary spermatocytes are to be considered. Testicular tumours associated with secondary spermatocytes or spermatids do not occur.

The following types of germ cell are recognized (Holstein & Roosen-Runge, 1981):

1. *Type A pale spermatogonium*

This cell normally rests with a broad base on the basal lamina of the seminiferous tubule (Fig. 3). It has a nucleus with finely granular karyoplasm and a relatively small nucleolus. The cytoplasm appears transparent. Rather long mitochondria, which are sometimes connected with one another by an electron-dense cement substance, lie near to the nucleus. This type of germ cell is always present in seminiferous tubules as long as spermatogenesis is taking place.

A special form of this type of spermatogonium, the type A long spermatogonium (Fig. 5) may be recognized. It has a rather long nucleus but otherwise has no special feature in the cytoplasm.

2. *Type A dark spermatogonium*

The second type of spermatogonium, occurring nearly as frequently as the A pale type, is a cell with a striking brightness within the karyoplasm and increased deposition of glycogen in the cytoplasm (Fig. 4). The cytoplasm therefore becomes more intensely stainable indicating the presence of more formed constituents. This type of spermatogonium is called 'A dark' because of the staining characteristics. However, the quantity of glycogen in the cytoplasm may vary considerably and sometimes membrane bound deposits of glycogen may even occur.

A presumably special form of type A dark spermatogonium is represented by the A cloudy type (Schulze, 1978) (Fig. 6). In such cells the karyoplasm has a flocculent or cloudy appearance.

Intercellular bridges are found in association with all type A spermatogonia.

3. *Type B spermatogonium*

The type B spermatogonium is recognizable by its nucleus which contains several nucleoli. Under the electron microscope the karyoplasm has a roughly granular appearance (Fig. 7). The mitochondria are round with cristate internal structures and are not connected with one another by cement substance. Vesicles of ER and granules of glycogen are distributed in the cytoplasm. The Golgi apparatus is not striking. B spermatogonia are mostly attached to the basal lamina but sometimes their nuclei have already shifted somewhat from their marginal location in the tubule towards a more central position.

Primary spermatocytes arise from the B spermatogonia. Whether or not the primary spermatocytes are involved in the formation of testicular tumours has to be doubted. In the literature there are tumours described as being 'spermatocytic seminomas' on the basis of light microscopy on paraffin sections. In the material at our disposal we have tissue from more than 400 patients with testicular tumours: all these have been thoroughly studied by means of semithin sections and electron microscopy but to date there has not been a single case showing tumour tissue which resembles spermatocytes. However, although we do not have material to substantiate the claims in the literature, the appearance of normal primary spermatocytes will now be described.

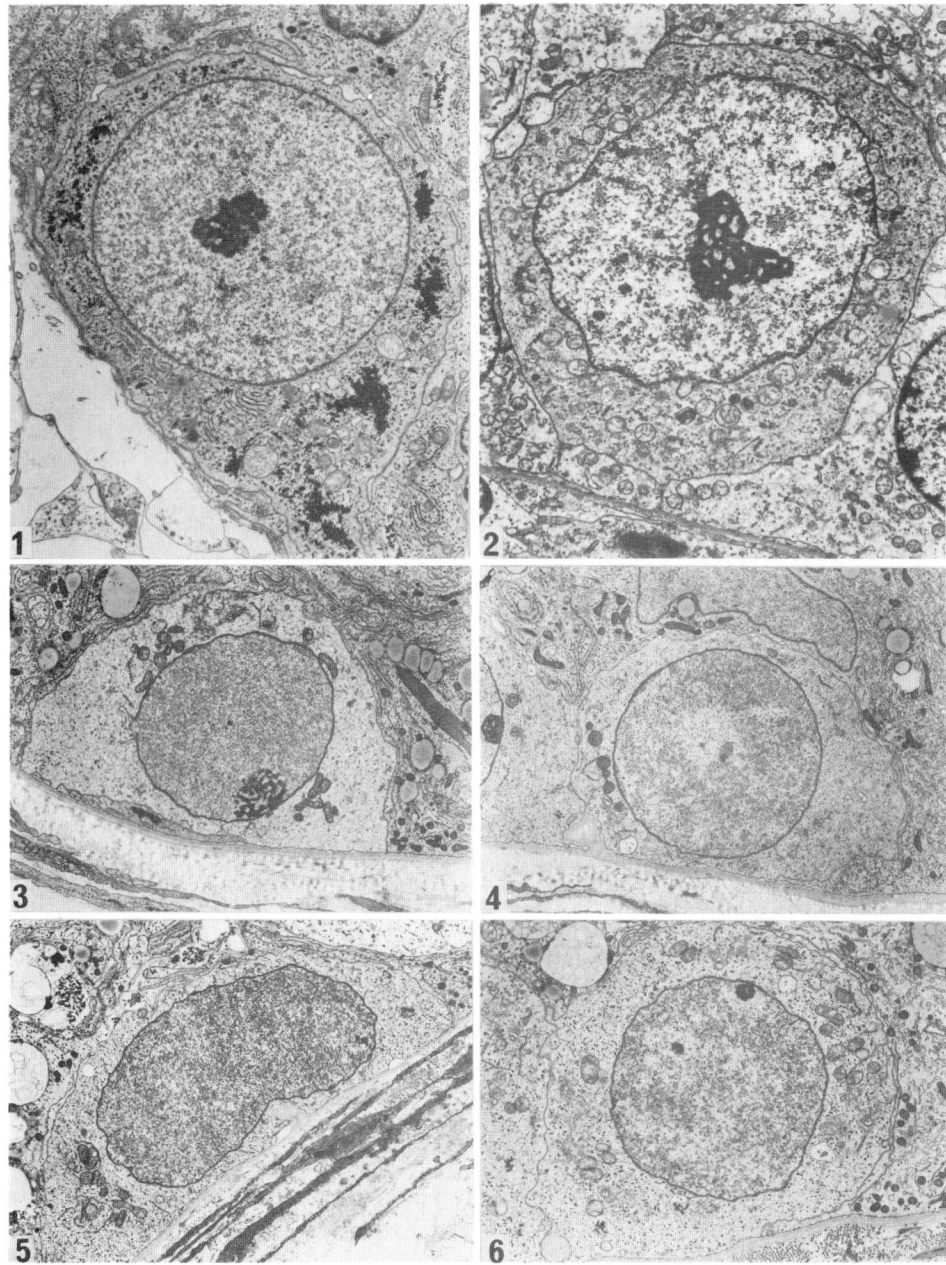

Fig. 1. Gonocyte in the testicular cord of an 8-week-old male embryo. ×5100.
Fig. 2. Prospermatogonium (fetal spermatogonium) of a 13-week-old male fetus. ×5100.
Fig. 3. Type A pale spermatogonium in the adult. ×4600.
Fig. 4. Type A dark spermatogonium. ×4600.
Fig. 5. Type A long spermatogonium. ×4600.
Fig. 6. Type A cloudy spermatogonium. ×4600.

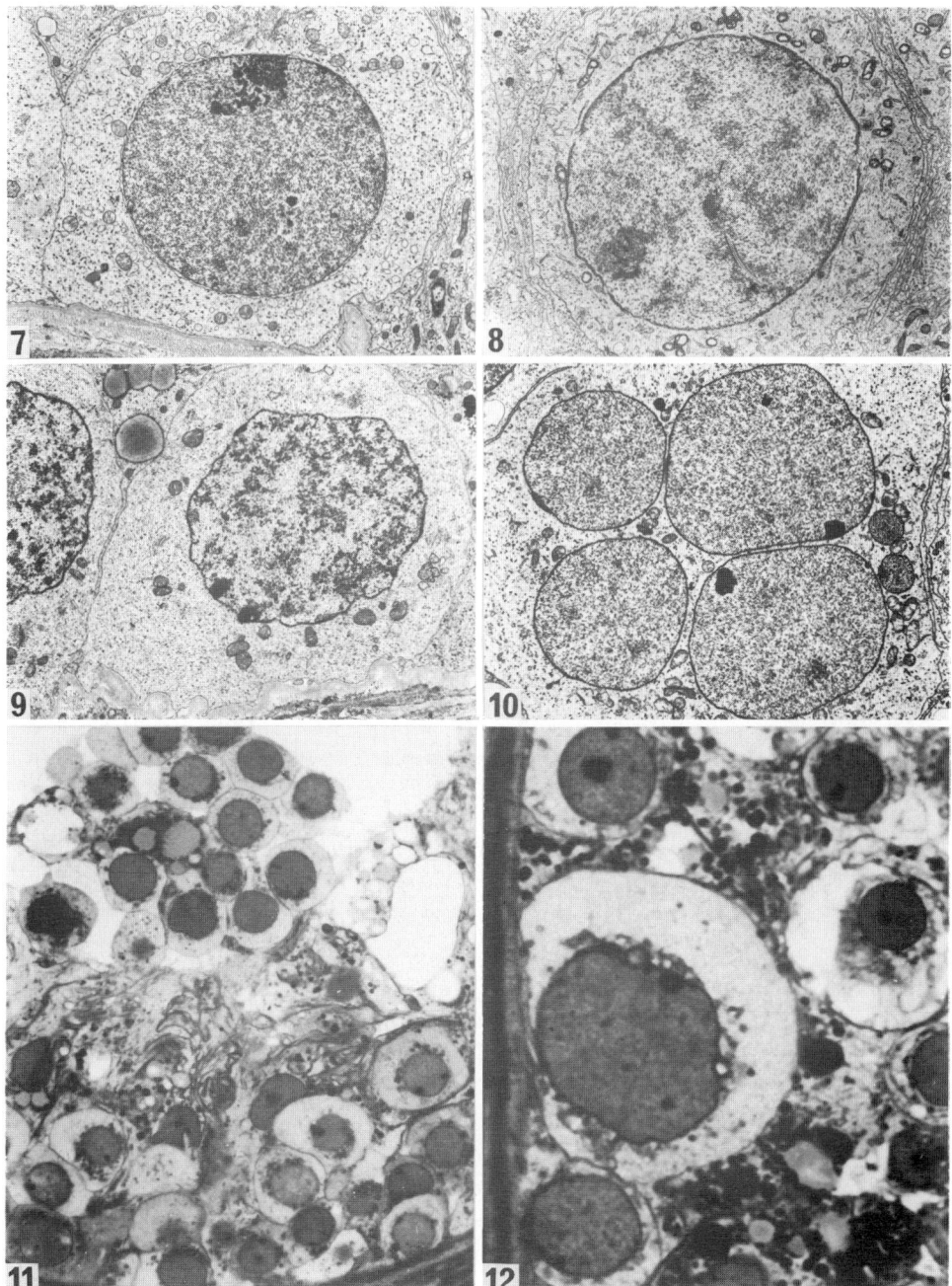

Fig. 7. Type B spermatogonium. ×4600.
Fig. 8. Primary spermatocyte. ×4600.
Fig. 9. Abnormal spermatogonium with atypical karyoplasm. ×4600.
Fig. 10. Multinucleated spermatogonium. ×4600.
Fig. 11. Multilayered type A spermatogonia in the basal compartment of the germinal epithelium and in the tubular lumen. ×840.
Fig. 12. Large, apparently polyploid spermatogonium. ×1600.

4. Primary spermatocyte

The primary spermatocytes are the largest cells in the germinal epithelium (Fig. 8). The chromosome pattern in the nucleus has many different forms corresponding to the various stages of meiotic prophase, from preleptotene to diplotene. Best recognized is the appearance of paired chromosomes each of which consists of two lateral elements and a central connection. This picture is most prominent during zygotene. In the subsequent stages of prophase the chromosomes shorten and are seen predominantly as dark strands of chromatin. Close to the perinuclear cistern there are further layers of flat cisterns of ER. Round mitochondria are found within the cytoplasm and these show widely dilated internal structures and are connected in groups by intermitochondrial cement substance. The Golgi apparatus is relatively large and in some spermatocytes there are already large vesicles resembling proacrosomal vesicles because they are filled with electron-dense substance.

Abnormal germ cells

Amongst the A spermatogonia and primary spermatocytes there are some abnormal cell forms which are certainly not tumour cells but might be mistaken for such. The recognition of these abnormal germ cells enhances the identification of the frankly neoplastic cells.

An uncommon histological picture of multilayering of the type A pale spermatogonia is sometimes seen in tubules of men of advanced age (Holstein, Bustos-Obregon & Hartmann, 1984) (Fig. 11). In addition, type A pale spermatogonia may appear in the tubular lumen after having passed the Sertoli cell barrier.

In some patients with disturbances of spermatogenesis, type A spermatogonia with large nuclei are found with greater frequency than under normal conditions. These nuclei are presumably polypoid. The large nuclei of such spermatogonia may look like type A pale nuclei, but other cells have nuclei with type A dark characteristics.

Abnormal patterns of karyoplasm may be observed in the nuclei of some spermatogonia (Fig. 9), their appearance resembling the prophase nuclei of primary spermatocytes. In such cases only electron microscopical investigation reveals that the cells are not in that stage of meiosis but have an abnormal framework of nuclear chromatin.

Commonly found are multinucleated spermatogonia (Fig. 10). Their nuclei may be all of the same type, either type A pale or type A dark. However, sometimes different types of nuclei are seen in one cell with type A pale and dark both being present, and sometimes even nuclear fragments within a symplasm are observed (Schulze, 1981).

Among the spermatocytes, there are three uncommon nuclear patterns which may be seen: (a) primary spermatocytes exhibiting nuclei without chromosomal strands; (b) megalospermatocytes (Holstein & Eckmann, 1986) with very large nuclei but without pairing of chromosomes; (c) primary spermatocytes with persistence of the zygonemal structures up to diplotene. These cells are the result of a disturbance during meiosis.

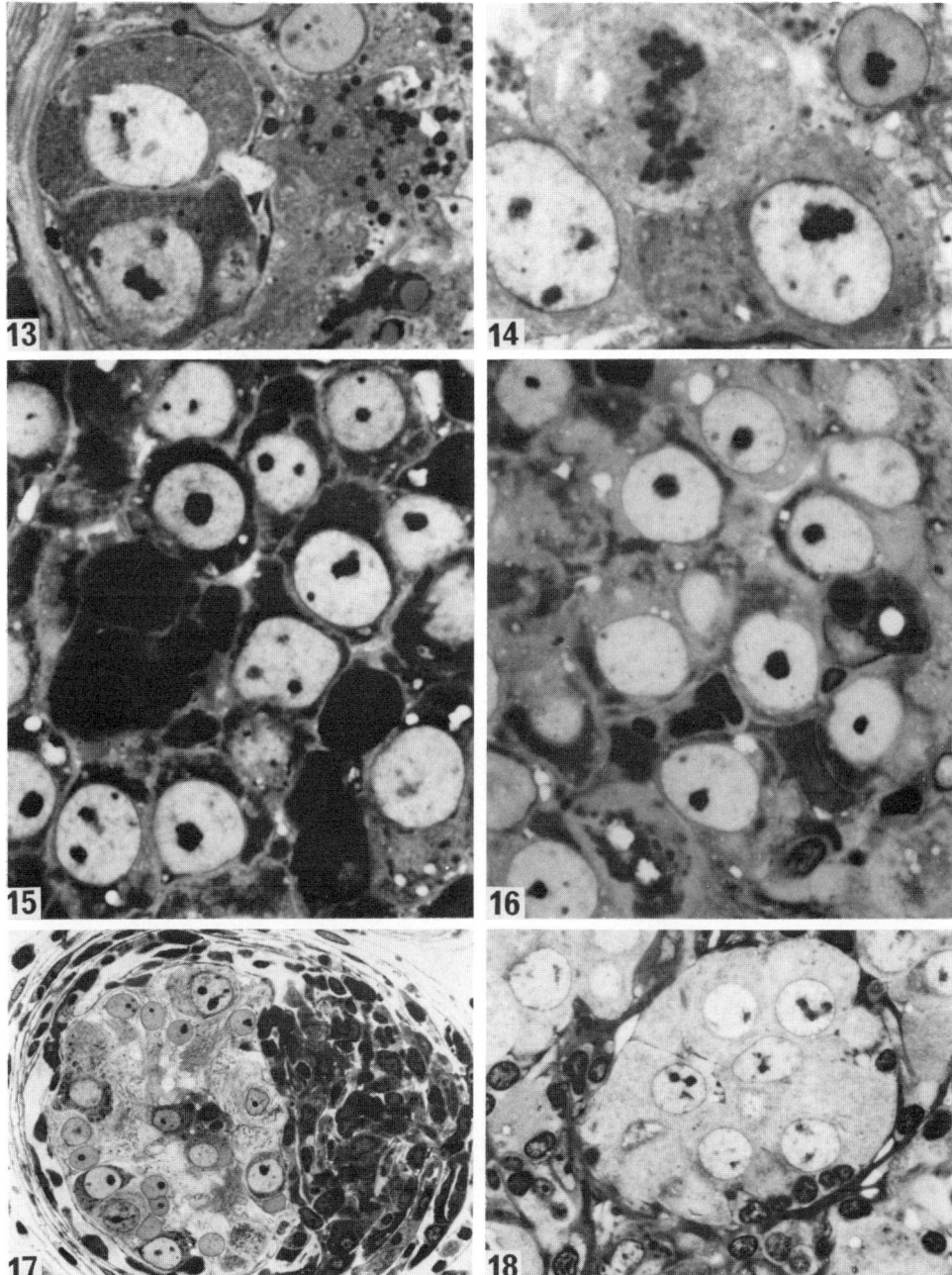

Fig. 13. Intratubular tumour cells (Tc 1). ×1400.
Fig. 14. Mitosis of intratubular tumour cells (Tc 1). ×1600.
Fig. 15. Tc 1 in the periphery of a solid seminoma. ×1400.
Fig. 16. Tc 2 in the centre of a solid seminoma. ×1400.
Fig. 17. Accompanying tissue (lymphocytes) in the lamina propria of a tubule showing Tc 1 in between Sertoli cells. ×420.
Fig. 18. Clusters of Tc 2 surrounded by lymphocytes. ×420.

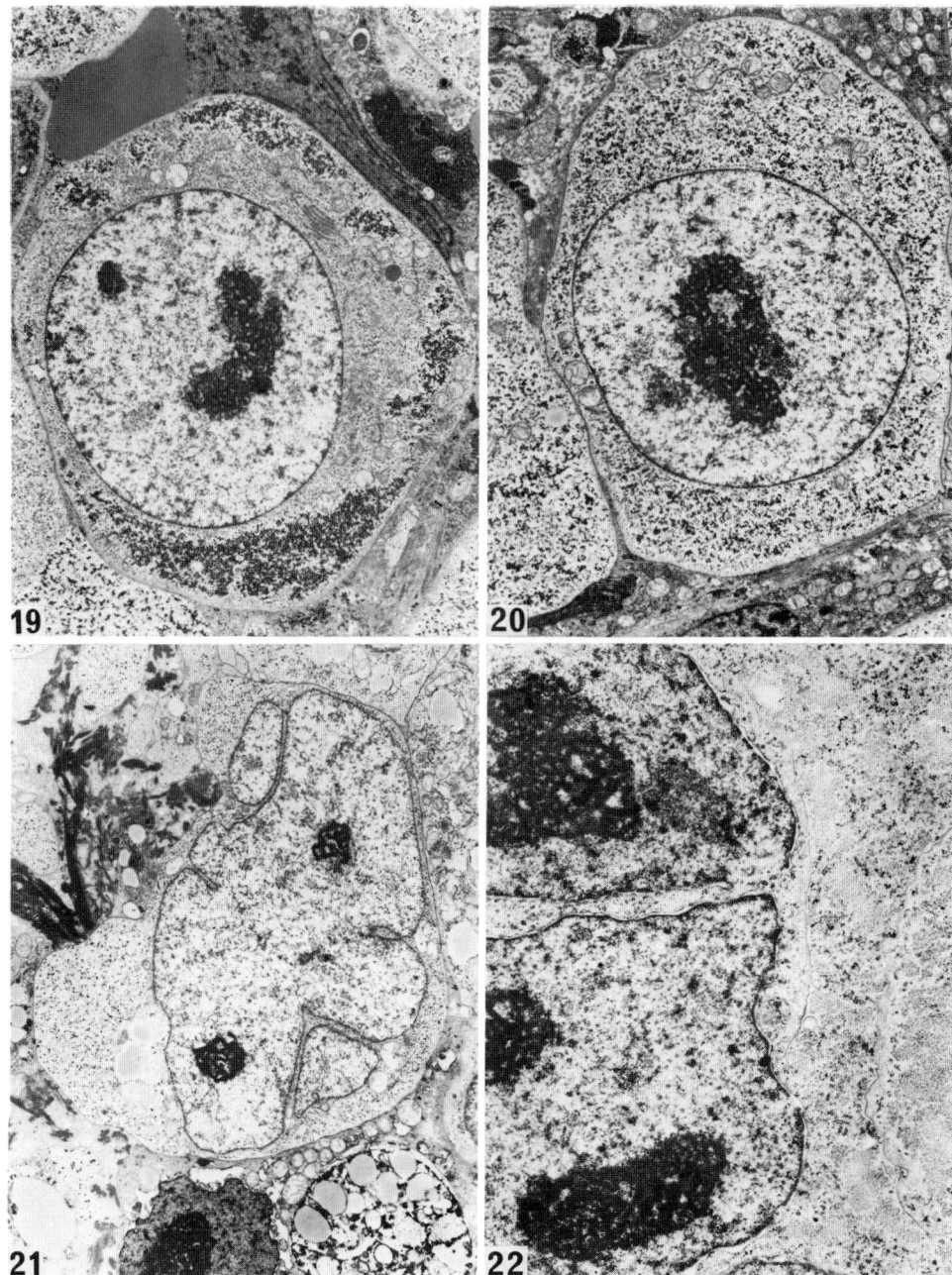

Fig. 19. Electron micrograph of Tc 1. ×3800.
Fig. 20. Electron micrograph of Tc 2. ×4200.
Fig. 21. Electron micrograph of Tc 3. ×3800.
Fig. 22. Part of syncytial Tc 4. ×9500.

Tumour cells with structural features of germ cells

It is possible to differentiate tumour cells unequivocally from the abnormal germ cells and their variants described above (Holstein & Körner, 1974). In the analysis of tumours it is of prime importance to demonstrate tumour cells which show some of the structural features of germ cells. Such cells will be designated 'Tc' (tumour cell) numbered 1–4. However, mention must also be made of other diverse tumour cell types and accompanying tissue since they also have a definitive part to play in defining the appearance of a tumour.

Tc 1. This is a tumour cell which exhibits a very large round nucleus with a very large nucleolus (Figs. 13–15 and 19). Large quantities of glycogen predominate in the cytoplasm and this can be demonstrated excellently by PAS staining of semithin sections. A subplasmalemmal margin of microfilaments is particularly characteristic and this even attracts attention in the semithin section, best seen as a light peripheral margin between neighbouring cells. The mitochondria mostly appear rounded and lack intermitochondrial cement substance. Numerous flat cisterns of ER are recognizable and sometimes annulated membranes are also seen. In addition, thin cytoplasmic processes containing microfilaments are evident.

The characteristics of Tc 1, glycogen and a peripheral margin of microfilaments with cytoplasmic processes, bear an extraordinary resemblance to the appearance of gonocytes during the embryonic period. The cytoplasmic processes suggest the capability of locomotion which is also a characteristic of early germ cells. The nuclei of the tumour cells, however, are significantly larger than the nuclei of gonocytes.

Tumour cells of the Tc 1 type may occur in seminiferous tubules where spermatogenesis is still present, either as solitary tumour cells or in larger numbers. At the sites where Tc 1 cells multiply within the seminiferous tubules, spermatogenesis will be eradicated by the displacement of type A spermatogonia which are shifted from the basal to the adluminal compartment and are finally released into the lumen of the tubule.

When Tc 1 cells are restricted to the basal compartment of the seminiferous tubules, the features are those of carcinoma-in-situ (CIS) (Skakkebaek & Berthelsen, 1981). However, Tc 1 cells may also penetrate the lamina propria of the seminiferous tubules to gain access to the interstitium (Schulze & Holstein, 1977). There they are located as single cells or cell clusters between the Leydig cells. They are always found at the invasive margin of solid sheets of seminoma.

Tc 1 cells appear to be tumour cells with a low rate of cell division. Within the seminiferous tubules and in the interstitium, ten mitotic figures are found for every thousand Tc 1 cells.

Tc 2. This is a tumour cell showing a very large round nucleus with a large nucleolus but with only a little, or no, glycogen scattered throughout the cytoplasm (Figs. 16, 18 and 20). Therefore the subplasmalemmal margin of microfilaments is only visible by electron microscopy because it is not well demarcated at the light microscopical level due to the absence of abundant glycogen. Relatively few organelles are present in the cytoplasm giving a very transparent appearance in semithin sections. Within the ER there are some flat cisterns and a sporadic occurrence of annulated membranes. The mitochondria are rounded and lack cement substance. The cells have only a few cytoplasmic processes.

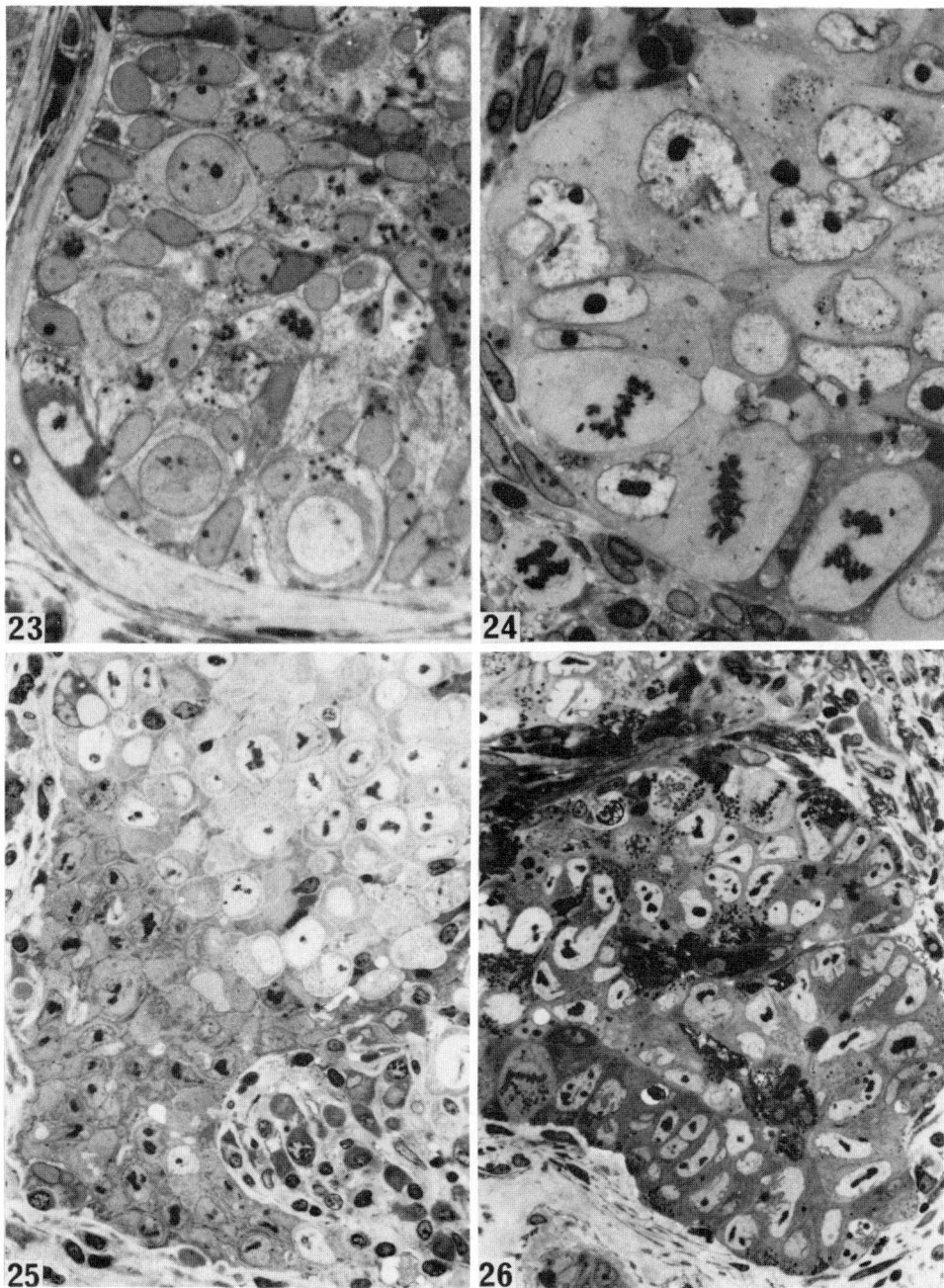

Fig. 23. Hypoplastic testicular tissue with tumour cells (Tc 1). ×840.
Fig. 24. Nodule of Tc 3. Mitoses are frequent. ×900.
Fig. 25. Connection between Tc 1 and Tc 4 (below). ×420.
Fig. 26. Nodule of Tc 3. The cells exhibit many granules. ×420.

Morphology of germ cells 11

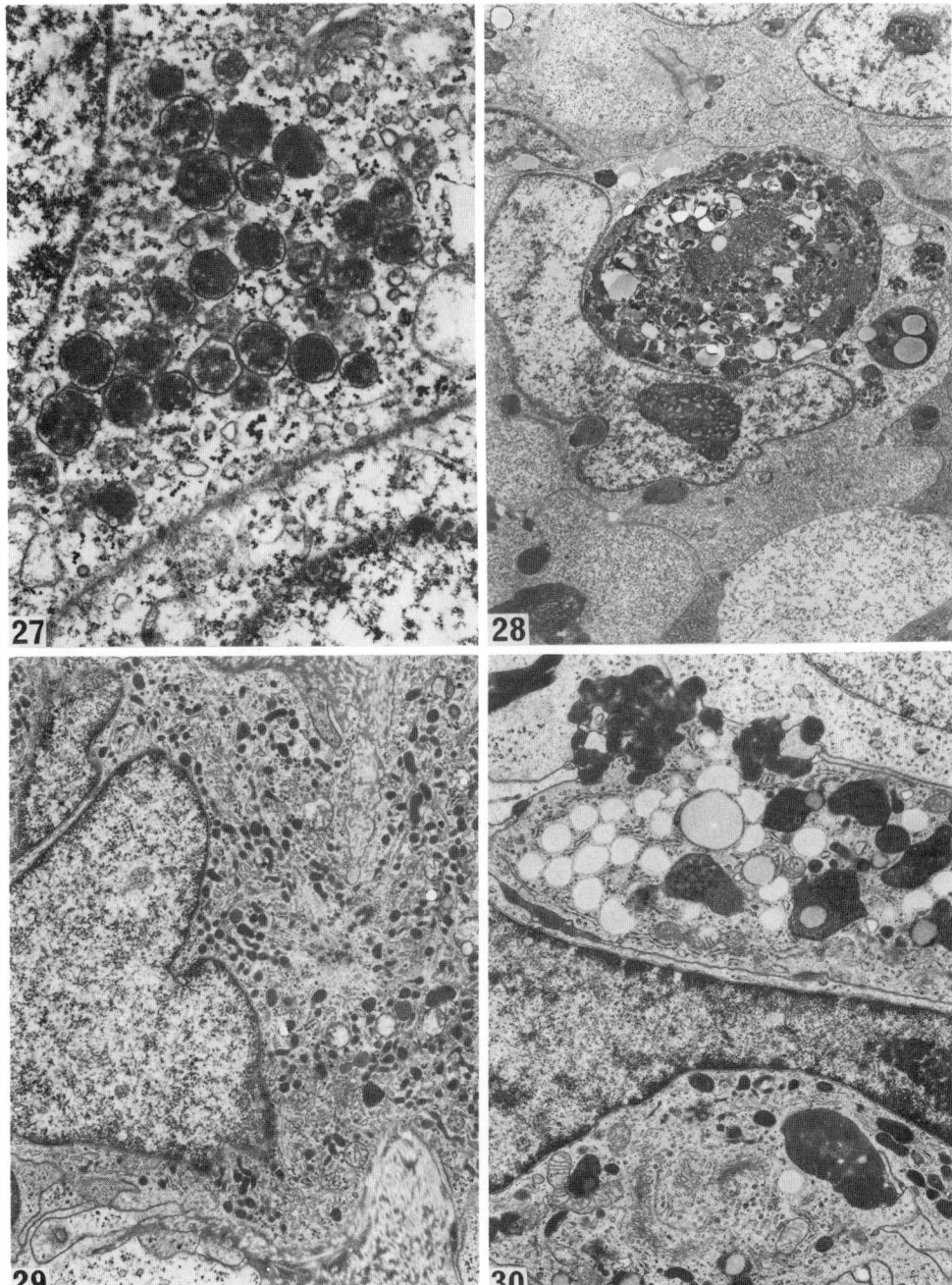

Fig. 27. Cytoplasmic vesicles of Tc 3 with floccular electron dense contents. ×20,000.
Fig. 28. Aggregated vesicles in the cytoplasm of Tc 3. ×3800.
Fig. 29. Many small electron-dense vesicles of Tc 3. ×8000.
Fig. 30. Large polymorphic vesicles with electron-dense material deliver their contents into intercellular spaces. ×8800.

Tc 2 cells do not appear frequently within seminiferous tubules. A gradual transition from Tc 1 to Tc 2 occurs, recognizable by the differing content of glycogen. Tc 2 cells are the predominant cell type in the centre of solid seminoma and are responsible for the typical seminoma appearance characterized light microscopically by 'uniform cells clear as water'. Tc 2 and Tc 1 have a similar rate of cell division with ten mitotic figures per 1000 tumour cells being identified.

Although Tc 2 cells are the predominant constituent of solid areas of seminoma, the tumour cells undergo different patterns of organization according to their relationships with accompanying tissues such as connective tissue, lymphocytes (Fig. 17), plasma cells and macrophages. Follicular, threadlike or other different patterns may be seen (Fig. 18). Central necrosis is not apparent even in large tumour masses.

Tc 3. This tumour cell has a very large, often distinctively lobed, nucleus with a very large nucleolus. Prominent nuclear polymorphism is obvious (Figs. 21, 24 and 26) and the cytoplasm appears relatively transparent. Glycogen is finely distributed throughout the cytoplasm and large masses of glycogen are lacking. The mitotic rate is significantly higher than Tc 1 and Tc 2, there being up to forty-five mitotic figures per 1000 tumour cells.

Tc 3 cells are mainly organized into tumour nodules and within these nodules there are further variants of tumour cells, obviously derived from Tc 3 (Fig. 26). They are characterized by well-developed Golgi apparatus and typical vesicles containing electron dense material. The following variants can be distinguished: (a) Cells with numerous small round or oval vesicles containing electron-dense material, resembling endocrine cells (Fig. 21). (b) Cells with numerous large polymorphic vesicles containing granular electron-dense material. These vesicles appear to arise from mitochondria (Fig. 30) and their content is released at the cell surface into the interstitial spaces. (c) Cells with round vesicles containing flocculent electron-dense material (Fig. 27). In some cells these vesicles coalesce to form larger complexes consisting of membrane bound granules, membranous figures and lipid droplets (Fig. 28).

Tc 3 cells are probably never found in CIS. In tumours containing Tc 3 cells there are almost always areas where there are also Tc 1 and Tc 2 cells.

Tc 4. This tumour cell has an angular, relatively small nucleus containing several nucleoli (Figs. 22 and 25). The cytoplasm is relatively dense and stains strongly in light microscopical preparations. The cell contains large quantities of glycogen and also has a subplasmalemmal margin of microfilaments. The cell borders between adjacent cells show a tendency to disintegrate. Persistent fragments of cell membrane are seen turning into vesicles, but elsewhere there is a deficiency of cell boundary thereby allowing partial confluence of the cytoplasm between adjacent cells.

Tc 4 areas are found in many seminomas at the periphery of solid nodules or cords of tumour. Tc 4 cells may also occur betwen the large Tc 1 and Tc 2 cells; however, they are difficult to identify not only light microscopically but even with the electron microscope. Sometimes islets of Tc 3 cells rest on cords of Tc 4 cells.

All the Tc 1 to Tc 4 tumour cells show features of embryonic germ cells. However, they can be recognized unequivocally as tumour cells because of their large or abnormal nuclei and their cellular organelles. It is difficult to describe exactly the features of tumour cells which support the deduction that they are derived from embryonic germ cells. Such characteristics as the amount of glycogen, subplasmalemmal microfilaments, annulated membranes, and finger-shaped cytoplasmic processes are all individually relatively nonspecific cellular features. However, the combination of these features in the tumour cells Tc 1 to Tc 4 is considered to be strong evidence of their derivation from germ cells.

Two hypotheses concerning the histogenesis of these tumours should be considered. Firstly, it may be possible that some germ cells survive in their embryonic state into adulthood then undergo neoplastic transformation. Alternatively, perhaps malignant transformation of type A spermatogonia is associated with dedifferentiation of the adult germ cells so that they revert structurally and functionally to more primitive precursor cells.

A different pattern is occasionally found in association with testicular tumours. Areas of hypoplastic seminiferous tubules resembling the germinal cords of the embryonic period may be seen between tubules containing CIS where component cells are of the Tc 1 subtype. These hypoplastic areas may even be recognizable with the naked eye as white regions on the cut surface of the testis. The hypoplastic cords consist of undifferentiated Sertoli cells with smooth oval nuclei, and may be devoid of germ cells or may show regions where relatively large germ cells are present. The large germ cells can be differentiated from early gonocytes not by their cellular structures but possibly on the basis of their larger nuclei. They contain

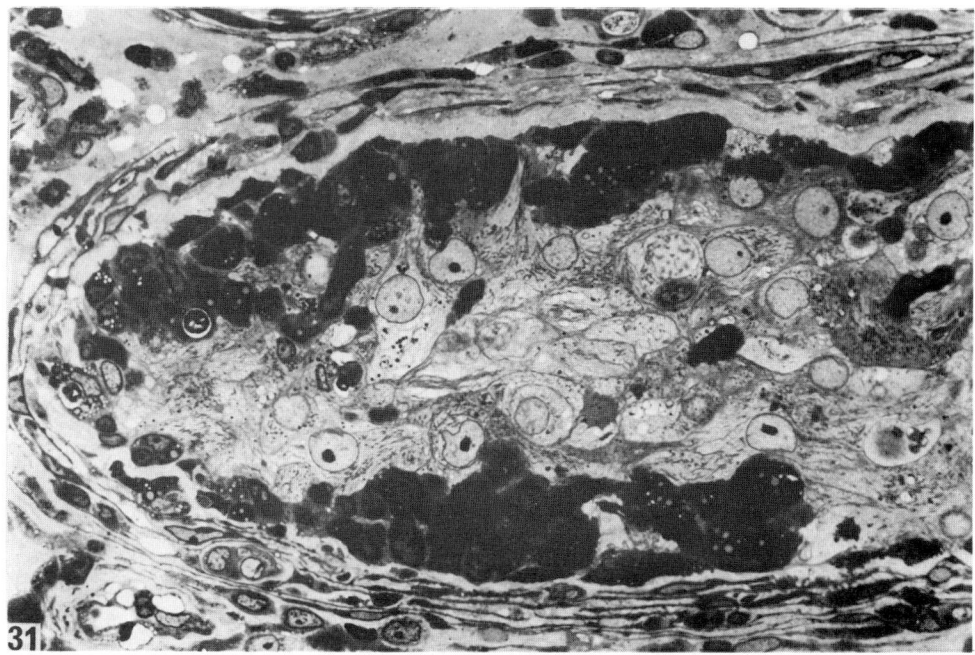

Fig. 31. Many heavily stained macrophages in the periphery of a seminiferous tubule affected with Tc 1. ×350.

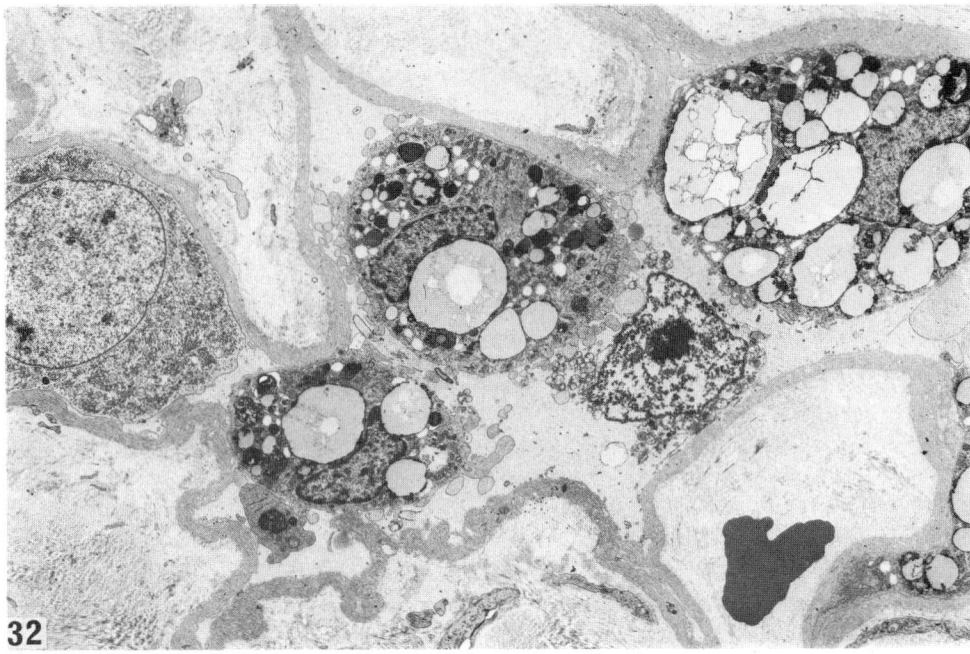

Fig. 32. Large macrophages heavily loaded with lipid droplets are surrounded by the shrunken basal lamina of the seminiferous tubule. Only one tumour cell (Tc 1) is visible, all other cellular components of the germinal epithelium have disappeared. ×2700.

large quantities of glycogen, a subplasmalemmal margin of microfilaments, rounded mitochondria, cisterns in the ER, annulated membranes and a small Golgi apparatus. Sporadically, these cells contain so much glycogen that they look like Tc 1 cells, supporting the assumption that Tc 1 cells are derivatives of early embryonic germ cells. This pattern in the testis demonstrates that tumour cells may be found not only in maldescended testes but also in hypoplastic areas of normally descended testes.

Further cell types which do not show characteristics of germ cells are found in many testicular tumours, these being: (1) Columnar epithelia of various types which are glycogen rich and may border large cavities, tubules or irregularly outlined spaces. (2) Syncytial cells with honey-combed cytoplasm and bizarre forms. (3) Smooth muscle cells or myofibroblasts occurring at the periphery of Tc 1 and Tc 2 tumour regions; these are also sometimes found in thick layers surrounding Tc 3 nodules. (4) Fibroblasts and fibrocytes in varying quantities; these are regular constituents of all testicular tumours, their amount and arrangement characterizing the histological appearance of testicular tumours giving solid areas of seminoma a lobular, alveolar, tubular or follicular appearance. (5) Lymphocytes in varying numbers are present in every testicular tumour. (6) Plasma cells: in advanced CIS, plasma cells are recognizable in the lamina propria of the seminiferous tubules filled with tumour cells. (7) Macrophages or their precursors, which are normally present in the interstitium of the testis. Niemi, Sharpe & Brown (1986) characterized such cells in rat testes by means of immunohistochemistry. Numerous

Morphology of germ cells 15

macrophages are recognizable in testicular tumours, and in CIS/intratubular seminoma where they are located in the lamina propria or within the tubules (Fig. 31). Presumably they are responsible for the appearance of large regions of tubular shadows in cases of early seminoma. They are capable of phagocytosing the tumour cells and the remaining Sertoli cells in the seminiferous tubules (Fig. 32). The final

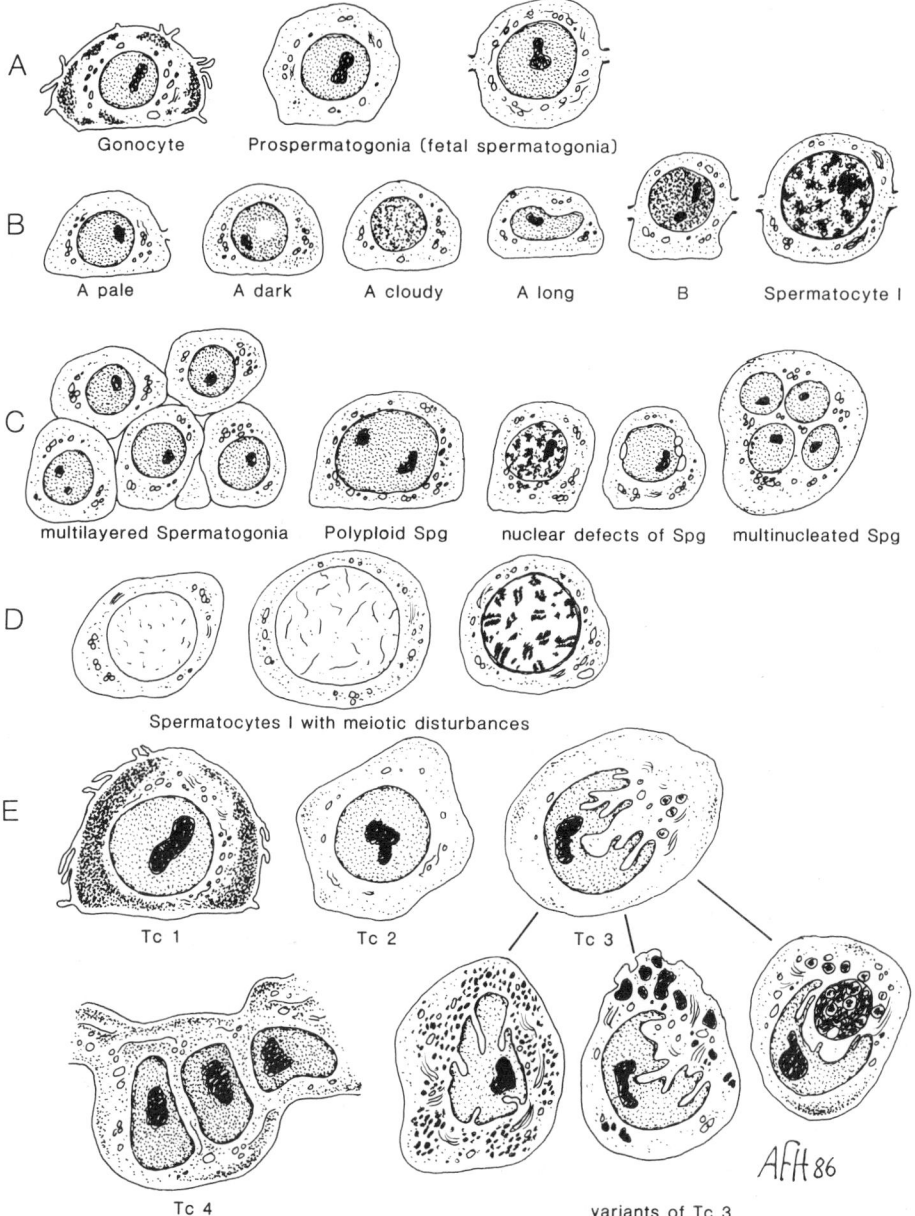

Fig. 33. Summarizing semischematic drawing based on ultrastructural investigations. (A) embryonic and fetal germ cells; (B) germ cells in the adult; (C) abnormal spermatogonia; (D) abnormal primary spermatocytes; (E) tumour cells (Tc 1–Tc 4) and variants of Tc 3.

outcome of this process is the appearance of empty tubules with a dense hyalinized lamina propria and a lumen lined exclusively by basal lamina. Macrophages are present throughout, between the tumour cells of solid nodules of seminoma, and in the interstitium intermingled with all tumour cells derived from germ cells. (8) Chondrocytes forming rounded or plate-shaped cartilagenous complexes.

On the basis of our material and the techniques we have used — light microscopy of semithin sections, and electron microscopy — a very reliable analysis of tumour cell types is obtained. The apparent abundance of ill-defined varieties of malignant cell forms can be categorized into a reduced number of specific cell types and their variants (Fig. 33). However, with only about 400 cases available for investigation, we had a limited quantity of material at our disposal in comparison to other authors. The so-called spermatocytic seminoma, for example, was not recognized in our series.

A seminoma can be diagnosed unequivocally. Likewise, teratoma can be identified without difficulty. All other diagnostic categories of testicular tumours depend on the quantities of the various cell types constituting the tumour (v. Hochstetter & Hedinger, 1982). Further diagnostic subdivisions of tumour types — mixed tumours — can be formulated without difficulty. This is accomplished not only on morphological grounds but also by using immunohistochemical techniques and measuring tumour markers (Javadpour, 1980; Jacobsen & Nørgaard-Pedersen, 1984; Miettinen, Virtanen & Talerman, 1985). The justification of such subclassification depends on the usefulness of making further discrimination between tumours, particularly with regards to the selection of presently available treatment protocols.

Acknowledgements

For translation of the manuscript we thank PD Dr Haide Breucker. Supported by Deutsche Forschungsgemeinschaft.

References

Gondos, B. (1977) Testicular development. In: *The Testis*, Vol. IV (ed. by A. D. Johnson and W. R. Gomes). Academic Press, New York.

v. Hochstetter, A. R. & Hedinger, Chr. E. (1982) The differential diagnosis of testicular germ cells tumours in theory and practice. A critical analysis of two major systems of classification and review of 389 cases. *Virchows Archives* [A], **396**, 247–277.

Holstein, A. F., Bustos-Obregon, E. & Hartmann, M. (1984) Dislocated type A spermatogonia in human seminiferous tubules. *Cell and Tissue Research*, **236**, 35–40.

Holstein, A. F. & Eckmann, Ch. (1986) Megalospermatocytes: indicators of disturbed meiosis in man. *Andrologia*, **18**, 601–609.

Holstein, A. F. & Körner, F. (1974) Light and electron microscopical analysis of cell types in human seminoma. *Virchows Archives* [A], **363**, 97–112.

Holstein, A. F. & Roosen-Runge, E. C. (1981) *Atlas of Human Spermatogenesis*. Grosse, Berlin.

Jacobsen, G. K. & Nørgaard-Pedersen, B. (1984) Placental alkaline phosphatase in testicular germ cell tumours and in carcinoma-in-situ of the testis. An immunohistochemical study. *Acta Pathologica, Microbiologica et Immunologica Scandinavica*, **92**, 323–329.

Javadpour, N. (1980) The role of biologic tumor markers in testicular cancer. *Cancer*, **45**, 1755–1761.

Miettinen, M., Virtanen, I. & Talerman, A. (1985) Intermediate filament proteins in human testis and testicular germ-cell tumors. *American Journal of Pathology*, **120**, 420–410.

Niemi, M., Sharpe, R. M. & Brown, W. R. A. (1986) Macrophages in the interstitial tissue of the rat testis. *Cell and Tissue Resarch*, **243**, 337–344.

Schulze, C. & Holstein, A. F. (1977) On the histology of human seminoma: development of the solid tumour from intratubular seminoma cells. *Cancer*, **39**, 1090–1100.

Schulze, W. (1978) Licht- und elektronenmikroskopische Studien an den A-Spermatogonien von Männern mit intakter Spermatogenese und bei Patienten nach Behandlung mit Antiandrogenen. *Andrologia*, **10**, 307–320.

Schulze, W. (1981) Normal and abnormal spermatogonia in the human testis. *Fortschritte der Andrologie*, **7**, pp. 33–45. Grosse, Berlin.

Skakkebæk, N. E. & Berthelsen, J. G. (1981) Carcinoma-*in-situ* of the testis and invasive growth of different types of germ cell tumours. A revised germ cell theory. *International Journal of Andrology*, Suppl. 4, 26–34.

Wartenberg, H. (1981) Differentiation and development of the testis. *The testis* (ed. by H. Burger and D. de Kretser), pp. 39–80. Raven Press, New York.

Wartenberg, H., Holstein, A. F. & Vossmeyer, J. (1971) Zur Cytologie der pränatalen Gonadenentwicklung beim Menschen. II. Elektronenmikroskopische Untersuchungen über die Cytogenese von Gonocyten und fetalen Spermatogonien im Hoden. *Zeitschrift für Anatomie und Entwicklungsgeschichte*, **134**, 165–185.

Discussion

Grigor Do the malignant cells within the tubules ever have the morphological characteristics of nonseminomatous germ cell tumour or do they always have the features of seminoma cells?

Holstein We have never seen intratubular malignant cells looking like nonseminomatous cells. We found only Tc 1 and Tc 2 within the seminiferous tubules.

M. Jacobsen Is it possible to characterize the microfilaments on Tc 1, 2, 4 any further, for example by using immunohistochemistry?

Holstein I think this could be possible, but we have not performed these investigations up to now.

Niemi Glycogen seems to be the most important single component which identified the tumour germ cells. However, glycogen content of the cytoplasm in tissue sections is dependent on the type and duration of fixation. Which fixative do you recommend for testicular biopsies?

Holstein In order to preserve glycogen in Tc 1 it is necessary to obtain the tumour material immediately after surgery. We fix the tissue by immersion in 5.5% glutaraldehyde in phosphate buffer. Postfixation is in OsO_4. Under these conditions most of the glycogen deposits are well preserved and can be demonstrated by modified PAS staining (Laczko & Levai, 1975, *Mikroskopie*, **31**, 1–4) and in electronmicrographs.

Niemi You say you have never seen spermatocytic seminoma among 400 cases of seminoma. I would like to ask the audience if such a tumour exists?

G. K. Jacobsen Spermatocytic seminoma does exist. In the first 5 years of the DATECA project, 13 cases of spermatocytic seminoma were diagnosed among the 1058 testicular germ cell tumours examined. This is 2.3% of all testicular germ cell tumours.

Skakkebæk I am not in any doubt that the spermatocytic seminoma does exist. However, I have recently seen several examples of misdiagnosis of this condition even by very experienced pathologists. Tumours which have originally been called spermatocytic seminoma have been reviewed and the diagnosis changed to classical seminoma. I am grateful to Dr Cameron in London for her help in the review of these cases.

Grigor Spermatocytic seminoma does occur and I have seen examples of it. I agree that it may sometimes not be recognized, and at other times may be over-diagnosed. If a definite diagnosis is to be made, the cellular detail must be seen clearly, but unfortunately fixation of testicular tumours is often inadequate and the histological detail is obscured by artifact. Poor fixation prevents recognition of the true nature of the tumour.

Müller Cytoplasmic glycogen content is a characteristic feature of the malignant cells. Some of your examples of abnormal spermatogonia contain glycogen. Is glycogen, therefore, a good marker of malignancy and premalignancy?

Holstein Normal spermatogonia, especially type A dark spermatogonia, contain glycogen granules. Intratesticular tumour cells (Tc 1 and Tc 2), however, exhibit large deposits of glycogen granules. These glycogen deposits result in a peripheral rim of negative staining where there is a clear subplasmalemmal microfilamentous web. The glycogen deposition in Tc 1 is only one characteristic of the tumour cell and in itself must not be considered as being diagnostic. Other features to be taken into consideration include the structure of the nucleus and the cytoplasm of these cells as visualised by semithin sections or electronmicrographs. The nucleus is large and a distinct nucleolus is seen. Annulated lamellae, typical mitochondria and other cell structures are also helpful.

Carcinoma-in-situ of the testis: possible origin from gonocytes and precursor of all types of germ cell tumours except spermatocytoma

N.E. SKAKKEBÆK,[1,2] J. G. BERTHELSEN,[3] A. GIWERCMAN[2] and J. MÜLLER[2]   [1]*University Department of Paediatrics, Hvidovre Hospital, Copenhagen,* [2]*Laboratory of Reproductive Biology, Rigshospitalet, Copenhagen, and* [3]*University Department of Gynaecology and Obstetrics, Herlev Hospital, Copenhagen, Denmark.*

Summary
Based on evidence from morphological and histochemical studies and from clinical experience, the following hypotheses are proposed: (1) carcinoma-in-situ (CIS) germ cells are malignant gonocytes; (2) these CIS gonocytes have some capacity to regress into more primitive, totipotent embryonic cells which can give rise to all types of nonseminomatous germ cell tumours; (3) the tumour germ cells of classical seminomas are malignant gonocytes derived from CIS gonocytes which have lost their ability to regress into totipotent embryonic cells; (4) the ability of CIS gonocytes to regress into totipotent embryonic cells decreases with age, whereas the capacity to form classical seminoma cells is preserved; (5) the transformation of CIS gonocytes into invasive tumours is dependent on factors such as gonadotrophins and/or testicular steroids; (6) the pathogenesis of classical and spermatocytic seminoma are unrelated.
As a consequence of these hypotheses an alternative nomenclature for carcinoma-in-situ, seminoma and dysgerminoma is suggested.

Key words. Carcinoma-in-situ testis, gonocytes, seminoma, nonseminoma, spermatocytoma, spermatocytic seminoma, histogenesis.

Introduction
The presence of atypical germ cells in seminiferous tubules adjacent to germ cell tumours of the testis (Wilms, 1896; Azzopardi, Mostofi & Theiss, 1961; Mark & Hedinger, 1965) has been observed since the end of the last century. It was generally believed that the presence of these cells resulted from effects of the tumour or represented spread from the tumour itself. Azzopardi *et al.* (1961) stated that 'the significance [of these abnormal intratubular germ cells] could not be established'.

Correspondence: Dr N. E. Skakkebæk, Laboratory of Reproductive Biology, Section 4052, Rigshospitalet, Copenhagen, Denmark.

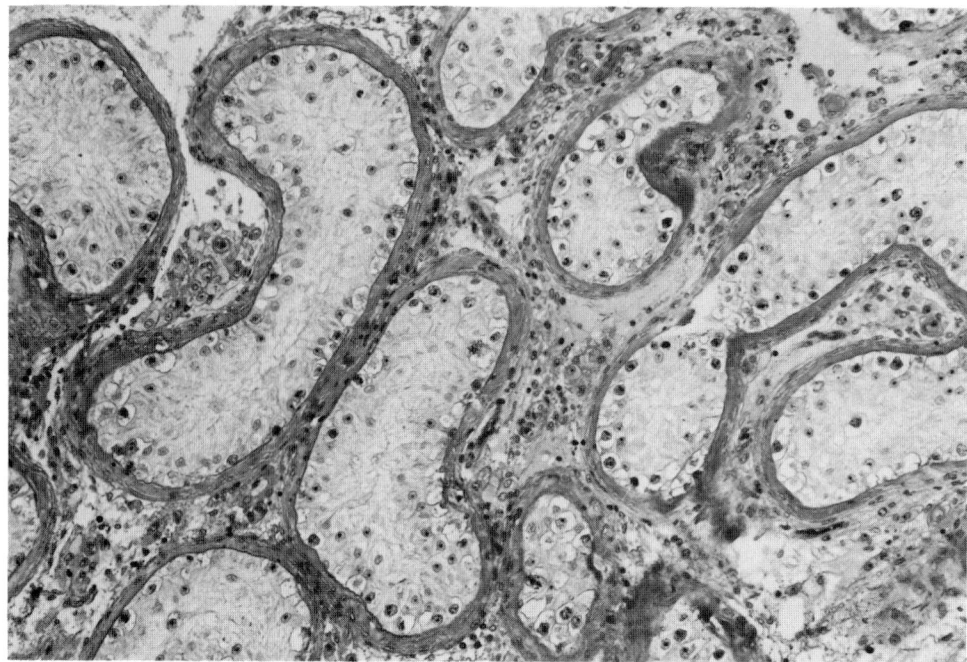

Fig. 1a. Section of testicular specimen showing carcinoma-in-situ in all tubules. Cleland's fixative, Iron-haematoxylin stain, original ×200.

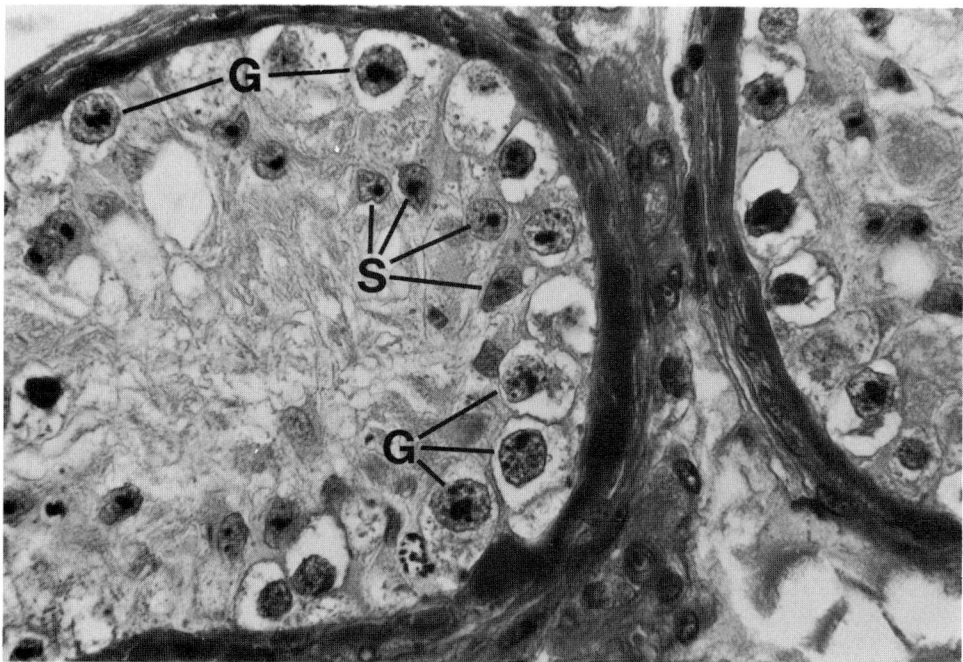

Fig. 1b. Same as Fig. 1a. Higher magnification. Note the carcinoma-in-situ germ cells (G) and the Sertoli cells (S). Note also the thickening of the tubular membrane. Original ×800.

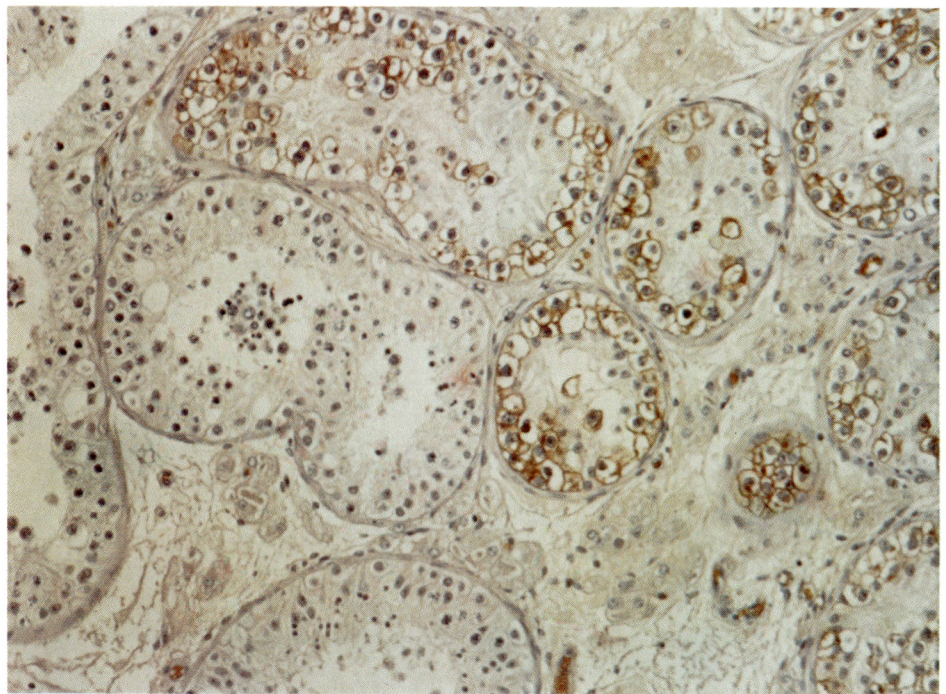

Fig. 2a. Section of testicular specimen showing carcinoma-in-situ. Immunoperoxidase demonstration of placental-like alkaline phosphatase (DAKO No. A 268) in CIS cells. PAP-technique. Stieve's fixative, original x160.

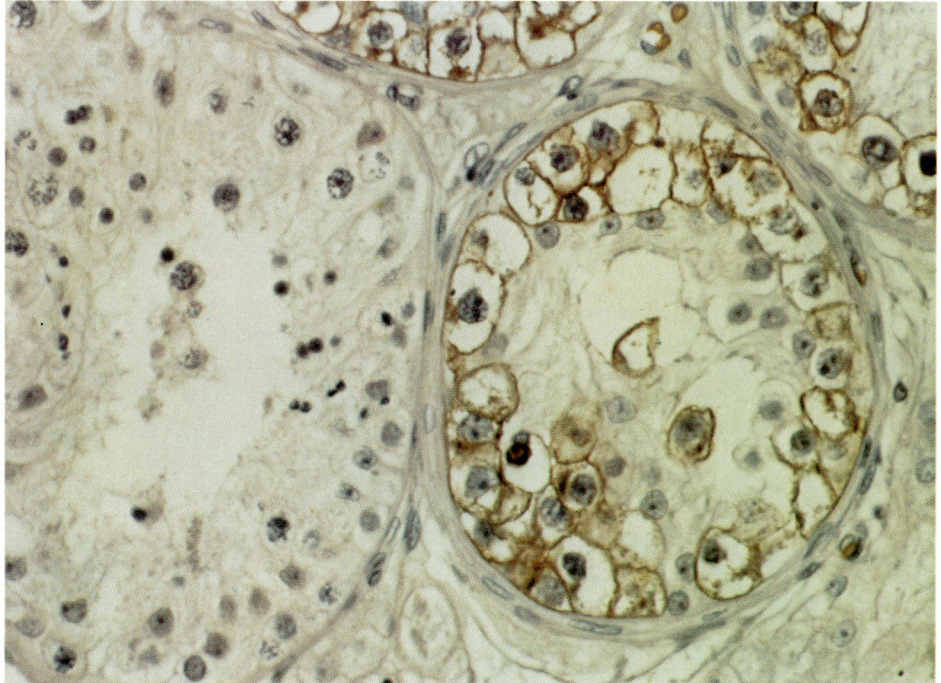

Fig. 2b. Same as Fig. 2a. Higher magnification. Note the normal tubule (left) and the CIS tubule (right). Note that the cellular membranes of the CIS cells show strongly positive reaction, original x400.

However, it is now generally recognized that the atypical germ cells in fact represent a carcinoma-in-situ (CIS) pattern (Skakkebæk, 1972a,b; Nielsen, Nielsen & Skakkebæk, 1974; Skakkebæk, 1975; Nüesch-Bachman & Hedinger, 1977; Skakkebæk, Berthelsen & Müller, 1982; Gondos, 1986) which gives rise to seminomas as well as nonseminomas.

In the following paper we shall give a short description of some biological features of the CIS germ cell and discuss its origin. In addition we shall propose an alternative to the present nomenclature for some germ cell tumours.

Morphological and histochemical aspects

The CIS germ cells (Fig. 1) are much larger than spermatogonia and have a significantly greater median nuclear diameter of 9.7 µm (range 9.2–10.5 µm) compared to 6.5 µm (range 5.7–7.1 µm) for spermatogonia. The chromatin pattern of the nuclei is coarse and several nucleoli are present. Rarely, CIS germ cells and normal germ cells including spermatogonia, spermatocytes and spermatids can be found within the same tubular cross section, representing a transition zone between CIS and normal seminiferous epithelium. In typical cases, the tubules with CIS are composed of a single row of CIS germ cells located between normal Sertoli cells and the basement membrane. In the CIS lesion of prepubertal testes, however, the CIS germ cells are normally distributed throughout the seminiferous tubules. The tubular membrane is thickened, and the morphology of both the Sertoli and Leydig cells is normal. Sometimes foci of lymphocytes are found in the interstitial tissue surrounding the seminiferous tubules. A detailed description of the histology of CIS has previously been reported (Skakkebæk, 1978; Müller *et al.*, 1985).

The CIS cells are rich in glycogen and placental-like alkaline phosphatase (PlAP) (Fig. 2) (Holstein & Körner, 1974; Nielsen *et al.*, 1974; Beckstead, 1983; Jacobsen & Nørgaard-Pedersen, 1984; Hustin, Collette & Franchimont, 1987).

CIS of the testis is a disperse process throughout the testis. Berthelsen & Skakkebæk (1981) found that a conventional surgical biopsy of approximately 3 mm in diameter usually is representative of the whole testicle.

The invasive potential of CIS germ cells

The malignant nature of the CIS cells has been confirmed in several studies. Most important in this respect are the results from investigations of adult patients with CIS which showed that CIS in approximately 50% of these cases will progress into invasive cancer within 5 years if orchidectomy is not performed (Skakkebæk & Berthelsen, 1978; Skakkebæk, Berthelsen & Visfeldt, 1981). This association between CIS and invasive cancer is also illustrated by the finding of seminiferous tubules with CIS in the testicular tissue adjacent to the majority of testicular tumours (Skakkebæk, 1975; Jacobsen, Henriksen & von der Maase, 1981). Several studies have shown that the CIS cells are precursors for both seminomas and nonseminomas except spermatocytic seminomas (Skakkebæk & Berthelsen, 1981a; Skakkebæk, Berthelsen & Müller, 1984).

Further evidence for the invasive potential of CIS germ cells was presented by Müller *et al.* (1984) who found a prepubertal CIS pattern in the undescended testis of a 10-year-old boy. He was followed with repeated biopsies showing the characteristic adult CIS lesion at the age of 13 years and invasive growth of malignant cells at the age of 21 years. At this time, examination of the orchidectomy specimen also revealed extension of the CIS germ cells to the rete testis.

Recently, we have had the opportunity to study a gonadoblastoma in a 9-year-old girl with 46,XY gonadal dysgenesis. Both the gonadoblastoma and the adjacent gonadal tissue contained cells which could not be distinguished from CIS cells with respect to nuclear morphology. Furthermore, all germ cells were PlAP-positive. Thus, the germinal component of gonadoblastomas may also arise from CIS germ cells.

The gonocyte characteristics of CIS germ cells
Even though the CIS germ cells and the spermatogonia are both located along the tubular wall, they have few characteristics in common. The morphology of the CIS cells is much more like gonocytes (primordial germ cells) (Fig. 3). Ultrastructural studies have also indicated a close resemblance of CIS cells to embryonal germ cells (Nielsen *et al.*, 1974; Schultze & Holstein, 1977; Albrechtsen *et al.*, 1982; Gondos, Berthelsen & Skakkebæk, 1983; Gondos, 1986; Holstein *et al.*, 1987). Furthermore, the CIS cells have histochemical features in common with gonocytes, both cell types being rich in glycogen and alkaline phosphatase (McKay *et al.*, 1953; Teilum, 1971; Beckstead, 1973; Holstein & Körner, 1974; Nielsen *et al.*, 1974; Jacobsen & Nørgaard-Pedersen, 1984; Hustin *et al.*, 1987), and both are extremely

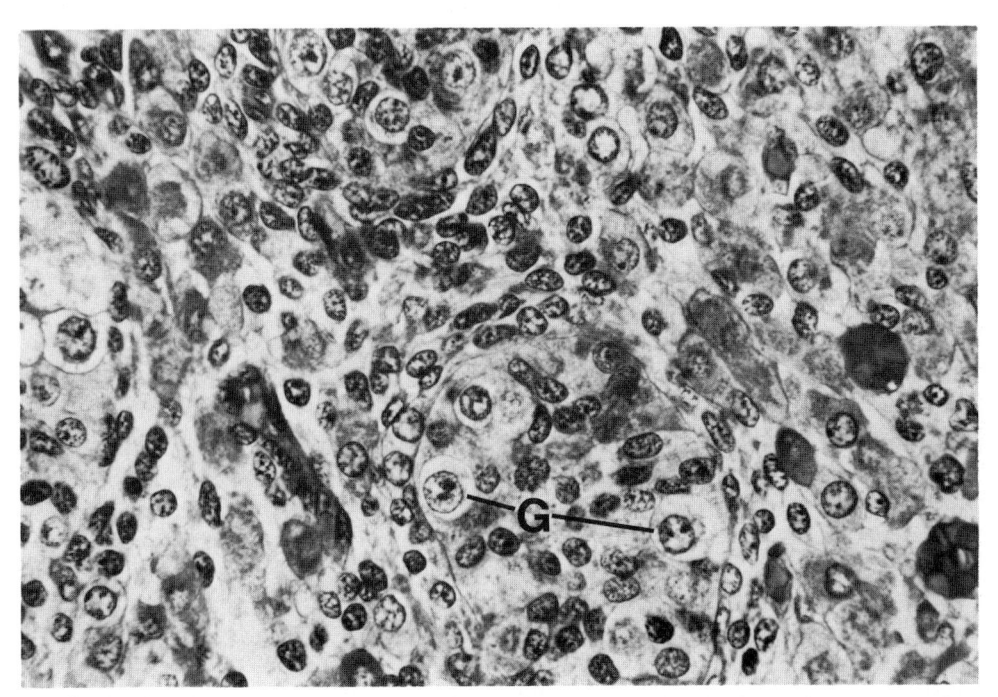

Fig. 3. Section of testis from a 3 month old fetus. Note the gonoctyes (G). Cleland's fixative, Iron-haematoxylin stain, original ×600.

sensitive to radiation (Mandl, 1964; Mandl et al., 1964; von der Maase, Giwercman & Skakkebæk, 1986) (see Fig. 1, p. 214, 215, this volume). The fact that CIS germ cells have been found in individuals only a few months old (Müller & Skakkebæk, 1984; Müller et al., 1985) also supports the assumption that these cells are of fetal origin.

Recent data (Damjanov et al., 1982; Damjanov, 1986) indicate that CIS cells express embryonic antigens.

Similarities and differences between the CIS cells and seminoma cells
Both morphology (Holstein & Körner, 1974; Gondos, 1986; Holstein et al., 1987) and histochemistry indicate a close relationship between CIS germ cells and the cells of classical seminoma. They are both rich in glycogen and alkaline phosphatase (McKay et al., 1953; Wahren, Holmgren & Stigbrandt, 1979), and both exhibit an aneuploid DNA pattern (Atkin, 1973; Müller & Skakkebæk, 1981). They also share their sensitivity to irradiation (Dixon & Moore, 1953; von der Maase et al., 1986).

However, ultrastructurally some differences exist between CIS and seminoma cells (Holstein et al., 1987).

Important functional differences have also been noted such as the capacity of CIS cells to develop into nonseminomatous tumours. This capacity may decrease with age, as nonseminomatous tumours are rare after the age of 40 (Schultz et al., 1984). It cannot be excluded that the conversion from CIS to nonseminoma passes through a stage of seminoma (Friedman, 1951). However, there is evidence suggesting that the conversion can occur directly from CIS to nonseminoma, as we have seen more than twenty cases of nonseminomas with CIS and found no evidence of a transition zone of seminoma between CIS and the tumour (Skakkebæk, 1975, unpublished). This finding is not in disagreement with the fact that widespread CIS lesions often develop into seminoma in one part, and nonseminoma in another part of the same testicle.

Thus, we believe that CIS germ cells are malignant gonocytes with the capacity to regress into more primitive embryonal cells, whereas seminoma cells are proliferative, malignant gonocytes which—possibly as an effect of ageing—have lost this transforming ability. The inability to assume embryonal characteristics may not always be complete: some seminomas contain a few syncytial giant cells which produce human chorionic gonadotropin (Skrabanek, Kirrane & Powell, 1979; Neville, 1979). However, such cells may be derived directly from CIS cells rather than from seminoma tumour cells.

The theory of a close association between the histogenesis of the classical seminoma and nonseminoma is indeed not new. In 1911 Ewing wrote: '. . . this study support[s] the view that all embryonal tumours [viz. seminomas and nonseminomas] of the testicle have an identical origin. Additional evidence of great value would be furnished by the discovery of very early stages of the tumours in question. No very early stages have yet been described.' His views were opposed by several authors, among those Thackray & Crane (1971), who wrote: 'Confusion arose from Ewing's interpretation of the seminoma as a one-sided development of a teratoma and his name of embryonal carcinoma for it'.

However, during the past 30 years more and more scientists have become aware of the close relationship between seminomas and nonseminomas. Friedman (1951, 1977) suggested that embryonal carcinoma develops from germinoma (seminoma), and more recently Raghavan *et al.* (1982) on the basis of investigations with tumour markers and experimental evidence have proposed that seminoma is the precursor for nonseminoma.

As indicated above, our present evidence would suggest that although seminomas may not directly give rise to nonseminomas, both types of tumours have a common cell of origin as Ewing (1911) suggested. We believe that this cell is the CIS germ cell.

Hormonal environment and invasive cancer
Endocrine factors may play a role in the development of invasive cancer of the testis, as germinal cancer seems to be related to the postnatal and the postpubertal increase in gonadotrophin and/or testosterone production (Skakkebæk & Berthelsen, 1981b). Thus, the yolk sac tumours of infancy may be related to the postnatal peaks of gonadotrophins and testicular steroids (Winter & Faiman, 1972; Forest, Cathiard & Bertrand, 1973), while the germ cell tumours of adulthood may depend on the pubertal rise of the same hormones.

Classical seminoma versus spermatocytic seminoma
The term 'seminoma' (from latin: semen) indicates an origin from spermatogenetic cells. While this is probably true with regard to the spermatocytic seminoma, the classical seminoma seems to originate from embryonal germinal cells, the gonocytes (see above). It is our opinion that the histogenesis of the two types of so-called 'seminoma' is completely different, even though leading pathologists still relate the histogenesis of the classical seminoma with that of the spermatocytic seminoma (Mostofi, 1980). Our viewpoint is emphasized by the fact that we were unable to find carcinoma-in-situ cells of the characteristic (gonocyte) type in the adjacent testicular tissue of a series of spermatocytic seminomas (Müller, Skakkebæk & Parkinson, 1987). Besides, the clinical features of the spermatocytic seminoma are at variance with those of the classical seminoma (Masson, 1946; Talerman, 1986).

We prefer the alternative term 'spermatocytoma' for the spermatocytic seminoma, a term which has previously been suggested by others (Masson, 1946; Friedman, 1951) (Table 1). As the classical seminoma, in our opinion, does not

Table 1. Nomenclature of germ cell neoplasia

Present	Proposed alternatives
Carcinoma-in-situ	Gonocytoma-in-situ
Seminoma (classical) and dysgerminoma	Gonocytoma (Teilum, 1971; Teter, 1960)
Intratubular seminoma	Intratubular gonocytoma
Spermatocytic seminoma	Spermatocytoma (Masson, 1946)
Nonseminomas	No change

originate from spermatogenetic cells, but from gonocytes, we suggest that the term 'gonocytoma' would be more appropriate. The term has previously been used by Teilum (1971). Teter (1960) used the same term for germ cell tumours in general. The dysgerminoma in the female, identical with the seminoma of the male, should according to the proposed nomenclature also be named gonocytoma.

As a consequence of the suggested alterations the term 'carcinoma-in-situ' should be replaced by 'gonocytoma-in-situ'.

Acknowledgement

This study was supported by The Danish Cancer Society, grants 84-007, 87-017, 86-044 and 86-065 and by P. Carl Petersen's fund, grant B1322.

References

Albrechtsen, R., Nielsen, M. H., Skakkebæk, N. E. & Wever, U. (1982) Carcinoma in situ of the testis. *Acta Pathologica et Microbiologica Scandinavica*, A, **90**, 301–303.
Atkin, N. B. (1973) High chromosome numbers of seminomata and malignant teratoma of the testis: a review of data on 103 tumours. *British Journal of Cancer*, **28**, 275–279.
Azzopardi, J. G., Mostofi, F. K. & Theiss, E. A. (1961) Lesions of testes observed in certain patients with wide-spread choriocarcinoma and related tumors. The significance and genesis of hematoxylin-staining bodies in the human testis. *American Journal of Pathology*, **38**, 207–225.
Beckstead, J. H. (1983) Alkaline phosphatase histochemistry in human germ cell neoplasms. *American Journal of Surgical Pathology*, **7**, 341–349.
Berthelsen, J. G. & Skakkebæk, N. E. (1981) Distribution of carcinoma-in-situ in testes from infertile men. *International Journal of Andrology*, Suppl. 4, 172–183.
Damjanov, I. (1986) Testicular germ cell tumors as model of carcinogenesis and embryogenesis. *Principles and Management of Testicular Cancer* (ed. by N. Javadpour), pp. 73–87. Thieme Inc., New York.
Damjanov, I., Knowles, B. B., Solter, D., Lange, P. H. & Fraley, E. E. (1982) Immunohistochemical localization of murine stage-specific embryonic antigens in human testicular germ cell tumors. *American Journal of Pathology*, **108**, 225–230.
Dixon, F. J. & Moore, R. A. (1953) Testicular tumours: clinicopathological study. *Cancer*, **6**, 427–454.
Ewing, J. (1911) Teratoma testis and its derivatives. *Surgical Gynaecology and Obstetrics*, **12**, 230–261.
Friedman, N. B. (1951) The comparative morphogenesis of extragenital and gonadal teratoid tumors. *Cancer*, **4**, 265–276.
Friedman, N. B. (1977) In: Braunstein, G. D., Friedman, N. B., Sacks, S. A. *et al*. Germ cell tumors of the testis. Interdepartmental Clinical Case Conference, University of California, Los Angeles (Speciality Conference). *Western Journal of Medicine*, **126**, 364.
Forest, M., Cathiard, A. M. & Bertrand, J. A. (1973) Evidence of testicular activity in early infancy. *Journal of Clinical Endocrinology and Metabolism*, **37**, 148–151.
Gondos, B., Berthelsen, J. G. & Skakkebæk, N. E. (1983) Intratubular germ cell neoplasia (carcinoma in situ): a preinvasive lesion of the testis. *Annals of Clinical and Laboratory Science*, **13**, 185–192.
Gondos, B. (1986) Intratubular germ cell neoplasia: ultrastructure and pathogenesis. *Pathology of the Testis and its Adnexa* (ed. by A. Talerman and L. M. Roth), pp. 11–28. Churchill Livingstone, New York.
Holstein, A. F. & Körner, F. (1974) Light and electron microscopical analysis of cell types in human seminoma. *Virchows Archiv*, A, **363**, 97–112.
Holstein, A. F., Schütte, B., Becker, H. & Hartmann, M. (1987) Morphology of normal and malignant germ cells. *International Journal of Andrology*, **10**, 1–18.
Hustin, J., Collette, J. & Franchimont, P. (1987) Immunohistochemical demonstration of placental alkaline phosphatase in various states of testicular development and in germ cell tumours. *International Journal of Andrology*, **10**, 29–35.
Jacobsen, G. K, Henriksen, O. B. & von der Maase, H. (1981) Carcinoma in situ of testicular tissue adjacent to malignant germ-cell tumors: a study of 105 cases. *Cancer*, **47**, 2660–2662.

Jacobsen, G. K. & Nørgaard-Pedersen, B. (1984) Placental alkaline phosphatase in testicular germ cell tumours and in carcinoma-in-situ of the testis. *Acta Pathologica Microbiologica et Immunologica Scandinavica*, A, **92**, 323–329.

von der Maase, H. Giwercman, A. & Skakkebæk, N. E. (1986) Radiation treatment of carcinoma-in-situ of testis. *Lancet*, **i**, 624–625.

Mandl, A. M. (1964) The radiosensitivity of germ cells. *Biological Reviews*, **39**, 288–371.

Mandl, A. M., Beaumont, H. M., Hughes, G. C. et al. (1964) The differential radiosensitivity of male primordial germ cells and spermatogonia. *Effects of Ionizing Radiation of the Reproductive System* (ed. by W. D. Carlson and F. X. Gassner), pp. 165. Pergamon Press, New York.

Mark, G. J. & Hedinger, C. (1965) Changes in the remaining tumor-free testicular tissue in cases of seminoma and teratoma. *Virchows Archiv*, A, **340**, 84–92.

Masson, P. (1946) Études dur le séminome. *Revue Canadienne de Biologie*, **5**, 361–387.

McKay, D. G., Hertig, A. T., Adams, E. C. & Danziger, S. (1953) Histochemical observations on the germ cells of human embryos. *Anatomical Record*, **117**, 201–219.

Mostofi, F. K. (1980) Pathology of germ cell tumors of the testis. *Cancer*, **45**, 1735–1754.

Müller, J. & Skakkebæk, N. E. (1981) Microspectrophotometric DNA measurements of carcinoma-in-situ germ cells in the testis. *International Journal of Andrology*, Suppl. 4, 211–221.

Müller, J. & Skakkebæk, N. E. (1984) Testicular carcinoma in situ in children with the androgen insensitivity (testicular feminisation) syndrome. *British Medical Journal*, **288**, 1419–1420.

Müller, J., Skakkebæk, N. E., Nielsen, O. H. & Græm, N. (1984) Cryptorchidism and testis cancer: atypical infantile germ cells followed by carcinoma in situ and invasive carcinoma in adulthood. *Cancer*, **54**, 629–634.

Müller, J., Skakkebæk, N. E., Ritzén, M., Plöen, L. & Petersen, K. E. (1985) Carcinoma in situ of the testis in children with 45,X/46,XY gonadal dysgenesis. *Journal of Pediatrics*, **106**, 431–436.

Müller, J., Skakkebæk, N. E. & Parkinson, C. (1987) The spermatocytic seminoma: views on pathogenesis. *International Journal of Andrology*, **10**, 147–156.

Neville, A. M. (1979) A new era in the classification of testicular tumours? *Investigative Cell Pathology*, **2**, 61.

Nielsen, H., Nielsen, M. & Skakkebæk, N. E. (1974) The fine structure of a possible carcinoma-in-situ in the seminiferous tubules in the testis of four infertile men. *Acta Pathologica et Microbiologica Scandinavica*, A, **82**, 235–248.

Nüesch-Bachmann, J. H. & Hedinger, C. (1977) Atypische Spermatogonien als Präkanzerose. *Schweizeriche Medizinische Wochenschrift*, **107**, 795–801.

Raghavan, D., Sullivan, A. L., Peckham, N. J. & Munro Neville, A. (1982) Elevated serum alphafetoprotein and seminoma: clinical evidence for a histologic continuum? *Cancer*, **50**, 982—989.

Schultz, H. P., et al. (1984) Testicular carcinoma in Denmark in 1976–1980. Stage and selected clinical parameters at presentation. *Acta Radiologica et Oncologica*, **23**, 249–253.

Schultze, C. & Holstein, A. F. (1977) On the histology of human seminoma. Development of the solid tumor from intratubular seminoma cells. *Cancer*, **39**, 1090–1100.

Skakkebæk, N. E. (1972a) Abnormal morphology of germ cells in two infertile men. *Acta Pathologica et Microbiologica Scandinavica*, A, **80**, 374–378.

Skakkebæk, N. E. (1972b) Possible carcinoma-in-situ of the testis. *Lancet*, **ii**, 516–517.

Skakkebæk, N. E. (1975) Atypical germ cells in the adjacent 'normal tissue' of testicular tumours. *Acta Pathologica et Microbiologica Scandinavica*, A, **83**, 127–130.

Skakkebæk, N. E. (1978) Carcinoma-in-situ of the testis: frequency and relationship to invasive germ cell tumours in infertile men. *Histopathology*, **2**, 157–170.

Skakkebæk, N. E. & Berthelsen, J. G. (1978) Carcinoma-in-situ of testis and orchidectomy. *Lancet*, **ii**, 204–205.

Skakkebæk, N. E. & Berthelsen, J. G. (1981a) Carcinoma-in-situ of the testis and invasive growth of different types of germ cell tumours. A revised germ cell theory. *International Journal of Andrology*, Suppl. 4, 26–33

Skakkebæk, N. E. & Berthelsen, J. G. (1981b) Carcinoma in situ testis and development of different types of germ cell tumours. *Advances in Andrology*, **7**, 89–93.

Skakkebæk, N. E., Berthelsen, J. G. & Visfeldt, J. (1981) Clinical aspects of testicular carcinoma-in-situ. *International Journal of Andrology*, Suppl. 4, 153–160.

Skakkebæk, N. E., Berthelsen, J. G. & Müller, J. (1982) Carcinoma-in-situ of the undescended testis. *Urologic Clinics of North America*, **9**, 377–385.

Skakkebæk, N. E., Berthelsen, J. G. & Müller, J. (1984) Histopathology of human testicular tumours: carcinoma-in-situ germ cells and invasive growth of different types of germ cell tumours. *Inserm*, **123**, 445–462.

Skrabanek, P., Kirrane, J. & Powell, D. (1979) A unifying concept of chorionic gonadotrophin production in malignancy. *Investigative Cell Pathology*, **2**, 75–85.

Talerman, A. (1986) Germ cell tumours, *Pathology of the Testis and its Adnexa* (ed. by A. Talerman and L. Roth), pp. 29–65. Churchill Livingstone, New York.

Teilum, G. (1971) *Special Tumours of Ovary and Testis and Related Extragonadal Lesions*. Munksgaard, Copenhagen.

Teter, J. (1960) A new concept of classification of gonadal tumours arising from germ cells (gonocytoma) and their histogenesis. *Gynaecologia*, **150**, 84–102.

Thackray, A. C. & Crane, W. A. J. (1971) Seminoma. *Pathology of the Testis* (ed. by R. B. C. Pugh), p. 164. Blackwell Scientific Publications, Oxford.

Wahren, B., Holmgren, P. A. & Stigbrandt, T. (1979) Placental alkaline phosphatase, alphafetoprotein and carcinoembryonic antigen in testicular tumors: tissue typing by means of cytologic smears. *International Journal of Cancer*, **24**, 749–753.

Wilms, M. (1896) Die tertoiden Geschwülste des Hodens, mit Einschluss der sog. Cystoide und Enchondrome. *Beitrage der Pathologisches Anatomie*, **19**, 233–366.

Winter, J. S. D. & Faiman, C. (1972) Pituitary–gonadal relations of testicular activity in early infancy. *Pediatric Research*, **6**, 125–135.

Discussion

Holstein I have many problems with the terms you used. The term 'atypical germ cells' was proposed many years ago on the basis of paraffin sections. You, yourself, were one of the first to point out that atypical germ cells might be tumour cells. This was a very important work. Today, however, by semithin sectioning and electron microscopy it is quite clear that these 'atypical germ cells' are tumour cells and not germ cells.

Your term 'CIS germ cell' is also misleading because I think that CIS tumour cells are not germ cells any longer. The term 'CIS gonocyte' could be misleading too. CIS tumour cells only *resemble* gonocytes, but in detail – the structure of the nucleus and some organelles – they are not gonocytes.

Please excuse these remarks but I think it is necessary to apply the correct nomenclature, especially for clinicians who are not very familiar with morphological facts.

Skakkebæk I agree with you that there are several problems with our current nomenclature. However, I think we should delay a decision on such matters until another occasion. We have no real difficulty in understanding the *meaning* of the terms which we use.

Grigor Do CIS cells differentiate into seminoma or nonseminoma within the tubules or after invasion has occurred?

Skakkebæk We have indicated previously (Skakkebæk et al., *International Journal of Andrology*, Suppl. 4, 26–34, 1981) that both possibilities exist. However, we have still not seen a single case of noninvasive CIS which has already differentiated into intratubular nonseminoma.

G. K. Jacobsen Could you please comment on the term 'intratubular neoplasia'. This is perhaps a better term than 'carcinoma-in-situ' because the cell of origin (germ cell) is not an epithelial cell.

Skakkebæk I do not think that 'intratubular neoplasia' is a practical term. It includes all types of tumour found within tubules including intratubular seminoma and extension of a tumour into the seminiferous tubules.

Grigor The term 'neoplasia' does not necessarily imply malignancy, whereas 'carcinoma' does. The cells we are talking about are clearly malignant, and I like the term 'carcinoma-in-situ'.

Immunohistochemical demonstration of placental alkaline phosphatase in various states of testicular development and in germ cell tumours

J. HUSTIN, J. COLLETTE* and P. FRANCHIMONT*

*Institute of Morphological Pathology, B-6280 Loverval, Belgium, and *Department of Radioimmunology, University of Liege, B-4000 Liège, Belgium*

Summary

Immunohistochemical localization of placental alkaline phosphatase (PlAP) has been performed on eighty-two samples of normal (embryonic, fetal, infantile or adult), cryptorchid or tumorous testicular tissue. The isoenzyme could be demonstrated at the cell membrane of primitive, embryonic germ cells but not in other normal tissues. In-situ carcinomas and seminomas were positively stained in 93% and 94% of cases respectively. The percentage of positivity decreased with tumour differentiation. It is suggested that PlAP is a marker of primitive germ cells and that it reappears in germ cell neoplasms by gene derepression.

Key words. Placental alkaline phosphatase, immunocytochemistry, embryonic testis, testicular carcinoma-in-situ, seminoma.

Introduction

Heat-stable alkaline phosphatase is an enzyme which is essentially characteristic of the mature, i.e. second and third trimester, placenta (Fishman *et al.*, 1976). This isoenzyme is being widely investigated: it has been shown that it could be produced by some tumours.

Interest has particularly focussed on germ cell tumours of the testis. In 1979, Wahren, Holmgren & Stigbrandt demonstrated that placental like alkaline phosphatase (PlAP) could be identified in a substantial number of seminomas. The study was quickly followed by others who also pointed to a highest frequency of elevated serum levels for seminoma (Lange *et al.*, 1982). Several papers dealing with tissue immunolocalization must also be noted. Uchida *et al.* (1981), Paiva *et al.* (1983) and Jacobsen & Nørgaard-Pedersen (1984) described the preferential labelling of seminomas as opposed to non-seminomatous germ cell tumours. Moreover, Jacobsen & Nørgaard-Pedersen (1984) have particularly commented on the frequent PlAP immunopositivity of carcinoma-in-situ (CIS) which is most frequently identified in the vicinity of infiltrative germ cells tumours.

We have also undertaken an immunohistological study of germ cell tumours and CIS and have confirmed the results of these authors. However, as data are somewhat conflicting as regards the immunostaining of normal testicular tissue, we conducted in parallel an immunocytochemical study of non-neoplastic testes obtained at various

Correspondence: Dr J. Hustin, Institute of Morphologic Pathology, Allee des Templiers 41, B-6280 Loverval, Belgium.

ages. We demonstrated that with the use of a polyclonal antibody displaying specificity for the heat-stable placental enzyme, primitive—i.e. embryonic—germ cells stain positively and that a link can thus be drawn between these embryonic cells and their adult malignant counterpart.

Materials and Methods

A total of eighty-two neoplastic and non-neoplastic specimens were investigated. The forty non-neoplastic group comprised twenty biopsies of normal testes, four neonatal and infantile testes, six embryonic gonads and ten samples of cryptorchid testes operated on after puberty. The tumour group consisted of forty-two cases: eighteen classical seminomas, one spermatocytic seminoma, twelve embryonal carcinomas, two choriocarcinomas and four immature teratomas. Two cases of testicular infiltration by malignant lymphoma were added as controls. All specimens were fixed in Bouin's fluid and embedded in paraplast. Several sections were obtained for immunocytochemistry. All series of PlAP immunostaining were run with representative sections of mature placenta as a positive control. The antibody used was polyclonal raised in the rabbit and purchased from Dakopatts a/s, Denmark (code no. A268). It was usually used at a 1/1000 dilution in phosphate buffered saline (PBS). Incubation was performed at 4°C overnight and was followed by an avidin–biotin revelation (Vectastain, Vector Labs, Burlingame, Calif.) with 3-3' diaminobenzidine as chromogen. Harris haematoxylin was used as a counterstain. For negative controls, non-immune rabbit serum was used in place of PlAP antibody. The intensity of reaction was graded by an arbitrary score from − to +++.

Results

1. Normal tissues

Immunostaining for PlAP was never encountered in infantile, prepubertal or normal adult testes. This absence of immunoreactivity was unequivocal. On the contrary, definite staining was present at the cell membrane of primitive germ cells in embryonic gonads. This finding was more conspicuous when the gonads had not yet undergone cord formation.

In one specimen of 7.5 mm crown–rump embryo, no definite gonad could be identified, but scattered PlAP positive germ cells were present alongside the genital ridge (Fig. 1).

In older embryos obtained during the second trimester of pregnancy, most of the germ cells were trapped within sex cords (Fig. 2). Immunopositivity decreased progressively and was completely negative in term specimens. It must be noted here that embryonic and fetal bones, intestine and liver were not immunostained.

Cryptorchid testes obtained during or after puberty were, as a rule, PlAP negative. In one case out of ten we disclosed two positive spermatogonia within an isolated tube. Positivity was again strictly limited to the cell membrane.

2. Germ cell tumours

The results of the immunocytochemical investigations are summarized in Table 1. The highest positivity (as a function of intensity of staining per cell and of the percentage of positive cells) was shared by carcinoma-in-situ, whether isolated or

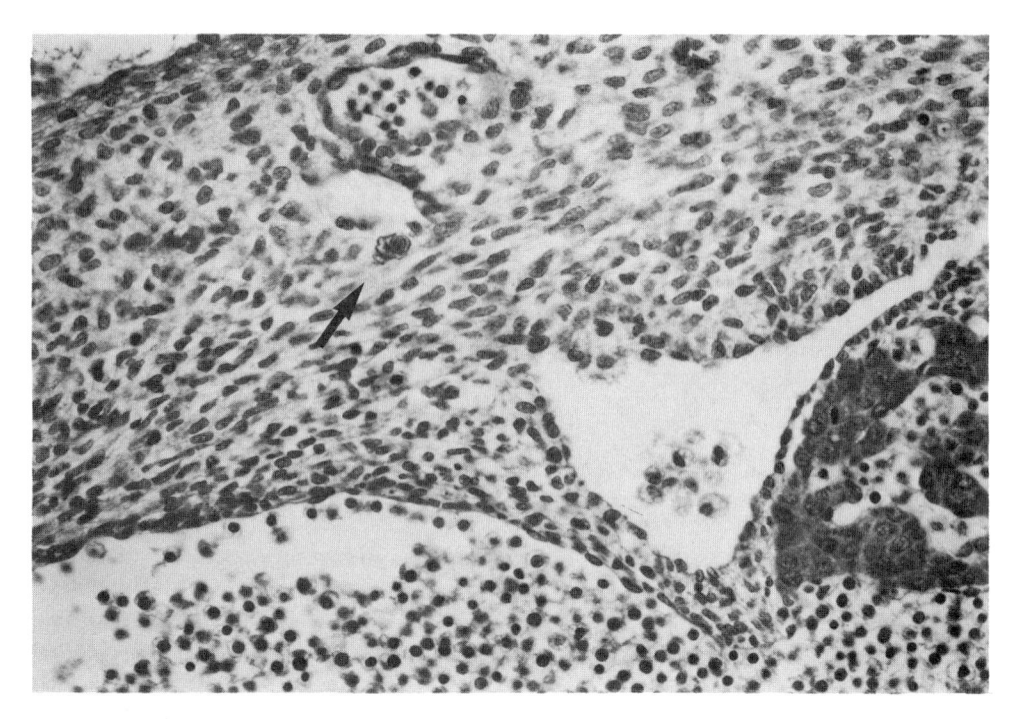

Fig. 1. Genital ridge, 7.5 mm embryo. An immunostained germ cell (arrow) is readily identified. (PlAP immunostaining + Harris haematoxylin counterstain, ×250.)

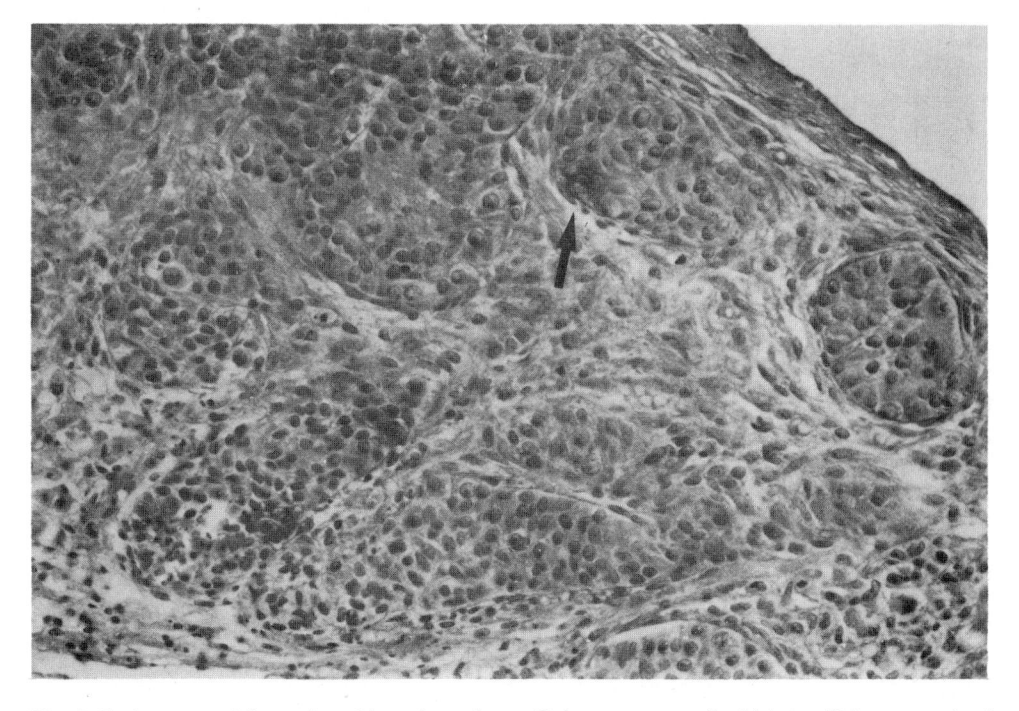

Fig. 2. Early sex cord formation. 14 weeks embryo. Only one germ cell which is still immunostained (arrow) is present in the field (PlAP immunostaining + Harris haematoxylin counterstain, ×250.)

Table 1. Germ cell tumours, PlAP immunostaining

	Intensity of staining				Total	Per cent positivity
	−	+	++	+++		
Carcinoma-in-situ (all cases)	1	4	7	3	15	93
Seminomas	1	6	9	2	18	94
Spermatocytic seminoma	1	−	−	−	1	0
Embryonal carcinomas	4	8	−	−	12	66
Choriocarcinomas	−	2	−	−	2	100
Immature teratomas	4	−	−	−	4	0

accompanying obvious tumours, and by seminoma (respectively 93% and 94% of cases) (Figs. 3 and 4).

Interestingly, the only case of spermatocytic seminoma was completely negative.

Intratubular atypical germ cells and seminoma cells displayed peripheral immunopositivity, ringing the entire cell membrane. Nearly 100% of CIS or seminoma cells were stained for PlAP. Two-thirds of embryonal carcinomas were PlAP positive. Usually the immunostaining was graded as + and restricted to a limited number of cells, usually less than 50%. Care had, however, to be exercised: most frequently areas of necrosis gave an impression of focal positivity but this was obviously pure artefact. The immunopositivity of both choriocarcinoma cases was in fact moderate, being more prominent on syncytio- rather than cytotrophoblast. In

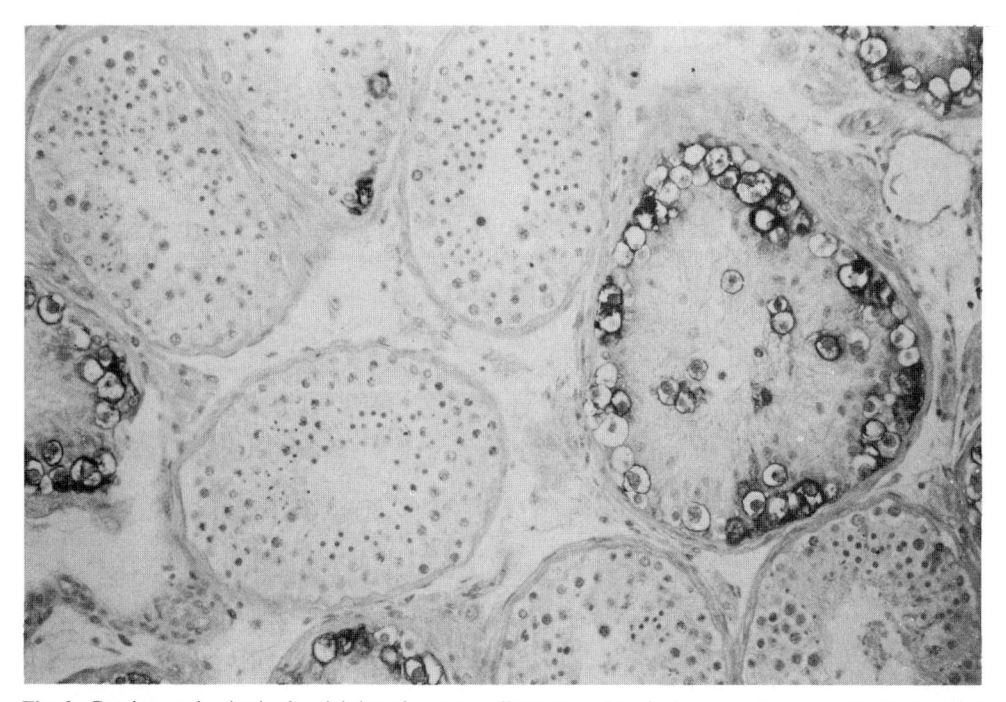

Fig. 3. Carcinoma-in-situ in the vicinity of a germ cell tumour. Atypical germ cells are markedly labelled at the cell membrane while tubes with normal spermatogenesis are not stained. (PlAP immunostaining + Harris haematoxylin counterstain, ×125.)

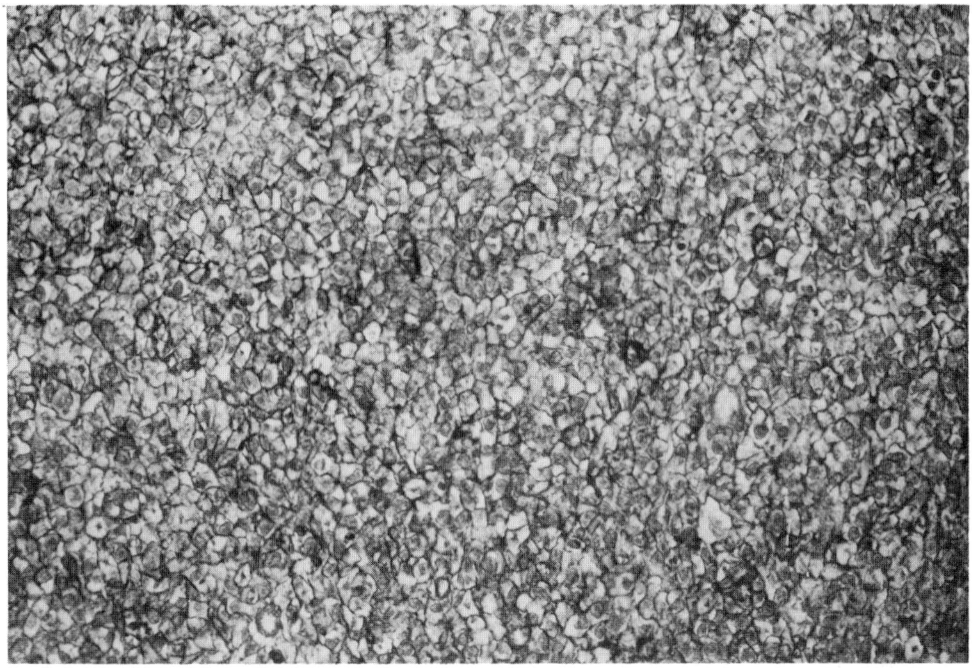

Fig. 4. Seminoma. All tumour cells are ringed by a distinct immunostaining. (PlAP immunostaining + Harris haematoxylin counterstain, ×125.)

contrast, immature teratomas with endodermal differentiation were strictly negative as were the two cases of testicular lymphoma.

Discussion

The immunoreactivity pattern obtained with our polyclonal antibody was characteristic of placental-type isoenzyme since it induced positive staining in third trimester placenta only, while embryonal and fetal liver cells, growing osteoblasts, and osteoclasts, intestinal mucosa and vascular endothelium were strictly negative. This contrasts with the manufacturer's description which stated cross-reactivity with intestinal alkaline phosphatase.

As regards the germ cell tumour series, our results correlate very well with those of Jacobsen & Nørgaard-Pedersen (1984). In particular, atypical germ cells of CIS were heavily immunostained, thus contrasting with normal spermatogonia, spermatocytes and spermatids. In fact atypical germ cells could be easily identified even at low magnification and we wonder whether the isolated finding of two positive germ cells in an otherwise negative cryptorchid testes, might have represented the very beginning of malignant transformation. A similar finding has been described by Beckstead (1983) who used histo-enzymatic demonstration of alkaline phosphatase without pointing to its possible placental nature. PlAP seems thus to be a very useful marker for *incipient* germ cell malignant transformation. PlAP staining is also very characteristic of seminoma cells (Wahren *et al.*, 1979) whereas in other types of germ cell tumours it is not more useful than staining for other classical markers such as hCG and AFP.

One may suggest that PlAP immunopositivity is restricted to undifferentiated germ cells. Indeed we have encountered more than one case of embryonal carcinoma which was weakly and irregularly positive or totally negative while surrounding CIS was heavily labelled. Moreover, immature teratomas were totally PlAP negative. Uchida *et al.* (1981) have demonstrated in such tumours an intestinal-like alkaline phosphatase positivity. These findings thus point to the concept of different isoenzyme production in the course of tumour differentiation.

Paiva *et al.* (1983) using monoclonal antibodies disclosed distinct immunofluorescence in normal adult or fetal testes as well as a positive reaction for enzyme histochemical demonstration of alkaline phosphatase. Neither Beckstead (1983) nor Uchida *et al.* (1981) nor Jacobsen & Nørgaard-Pedersen (1984) could confirm such results. In this study we were also unable to find any immunopositivity in normal adult or infantile or neonatal testes, but embryonic gonads were characterized by PlAP positivity of primitive germ cells. These were also immunostained during their early migration towards the genital ridge and interestingly were the sole cells to be immunostained in the whole embryo.

During progressive embryonic and fetal development, germ cells were progressively confined to the inner part of sex cords and PlAP progressively decreased and eventually disappeared. This finding is suggestive of an important function of PlAP during testicular morphogenesis. It has been postulated (Risk & Johnson, 1985) that PlAP could be a regulator of cell growth. Indeed, it is totally absent from first trimester placenta when active trophoblastic proliferation takes place, but it is readily demonstrated in second and third trimester specimens when placental growth is under closer control.

During testicular development, a similar mechanism might be suggested. PlAP is present at the cell membrane of germ cells as long as they are not enclosed within cords or tubules, thus preventing any disorderly growth. Spermatogonia either quiescent or involved in the active process of spermatogenesis are PlAP negative probably because of gene repression: cell growth at this moment is no longer regulated.

In conclusion, placental-like alkaline phosphatase is defined at the cell membrane of primitive embryonic and tumorous undifferentiated germ cells. The presence of this isoenzyme could be linked to a control of cell growth during embryonic development and to a gene derepression during tumorigenesis. Its almost constant demonstration in CIS indicates that it is a very sensitive marker of early malignant transformation.

With a 93% frequency of massive positivity in seminoma, PlAP is up to now the best marker of this type of neoplasm.

References

Beckstead, J. H. (1983) Alkaline phosphatase histochemistry in human germ cell neoplasms. *American Journal of Surgical Pathology*, **7**, 341–349.

Fishman, L., Miyayama, H., Driscoll, S. G. & Fishman, W. H. (1976) Developmental phase-specific alkaline phosphatase isoenzymes of human placenta and their occurrence in human cancer. *Cancer Research*, **36**, 2268–2273.

Jacobsen, G. K. & Nørgaard-Pedersen, B. (1984) Placental alkaline phosphatase in testicular germ cell tumours and in carcinoma-*in-situ* of the testis. *Acta Pathologica Microbiologica et Immunologica Scandinavica*, Sect. A, **92**, 323–329.

Lange, P. H., Millan, J. L., Stigbrandt, T., Vessella, R. L., Ruoslahti, E. & Fishman, W. H. (1982) Placental alkaline phosphatase as a tumor marker for seminoma. *Cancer Research*, **42**, 3244–3247.

Paiva, J., Damjanon, I., Lange, P. H. & Harris, H. (1983) Immunohistochemical localization of placental like alkaline phosphatase in testis and germ-cell tumors using monoclonal antibodies. *American Journal of Pathology*, **111**, 156–165.

Risk, J. M. & Johnson, P. M. (1985) Antigen expression by human trophoblast and tumour cells: models for gene regulation. *Contributions to Gynecology and Obstetrics*, Vol. 14: *Immunology and Immunopathology of Reproduction* (ed. by V. Toder and A. E. Beer), pp. 74–82. Karger, Basel.

Uchida, T., Shimoda, T., Miyata, H., Shikata, T., Iino, S., Suzuki, H., Oda, T., Hirano, K. & Sugiura, M. (1981) Immunoperoxidase study of alkaline phophatase in testicular tumor. *Cancer*, **48**, 1455–1462.

Wahren, B., Holmgren, P. A. & Stigbrandt, T. (1979) Placental alkaline phosphatase, alphafetoprotein and carcinoembryonic antigen in testicular tumors tissue typing by means of cytologic smears. *International Journal of Cancer*, **24**, 749–753.

Discussion

Grigor Which cells in the normal human placenta stain for PlAP and do yolk sac tumours contain PlAP?

Hustin Only the syncytiotrophoblastic border of the chorionic villi stains for PlAP, and only in the mature placenta, that is in the second and third trimesters. The area of positivity is membrane-bound and is seen especially in the microvillous area. Cytotrophoblast is not stained.

We have not examined infantile yolk sac tumours.

G. K. Jacobsen The Dakopatts antibody against PlAP is polyclonal and therefore various subtypes of placental alkaline phosphatase may be demonstrated. Did you study any of your embryos or testicular tumour sections with monoclonal antibodies against the testicular subtype of PlAP?

Hustin Up to the present time we have only studied 10 germ cell tumours with a battery of monoclonal antibodies against PlAP, in collaboration with Professor M. de Broe in the department of Nephrology, University of Antwerp, Belgium. Seminomas are heavily stained but our results are still fragmentary. Our study with embryos is only beginning, but obvious difficulties are encountered because of the specific technical requirements.

Immunohistochemical identification of macrophages, lymphoid cells and HLA antigens in the human testis

P. PÖLLÄNEN *and* M. NIEMI   Department of Anatomy, University of Turku, Turku, Finland

Summary

The presence and distribution of macrophages, several subtypes of lymphocytes and HLA antigens in the human testis were studied using monoclonal antibodies and immunocytochemical staining. Cells identified as tissue macrophages were relatively abundant. They were dispersed individually in the interstitium and were often included in Leydig cell clusters. Occasional macrophages were observed in the tubular wall, but never in the seminiferous tubules. Very few lymphocytes were found in the testicular interstitium. These were mainly T lymphocytes. T helper/inducer and T cytotoxic/suppressor cells were extremely scarce. B1+ cells were not observed, but occasional Leu-14+ cells could be seen. NK cells were not found. The number of T lymphocytes in the tunica albuginea was considerably higher than in the interstitial tissue. HLA-ABC and HLA-DR antigens could be observed in the endothelial cells and macrophages which were both strongly positive. The myoid cells and the Leydig cells expressed these antigens only weakly. Neither of the HLA antigens was expressed in the germinal epithelium.

Key words.   Macrophages, lymphocytes, leukaemia, human testis.

Introduction

The human testicular interstitium is composed of relatively abundant connective tissue, in which the Leydig cells are embedded (Fawcett, Neaves & Flores, 1973). As loose connective tissue elsewhere in the body, the testicular interstitium should contain a variety of single cells, including leucocytes. However, in the literature concerning human testicular cytology, cells other than the Leydig cells are only seldom mentioned (Holstein, 1978; Suominen & Söderström, 1982; Ritchie *et al.*, 1984). Macrophages, mast cells, lymphocytes and fibroblasts have been identified in the interstitium of other mammalian species (Christensen, 1975; Ohata, 1979; Niemi, Sharpe & Brown, 1986).

  Testis, together with bone marrow and brain, is a common place of relapse in childhood acute lymphocytic leukaemia (Pinkel, 1971; Kuo, Tschang & Chu, 1976; Saiontz *et al.*, 1978). Why testis provides an advantageous environment for the leukaemic cells to survive, is not known. It has been suggested that the cytotoxic drugs do not penetrate to the testis. Another explanation might be that the immunological environment of the testis is unusual and contributes to the generation of relapses.

Correspondence: Dr Pasi Pöllänen, Department of Anatomy, University of Turku, SF-20520 Turku, Finland

The observation that allografts survive in the testicular interstitium (Aron, Marescaux & Petrovic, 1957; Ferguson & Scothorne, 1977; Head, Neaves & Billingham, 1983a; Maddocks, Oliver & Setchell, 1984) indicates that the testis exhibits special immunological features that make it a privileged site for transplantation.

We have sought an explanation for these unusual types of reaction in the testis by the means of an immunohistochemical study, and investigated the presence of macrophages, several subtypes of lymphocytes and HLA antigens in the human testis.

Materials and Methods

The testis tissue samples were obtained at autopsy from three healthy men who had died in accidents no more than 24 h previously. All the specimens were histologically normal.

Pieces cut from the freshly removed testes were frozen in liquid nitrogen and sectioned in a cryostat. The sections (5 μm) were first dried at room temperature for 45 min and then fixed in cold acetone ($-15°C$) for 15 min.

Immunocytochemistry

The antibodies used are shown in Table 1. Both the indirect immunoperoxidase method and the biotin–avidin staining method were applied. Before incubation with the primary antibodies in the former method, the endogenous peroxidase was blocked by incubating the sections in fresh 0.5% H_2O_2 in methanol for 15 min. Non-specific binding sites were blocked by incubating the sections with 5% normal rabbit serum for 15 min. Peroxidase-conjugated rabbit-anti-mouse immunoglobulins (Dakopatts, Copenhagen, Denmark) were used as the second antibody in the indirect immunoperoxidase staining, and biotin-conjugated goat-anti-mouse immunoglobulins (Becton Dickinson, Mountain View, California) in the biotin–avidin staining. The third conjugate in the biotin–avidin method was horseradish

Table 1. Antibodies used in the study

Antibody	Specificity of antibody	Reference
T4	Inducer T cell subset	Coulter*
T8	Cytotoxic and suppressor lymphocytes	Coulter
T11	All T lymphocytes	Coulter
B1	B cells	Coulter
MY4	Monocytes, some granulocytes	Coulter
Anti-Leu-1	All T cells	Becton Dickinson[†]
Anti-Leu-2a	Cytotoxic/suppressor T cells	Becton Dickinson
Anti-Leu-3a+3b	Helper/inducer T cells, macrophages	Becton Dickinson
Anti-Leu-4	All T cells	Becton Dickinson
Anti-HLA-DR	HLA-DR (non-polymorphic)	Becton Dickinson
Anti-Leu-M5	Monocytes, tissue macrophages	Becton Dickinson
Anti-Leu-11	NK cells	Becton Dickinson
Anti-Leu-14	B cells	Becton Dickinson
DA2	HLA-DRw (non-polymorphic)	Brodsky et al., 1979[‡]
PA2.6	HLA-ABC	Parham & Bodmer, 1978[‡]

* Coulter Cline, Hialeah, Florida.
† Becton Dickinson, Moutain View, California.
‡ Gift from Dr Goodfellow, Imperial Cancer Research Fund.

peroxidase-conjugated avidin (Becton Dickinson). The peroxidase activity was demonstrated with diaminobenzidine.

Results

Macrophages

Cells identified as tissue macrophages on the basis of their MY4 and Leu-M5 antigens were relatively abundant in the intertubular tissue of human testis (Figs. 1 and 2). They were dispersed individually in the interstitium and were often included in Leydig cell clusters. They could also be observed in the lamina propria of the seminiferous tubules (Fig. 3). Macrophages were never present in the seminiferous tubules.

Lymphocytes

Very few lymphocytes were found in the testicular interstitium. These were mainly T lymphocytes (T11+, Leu-1+), which were scattered throughout the interstitial tissue (Fig. 4). T helper/inducer (T4+, Leu-3a+3b+) and T cytotoxic/suppressor cells (T8+, Leu-2a+) were extremely scarce. B1+ cells were not observed, but occasional Leu-14+ cells could be seen. NK cells (Leu-11+) were not found. The number of T11+ lymphocytes in the tunica albuginea was considerably higher than in the interstitial tissue of testis.

HLA antigens

HLA-ABC antigen could be observed in the endothelial cells and macrophages which were both strongly positive. The myoid cells and the Leydig cells expressed this antigen only weakly (Fig. 5). The HLA-DR antigen was found in the same sites as the HLA-ABC antigen (Fig. 6). Neither of the HLA antigens was expressed in the germinal epithelium.

Discussion

The results of the present study show that all the cells required for cellular immunity are present in the normal human testicular interstitium. The seminiferous tubules, on the other hand, are devoid of these cell types. The number of lymphocytes in the interstitial tissue, however, is low in comparison to the connective tissue of many other organs like the ovary (unpublished observation). The lymphocytes in the human testis seem to be mainly of the T type. Among the subclasses of T-cells, the number of T inducer cells seems to be particularly low in the testicular interstitium. The dominance of the T lymphocytes may be due to the greater propensity of T cells to migrate to the tissue (Bhan *et al.*, 1985). Our observation may explain the fact that early testicular relapse occurs particularly in T cell disease (Hustu & Aur, 1978; Kim *et al.*, 1981).

The considerably smaller number of lymphocytes in the testis than in several other organs containing ordinary loose connective tissue may indicate that the lymphocytes do not migrate through the testicular blood vessels as easily as through vessels in other sites. Our present observations demonstrate that there may be differences in the permeability of microvessels to lymphocytes even between the testicular interstitium and the tunica albuginea.

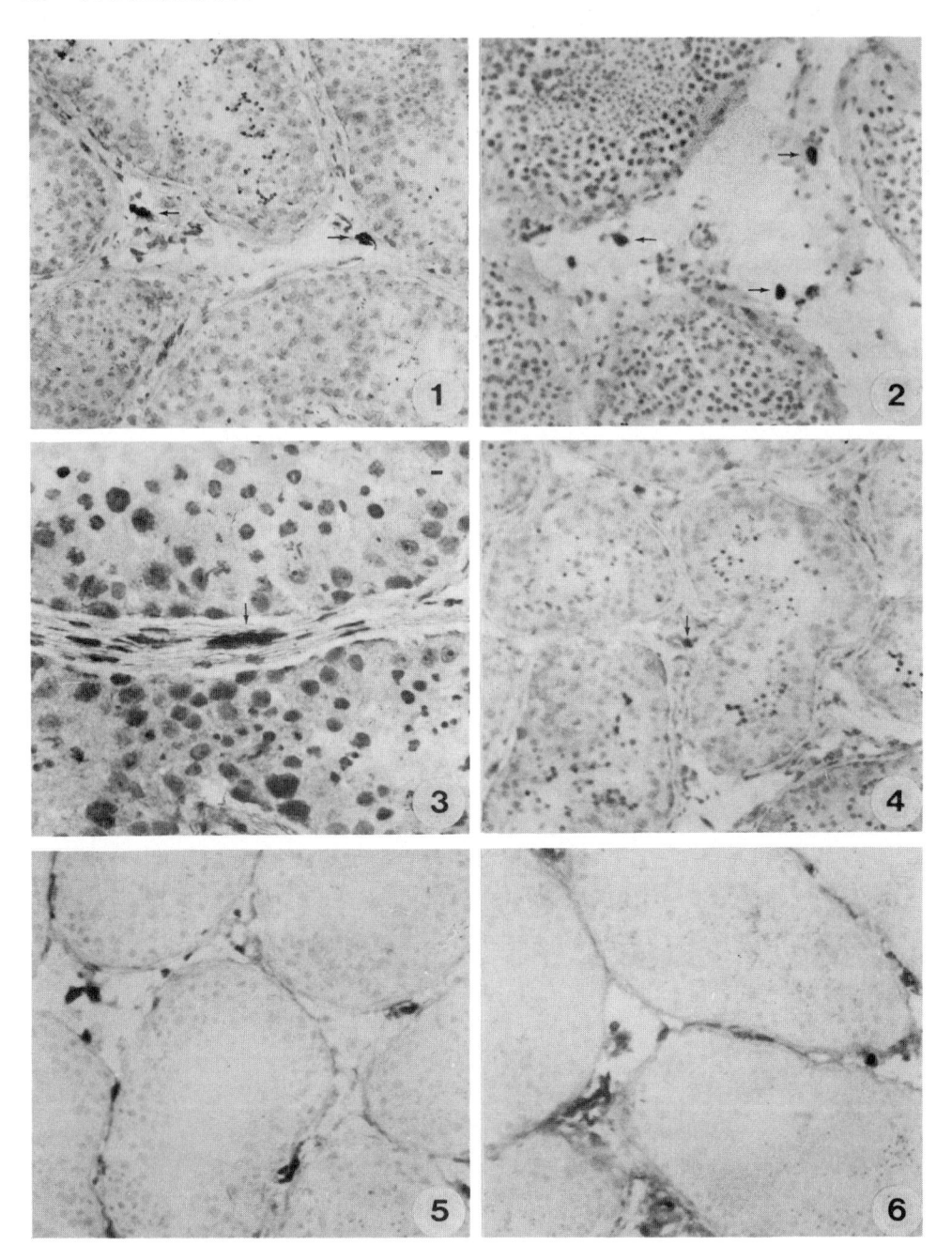

Fig. 1. Biotin−avidin staining for Leu-M5+ macrophages (arrows) in a frozen section of human testis. ×1520.
Fig. 2. Indirect immunoperoxidase staining for MY4+ macrophages (arrows) in a frozen section of human testis. ×1520.
Fig. 3. A Leu-M5+ macrophage (arrow) in the lamina propria of a seminiferous tubule. Biotin−avidin staining in a frozen section of human testis. ×3800.
Fig. 4. Biotin−avidin staining for Leu-1+ lymphocytes (arrow) in a frozen section of human testis. ×1520.
Fig. 5. Indirect immunoperoxidase staining for HLA-ABC antigen in a frozen section of human testis. ×1520.
Fig. 6. Indirect immunoperoxidase staining for HLA-DR antigen in a frozen section of human testis. ×1520.

The absence of class I and class II MHC molecules from the seminiferous epithelium probably protects the cells of the spermatogenic series from destruction by T lymphocytes. On the other hand, the absence of these antigens may impair the immunosurveillance of tumours derived from germ and Sertoli cells, supposing that the tumour cells do not carry these antigens on their surface. Because the testicular macrophages were positive to the class II molecule, presentation of processed foreign antigens to the T inducer lymphocytes should be possible in the human testis.

Although the testis is known to be an immunologically privileged site for auto- and allografts in the rodents, nothing is known about the behaviour of the human testis in equal situations. Recent observations show that differences in the lymphatic drainage and composition of the interstitial mononuclear cells may influence the survival of the transplants in the testis (Pöllänen, Maddocks & Niemi, unpublished results). The human testis takes an intermediate position in its number of macrophages between the ram and the rat, but it has similar lymphatic drainage as the ram testis (Fawcett et al., 1973), in which the allografts do not survive (Maddocks, Cormack & Setchell, 1985). The lymphocyte counts in the human testis are similar to those in the rat and the ram testis.

The reasons for testis being one of the first sites of relapse after a long-time remission in acute lymphocytic leukaemia are not known. Many factors may be involved, including the poor penetration of drugs to the testis, but the special immunological environment of the testis and the immunosuppressive effects of drugs used in the therapy may play an important role. Although the present observations do not explain the unusual behaviour of the testis in childhood acute lymphocytic leukaemia, they clearly demonstrate that the testicular interstitium is unusually constituted regarding its immunoreactive cytology.

Acknowledgement

We are grateful to Dr Goodfellow and Dr Uksila for some of the antibodies used.

References

Aaron, M., Marescaux, J. & Petrovic, A. (1957) Greffes homoplastiques chez le mammifères. *Colloques Internationales du C.N.R.S.* **78**, 25–33

Bhan, A. K., Reinisch, C. L., Levey, R. H., McCluskey, R. T. & Schlossman, S. F. (1975) T-cell migration into allografts. *Journal of Experimental Medicine*, **14**, 1210–1219.

Brodsky, F. M., Parham, P., Barnstable, C. J., Crumpton, M. J. & Bodmer, W. F. (1979) Monoclonal antibodies for analysis of the HLA system. *Immunological Reviews*, **47**, 3–61.

Christensen, A. K. (1975) Leydig cells. *Handbook of Physiology*, Section 7, Vol. 5, pp. 57–94. American Physiological Society, Washington D.C.

Fawcett, D. F., Neaves, W. B. & Flores, M. N. (1973) Comparative observations of intertubular lymphatics and the organization of the interstitial tissue of the mammalian testis. *Biology of Reproduction*, **9**, 500–532.

Ferguson, J. & Scothorne, R. S. (1977) Extended survival of pancreatic islet allografts in the testis of guinea pigs. *Journal of Anatomy*, **124**, 1–8.

Head, J. R. & Billingham, R. E. (1985) Immune privilege in the testis. II. Evaluation of potential local factors. *Transplantation*, **40**, 269–275.

Head, J. R., Neaves, W. B. & Billingham, R. E. (1983) Immune privilege in the testis. I. Basic parameters of allograft survival. *Transplantation*, **36**, 423–431.

Holstein, A. F. (1978) Spermatophagy in the seminiferous tubules and excurrent ducts of the testis in rhesus monkey and in man. *Andrologia*, **10**, 331–352.

Hustu, H. O. & Aur, R. J. A. (1978) Extramedullary leukaemia. *Clinics in Haematology*, **7**, 313–337.

Kim, T. H., Hargreaves, H. K., Brynes, R. K., Hawkins, H. K., Lui, V. K.-S., Woodward, J. & Ragab, A. H. (1981) Pretreatment testicular biopsy in childhood acute lymphocytic leukaemia. *Lancet*, **ii**, 657–658.

Kuo, T.-T., Tschang, T.-P. & Chu, J.-Y. (1976) Testicular relapse in childhood acute lymphocytic leukaemia during bone marrow remission. *Cancer*, **38**, 2604–2612.

Maddocks, S., Oliver, J. R. & Setchell, B. P. (1984) The survival and function of isolated pancreatic islets of Langerhans transplanted into the testis of adult rats and their effect on the testis. *Inserm*, **123**, 497–502.

Maddocks, S., Cormack, J. & Setchell, B. P. (1985) The failure of thyroid allografts in the ovine testis. *Proceeding of the Australian Society of Reproductive Biology*, **17**, 51–59.

Niemi, M., Sharpe, R. M. & Brown, W. R. A. (1986) Macrophages in the interstitial tissue of the rat testis. *Cell and Tissue Research*, **243**, 337–344.

Ohata, M. (1979) Electron microscopic study on the testicular interstitial cells in the mouse. *Archivum Histologicum Japonicum*, **42**, 51–79.

Parham, P. & Bodmer, W. F. (1978) Monoclonal antibody to a human histocompatibility alloantigen, HLA-A2. *Nature*, **276**, 397–399.

Pinkel, D. (1971) Five-year follow-up of 'total therapy' of childhood lymphocytic leukaemia. *Journal of the American Medical Association*, **216**, 648–652.

Ritchie, A. W. S., Hargreave, T. B., James, K. & Chisholm, G. D. (1984) Intraepithelial lymphocytes in the normal epididymis. A mechanism for tolerance to sperm auto-antigens. *British Journal of Urology*, **56**, 79–83.

Saiontz, H. I., Gilchrist, G. S., Smithson, W. A., Burgert, E. O., Jr & Cupps, R. (1978) Testicular relapse in childhood leukaemia. *Mayo Clinic Proceedings*, **53**, 212–216.

Suominen, J. & Söderström, K.-O. (1982) Lymphocyte infiltration in human testicular biopsies. *International Journal of Andrology*, **5**, 461–466.

Discussion

Hargreave We have conducted similar studies in Edinburgh (Ritchie *et al.*, 1982, *British Journal of Urology*; El Demiry *et al.*, 1985, *British Journal of Urology*) and agree with your findings in normal human testicular tissue, but this is not necessarily so in abnormal human testis. Testicular biopsies from infertile men contain increased numbers of T cells and in some cases intratubular T cells. What is the source of your 'normal' tissue and are you sure it was normal?

Pöllänen We used autopsy material from men under the age of 40 years, who had died accidentally not more than 24 hours previously. The testes were histologically normal.

Müller The problem of late testicular relapse of lymphoblastic leukaemia is largely confined to children. Have you investigated this age group?

Pöllänen No

Skakkebæk Carcinoma-in-situ of the testis is often associated with a focal infiltrate of lymphocytes. Is it a result of an immunological process and would you like to speculate on the function of this reaction?

Pöllänen It may be possible that an immunological response is generated against the CIS cells in the human testis. However, there is no available data on the response of the human testis against foreign cells such as CIS cells or transplant cells.

The function of the primordial germ cell in extragonadal tissues

N. B. FRIEDMAN   *Departments of Pathology, Cedars Sinai Medical Center, Los Angeles, California 90048, and University of Southern California, U.S.A.*

Summary

The identity of the germ cell tumours of the pineal and the thymus with those of the testis and ovary suggests that the widely disseminated primordial germ cells might subserve some special function in these sanctuaries. It is proposed that thymic localization might be required for the conveyance of genetic haematological and immunological information and that the pineal–diencephalic localization could programme neuroophthalmic tissues prior to the development of the blood–brain barrier. The latter speculation was tested by producing allergic encephalomyelitis in thymectomized, bursectomized and thymobursectomized chickens. It was found that although thymectomy and, to a lesser extent, bursectomy decreased the severity of the experimental encephalomyelitis the combined procedure resulted in more severe inflammatory lesions. This may be due to release of suppressed intraneural immunological mechanisms in the somatically impaired bird.

Key words.   Germ cells, thymus, pineal, allergic experimental encephalomyelitis.

In this study it is proposed to apply the results of embryological and haematological studies to the nature of extragonadal germ cell tumours in man. Since the retroperitoneal site generally proves metastatic and the sacrococcygeal growths may not be germinal, emphasis will be placed on the pineal and thymus.

Ever since it was realized that germ cells did not arise from the 'germinal' epithelium of the gonad but originated from extraembryonic primordial germ cells (Beard, 1900), their occurrence in tissues outside the gonad has piqued the curiosity of investigators. Migration to the developing gonad in the urogenital ridge is necessary in order to transmit genetic information for the next generation to the new gametes. Although it has been recognized for a long time that these primordial elements could be found widely scattered in the developing embryo (Witschi, 1948), no functional significance was ascribed to them. Subsequently it was recognized that such cells could give rise to germ cell tumours in extragonadal sites, notably the pineal (Russell, 1944), as well as in the hypothalamus, posterior pituitary and diencephalon. The mediastinal teratoid growths were the next to be

Correspondence: Dr Nathan B. Friedman, Department of Pathology, Cedars Sinai Medical Center, Los Angeles, California 90048, U.S.A.

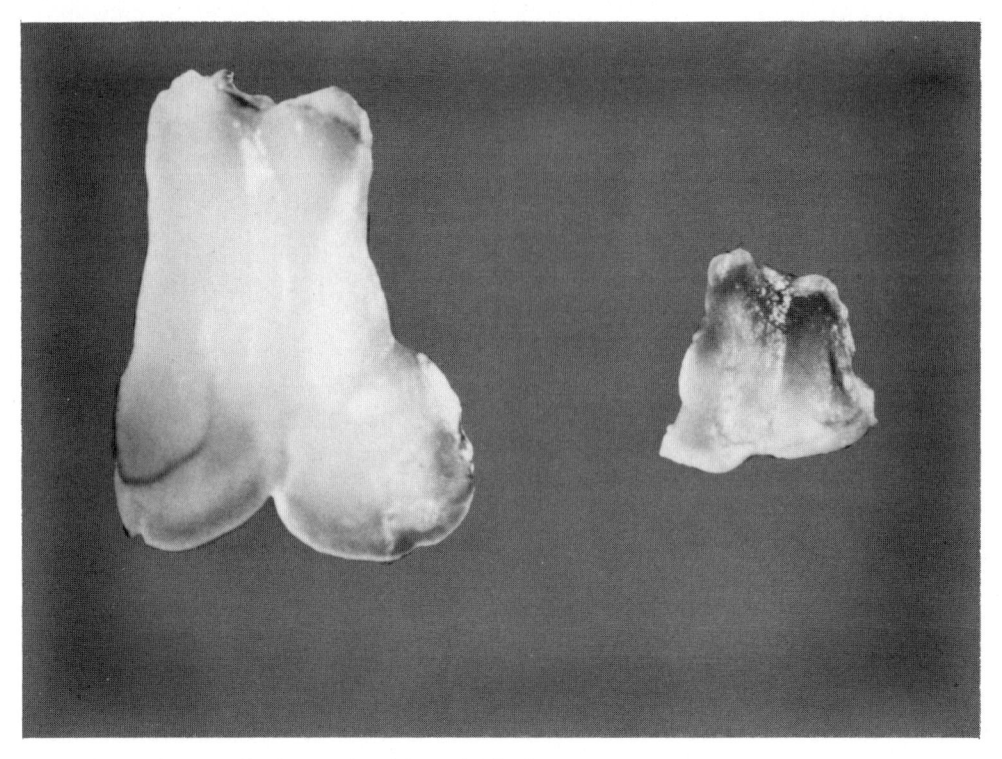

Fig. 1. Gross photograph of control and hypoplastic thymus.

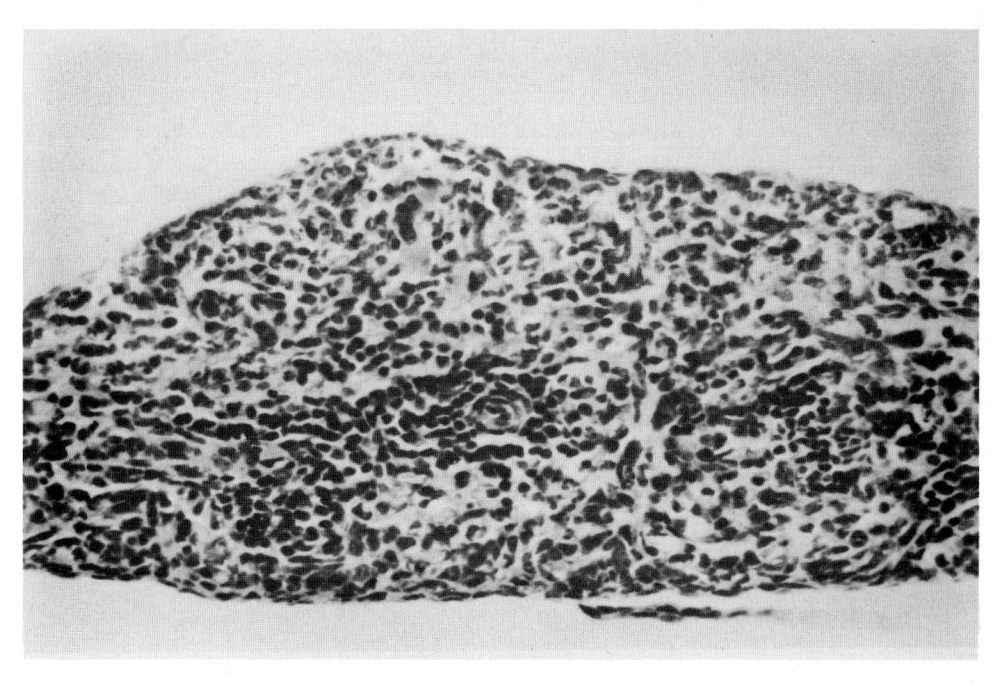

Fig. 2. Photomicrograph of tiny hypoplastic spleen. (Original × 420.)

incorporated into the scheme with the recognition of their thymic localization (Schlumberger, 1946) and the identification of thymic germinoma (Friedman, 1951).

Why do primordial germ cells survive in both pineal and thymus as they must in order for germinoma and the entire spectrum of teratoid tumours to appear in these particular sites? Both organs are known to be sanctuaries (Friedman & Van de Velde, 1981) and it seems only reasonable that some function must be served.

The role of the thymus in the production of specialized lymphocytes can be related to stem cell migration to that organ (Moore & Owen, 1967). A corollary could be that germ cells programme the thymus with immunological information (Friedman, 1967; Friedman & Van de Velde, 1974, 1981). Certain primitive elements not clearly identified as haematopoietic have been described not only in the yolk sac but also in retrosternal locations near the thymus (Kelemen, Calvo & Fliedner, 1979). Furthermore the suggestion has been made that primordial germ cells and thymic stem cells have interesting similarities (Auerbach, 1970).

This association of haemic and germinal elements is clearly seen in certain strains of mice, such as those with mutant genes at the W locus (Mintz & Russell, 1957). On the basis of unitary gene action (Metcalf & Moore, 1971), common regulatory factors must affect haematopoietic stem cells and primordial germ cells as well as melanoblast precursors. In addition to the gonadal and marrow defects a poorly developed thymus (Fig. 1) and spleen (Fig. 2) and deficient haematopoiesis in fatty livers (Fig. 3) characterize these animals.

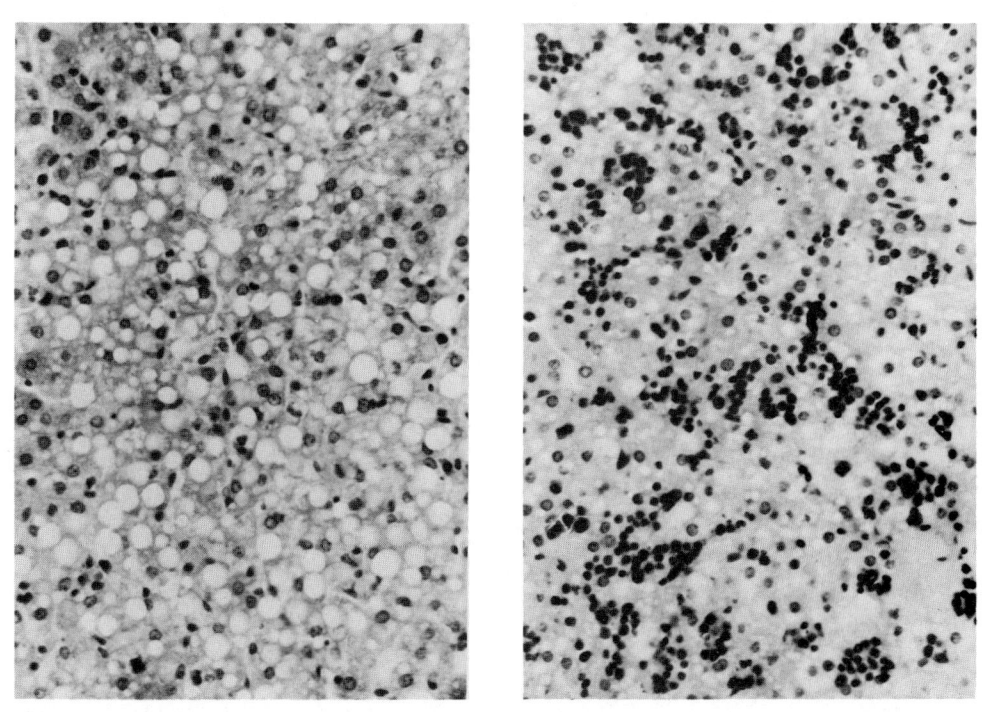

Fig. 3. (A) Photomicrograph of fatty liver with deficient haematopoiesis. (Original × 420.) (B) Photomicrograph of control liver. (Original × 420.)

The recent reports recognizing an association between germ cell tumours of the thymus and haematological neoplasia (Goldman, 1985; Nichols et al., 1985; Reynoso et al., 1986) would seem to confirm the suggested relationship between primordial germ cells and haematopoietic stem cells (Friedman & Van de Velde, 1974). The association with the Klinefelter syndrome of thymic germ cell tumours reported by Nichols et al. (1986) almost suggests a human parallel to the WW mice. Even lymphomas of the thymus have been encountered in some of the WW mice studied in our laboratory. The haematopoietic potential of teratocarcinoma (Cudennec & Johnson, 1981) and the occurrence of fetal haemoglobin in testicular germinal tumours (Jacobsen & Jacobsen, 1983) are compatible with this viewpoint.

A speculation to account for the pineal–diencephalic localization of germ cells led to studies of experimental allergic encephalomyelitis in bursectomized and thymectomized chickens. It was hypothesized that genetic immunological data might be required by brain and eye before the blood–brain barrier is set up. It was expected that chickens subjected to both bursectomy and thymectomy would manifest less inflammatory reaction in the neural tissues than controls. Although thymectomized birds showed diminution of the reaction the double operated subjects manifested more inflammatory changes than the controls (Fig. 4) (Friedman, Schainen & Lee, 1983). This could be interpreted as due to a release of intrinsic neural immunological factors whose existence has been suggested in relation to multiple sclerosis (Tourtelotte & Booc, 1978).

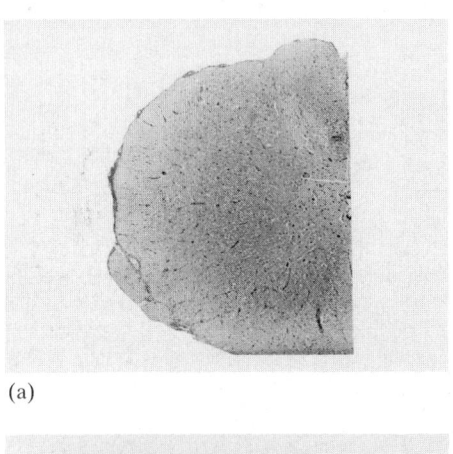

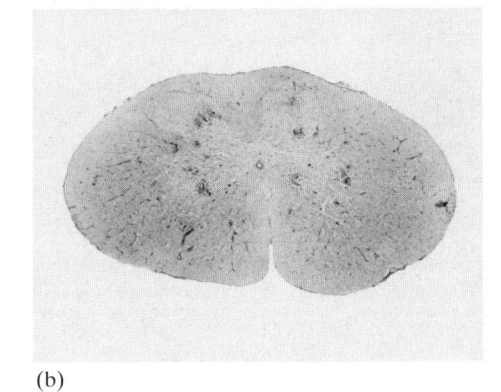

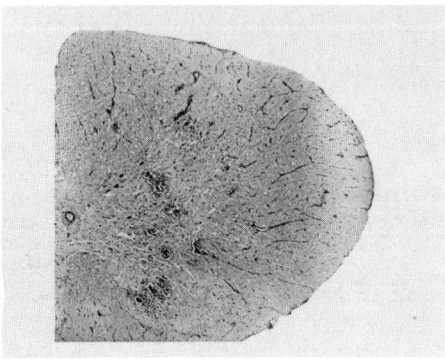

Fig. 4. Allergic encephalomyelitis. (a) Spinal cord of thymectomized chicken. (Original × 50.) (b) Spinal cord of thymobursectomized chicken. (Original × 20.) (c) Spinal cord of thymobursectomized chicken. (Original × 50.)

Extragonadal germ cells 47

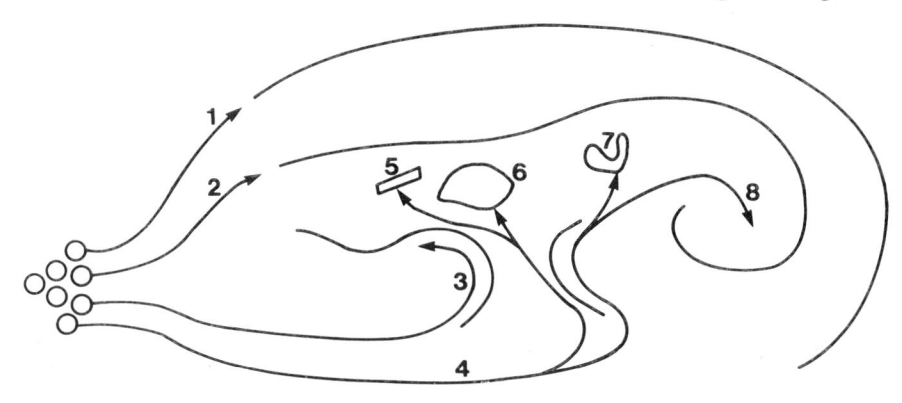

Fig. 5. Shows germ and stem cell lines and migrations. (See text and also Fig. 6.)

The pathways of migratory elements from the yolk sac to their final destinations are shown diagrammatically in Fig. 5. Germ cells travel to the gonadal blastema (3), extragonadal germ cells and haematopoietic stem cells (4) to thymus (7), brain (8), liver (6) and marrow (5). The primordial germ layers, instead of the traditional somatic ectoderm–mesoderm–entoderm triad, can be viewed as extraembryonic (placenta, membranes) (1), somatic (2) and germinal-haematopoietic (3, 4). The yolk sac is a blend of somatic and extraembryonic tissue and serves as a protective holding organ for the germ line and the stem cells (Friedman & Van de Velde, 1981).

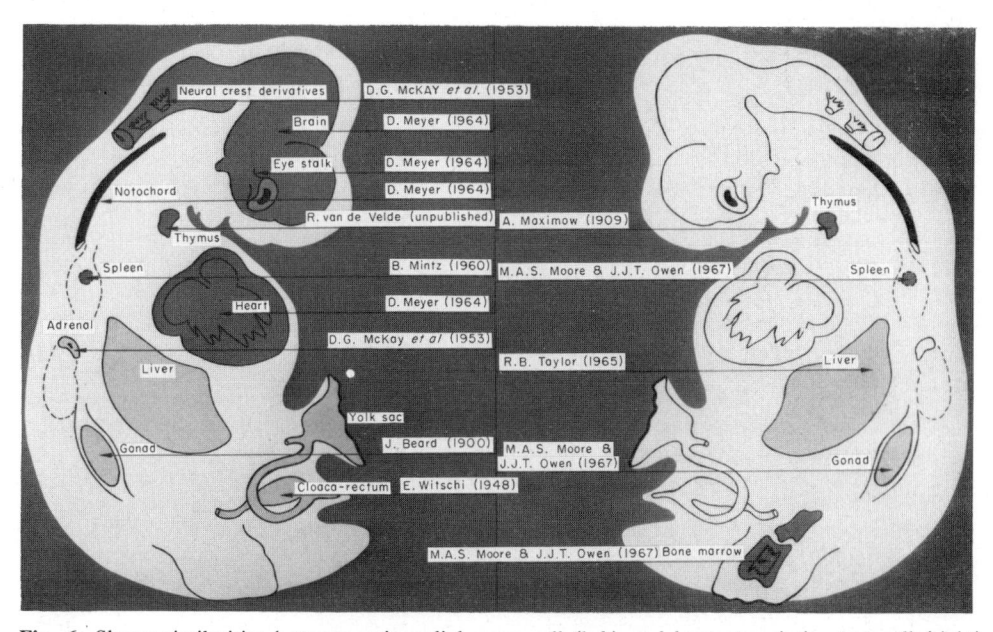

Fig. 6. Shows similarities between primordial germ cell (left) and haematopoietic stem cell (right) localizations. (This diagram is a photograph of an exhibit which was presented at the Western Section, American Urological Association meeting in Las Vegas, Nevada, in April 1971, where it was awarded the first prize.)

These concepts are not only useful in the understanding of ectopic germ cell tumours but can be employed as working speculations in designing models for experimental attacks on a variety of neoplastic and immunological disorders.

References

Auerbach, R. (1970) Toward developmental theory of antibody formation: the germinal theory of immunity. In: *Development Aspects of Antibody Formation and Structure* (ed. by Sterzl, J. & Riho, I.). Academic Press Inc., New York.

Beard, J. (1900) The morphological continuity of the germ cells in Raja Batis. *Anatomischer Anzeiger (Jena)*, **18**, 465.

Cudennec, C. A. & Johnson, G. R. (1981) Presence of multipotential hemopoietic cells in teratocarcinoma cultures. *Journal of Embryology and Experimental Morphology*, **61**, 51–59.

Friedman, N. B. (1951) The comparative morphogenesis of extragenital and gonadal teratoid tumours. *Cancer*, **4**, 264–276.

Friedman, N. B. (1967) Tumours of the thymus. *Journal of Thoracic and Cardiovascular Surgery*, **53**, 163–182.

Friedman, N. B., Schainen, J. S. & Lee, W. (1983) Enhancement of allergic encephalomyelitis in chickens by combined thymobursectomy. *Federation Proceedings*, **42**, 1213.

Friedman, N. B. & Van de Velde, R. L. (1974) Germinomas in Man and Hemogonadal Defects in Mice. *Proceedings of 10th International Congress of International Academy of Pathology*, p. 45. Hamburg, Germany.

Friedman, N. B. & Van de Velde, R. L. (1981) Germ cell tumors in man, pleiotropic mice, and continuity of germplasm and somatoplasm. *Human Pathology*, **12**, 772–776.

Goldman, R. L. (1985) Germ cell tumors of hematologic diseases. *American Journal of Surgical Pathology*, **9**, 905.

Jacobsen, G. K. & Jacobsen, M. (1983) Immunohistochemical demonstration of hemoglobin F (HbF) in testicular germ cell tumors. *Oncodevelopmental Biology and Medicine*, **4**, C45–C51.

Kelemen, E., Calvo, W. & Fliedner, T. M. (1979) *Atlas of Human Hemopoietic Development*. Springer, Heidelberg.

Maximow, A. (1909) Untersuchungen über Blut und Bindegewebe. II. Über die Histogenese der Thymus bei Saügetieren. *Archiv für Mikrobiologie und Anatomie*, **74**, 525.

McKay, D. G., Hertig, A. T., Adams, E. & Danziger, S. (1953) Histochemical observation on the germ cells of human embryos. *Anatomical Record*, **117**, 201.

Metcalf, D. & Moore, M. A. S. (1971) *Haemopoietic Cells*. North-Holland, Amsterdam, The Netherlands.

Meyer, D. B. (1964) The migration of primordial germ cells in the chick embryo. *Developmental Biology*, **10**, 154.

Mintz, B. (1960) Embryological phases of mammalian gametogenesis. *Journal of Cellular and Comparative Physiology*, **56**, 31.

Mintz, B. & Russell, E. (1957) Gene induced embryological modifications of primordial germ cells in the mouse. *Journal of Experimental Zoology*, **134**, 207.

Moore, M. A. S. & Owen, J. J. (1967) Experimental studies on the development of the thymus. *Journal of Experimental Medicine*, **126**, 715.

Nichols, C., Palmer, C., Heerema, N., Williams, S., Loehrer, P. & Einhorn, L. (1986) Primary mediastinal germ cell tumour (PMGCT) associated with Klinefelter syndrome (KS). *Proceedings of the American Society of Clinical Oncology*, **5**, 107.

Nichols, C. R., Hoffman, R., Einhorn, L. H., Williams, S. D., Wheeler, L. A. & Garnick, M. B. (1985) Hematologic malignancies associated with primary mediastinal germ cell tumors. *Annals of Internal Medicine*, **102**, 603–609.

Reynoso, E., Yau, J., Shepherd, D., Bailey, D., Evans, W. & Baker, M. (1986) Acute leukemia and mediastinal teratocarcinoma. *Proceedings of the American Society of Clinical Oncology*, **5**, 97.

Russell, D. S. (1944) The pinealoma: its relationship to teratoma. *Journal of Pathology and Bacteriology*, **56**, 145.

Schlumberger, H. G. (1946) Teratoma of the anterior mediastinum in the group of military age: a study of 16 cases and a review of theories of genesis. *Archives of Pathology*, **41**, 398.

Taylor, R. B. (1965) Pluripotential stem cells in mouse embryo liver. *British Journal of Experimental Pathology*, **46**, 376.
Tourtelotte, W. W. & Booc, I. M. (1978) Multiple sclerosis: the blood–brain barrier and the measurement of *de novo* central nervous system IgG synthesis. *Neurology*, **28**, 76.
Witschi, E. (1948) Migration of the germ cells of human embryos from the yolk sac to the primitive gonadal folds. *Contributions to Embryology*, **32**, 67.

Discussion

Grigor A question on terminology. Is 'gonocyte' synonymous with 'primordial germ cell'?

Friedman Primordial germ cells are the original germ cells described by John Beard in 1900 (Beard, 1900, *Anatomischer Anzeiger*, **18**, 465), and I think these are the precursors of gonocytes.

Grigor Are there migrating cells which are common precursor cells of the germ cell and immunological and haematological cell lines?

Friedman I think they probably are.

Intermediate filament proteins as tissue specific markers in normal and neoplastic testicular tissue

W. F. J. FEITZ,[1,3] F. M. J. DEBRUYNE[1] and
F. C. S. RAMAEKERS[2]   Departments of [1]Urology and
[2]Pathologic Anatomy, Radboud University Hospital, Nijmegen,
and [3]Department of Surgery, Deventer Hospitals, Deventer,
The Netherlands

Summary

Normal testicular tissue and primary and metastatic testicular germ cell tumours were examined for their intermediate filament protein (IFP) expression. Seminomas were shown to react with antibodies to vimentin, while non-seminomatous germ cell tumours were strongly positive with antibodies to cytokeratin. In the case of teratocarcinoma, several components of the tumour can be distinguished using a combination of monoclonal and polyclonal antisera in the double-label immunofluorescence technique. We conclude that antibodies to cytokeratin and vimentin can be helpful in the diagnosis of testicular germ cell tumours, especially in the differentiation between seminomas and non-seminomatous testis tumours.

Key words. Intermediate filaments, cytokeratin, vimentin, desmin, testis tumours.

Introduction

Immunocytochemical techniques have become valuable tools in many fields of clinical pathology and medical research. One of the most promising types of tissue specific markers so far is represented by the intermediate filament proteins. Five types of intermediate filament protein (IFP) have been recognized and analysed by biochemical and immunohistochemical techniques (Moll *et al.*, 1982; Ramaekers *et al.*, 1983; Cooper, Schermer & Sun, 1985). These five types are formed by the vimentin, desmin and neurofilament proteins, glial fibrillary acidic protein, and the cytokeratins. These latter polypeptides, the cytokeratins, are specific for epithelial tissues and occur in cell-type specific combinations (Moll *et al.*, 1982; Cooper, Schermer & Sun, 1985). The cytokeratin patterns of epithelial tumours are either identical to, or at least closely related to, the cytokeratin pattern present in the cell of origin (Moll *et al.*, 1982, 1983). Several conventional antisera as well as monoclonal antibodies have been raised against IFPs, and most of them have been shown to react in a tissue specific manner. Since normally IFPs are retained in a cell upon

Correspondence: Dr W. F. J. Feitz, Department of Urology, University of Nijmegen, Geert Grooteplein Zuid 16, 6525 GA Nijmegen, The Netherlands.

malignant transformation, such antibodies can be exploited in surgical pathology to assist in the final tumour diagnosis (Osborn & Weber, 1983; Ramaekers et al., 1983).

Normal testicular tissue

When frozen or paraffin sections of normal human testis (Fig. 1a–f) are incubated with the antisera to cytokeratin, a strong positive reaction is only seen in the epithelial cells lining the ductus efferens and the rete testis (Fig. 1e). No other cell types are positive to cytokeratin (Fig. 1a), except for one case where we have found some cytokeratin positive cells in the seminiferous tubules (Fig. 1b). This case, however, represented testis tissue in which spermatogenesis was lacking because of the presence of a tumour (see also Damjanov & Andrews, 1983; Miettinen, Virtanen & Talerman, 1985). From the use of cytokeratin-polypeptide-specific monoclonal antibodies described above and two-dimensional gel electrophoresis (Achtstaetter et al., 1982) it can be concluded that the cells lining the rete testis contain cytokeratins 7, 8, 18 and 19 while the epithelium of the ductus efferens in addition contains cytokeratin 5. The epididymis, ductus deferens and seminal vesicles also contain cytokeratins 5, 7, 8, 18, 19 and may contain cytokeratin 17. The antibodies to vimentin do not stain the epithelial cells of the ductus efferens. Strikingly, however, a considerable percentage of the epithelial cells of the rete testis are positive for vimentin (Fig. 1f). Double-labelling experiments clearly proved this co-expression of cytokeratin and vimentin in rete testis lining epithelial cells (compare Figs. 1e and 1f and Ramaekers et al., 1986). Also in the cytokeratin positive cells present in the seminiferous tubules described above, co-expression of cytokeratins and vimentin is seen (not shown). Furthermore, a positive reaction with the vimentin antibodies is found in Sertoli cells and in Leydig cells (Fig. 1c). The Leydig cells, however, show a variable reaction, with some cells negative for vimentin and others containing perinuclear clusters of this antigen. Fibroblasts and blood vessels are also stained with the antivimentin antibody. We could not find any staining reaction with any of the antibodies in spermatozoa. Virtanen et al. (1984), however, could show that human spermatozoa have a highly specialized cytoskeletal organization with vimentin forming band-like structures in the sperm head. Myoid cells surrounding the seminiferous tubules are strongly positive with the antibodies to desmin (Fig. 1d). Some of these myoid cells could be shown to co-express desmin and vimentin as demonstrated in the double-label indirect immunofluorescence technique (Ramaekers et al., 1986). The desmin antibodies did not stain any cell type other than muscle cells. Neurofilament antibodies stained only nerve cells.

Seminomas

Classical seminomas, anaplastic seminoma in the testis and metastases of anaplastic seminomas are positive for vimentin. This staining reaction is, however, usually observed in a variable number of the tumour cells (Fig. 1h). When incubated with polyclonal or monoclonal antibodies to cytokeratins almost all cases are negative (Fig. 1g and Battifora et al., 1984) although in some of these cases few cytokeratin

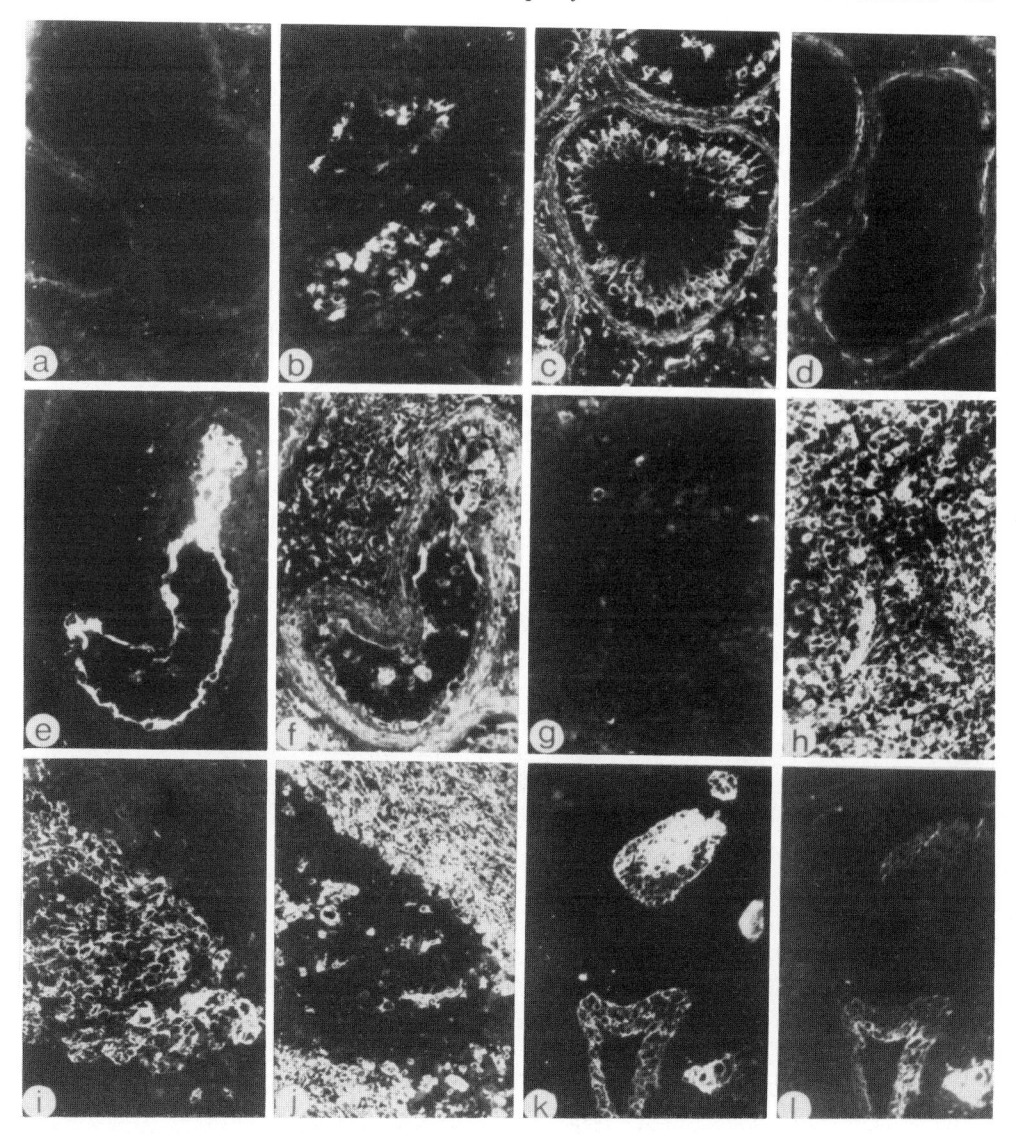

Tissue specific markers in testicular cancers 53

Fig. 1. Immunofluorescence micrographs of normal and malignant testicular tissues. Normal human testis (a–f) shows strong positive reaction with cytokeratin antibodies in the epithelial cells lining the ductus efferentes and rete testis (e) and except for occasionally positive cells in some seminiferous tubules (b) no other cells are cytokeratin positive (a). A vimentin positive reaction is found in Sertoli and Leydig cells (c). Myoid cells surrounding the seminiferous tubules were strongly positive with the antibodies to desmin (d). Co-expression of cytokeratin (e) and vimentin (f) can be seen in the epithelial cells of the rete testis (e, f). Classical and anaplastic seminomas are positive for vimentin (h) and negative for cytokeratin (g) although a few cytokeratin positive cells can occasionally be seen in such tumours. Non-seminomatous testicular tumours such as embryonal cell carcinomas show a positive reaction with cytokeratin antibodies in the tumour cells (i) but not with the vimentin antibodies (j), which stain only the stromal component. In teratocarcinomas (k, l) a differentiation can be made between the glandular and squamous components using a monoclonal antibody to cytokeratin 18 (l) in combination with the polyclonal keratin antiserum (k). (a–l: × 150). (a) Normal testis: cytokeratin. (b) Normal testis: cytokeratin. (c) Normal testis: vimentin. (d) Normal testis: desmin. (e) Rete testis: cytokeratin. (f) Rete testis: vimentin. (g) Seminoma: cytokeratin. (h) Seminoma: vimentin. (i) Embryonal carcinoma: cytokeratin. (j) Embryonal carcinoma: vimentin. (k) Teratocarcinoma: keratin (polyclonal). (l) Teratocarcinoma: cytokeratin.

positive cells scattered through the tumour tissue sections were seen (Miettinen *et al.*, 1985).

Non-seminomatous testicular tumours
Non-seminomatous testicular tumours, including primary and metastatic embryonal cell carcinomas, primary and metastatic endodermal sinus tumour, choriocarcinomas and teratocarcinomas react with cytokeratin antibodies but not with vimentin antisera (Battifora *et al.*, 1984; Miettinen *et al.*, 1985; Ramaekers *et al.*, 1986). Only stromal components of the tumour are positive for vimentin. Double-label immunofluorescence microscopy shows that the vimentin and cytokeratin reaction patterns are mutually exclusive in these tumours (compare Fig. 1i, j). Different types of epithelial differentiation in teratocarcinomas can be identified using the different monoclonal cytokeratin antibodies. For example, with a monoclonal antibody to cytokeratin 18 (RGE53) a distinction can be made between the glandular and the squamous component of the tumour (Fig. 1k, l). Haugen & Taylor (1984) and Trojanowski & Hickey (1984) have shown the presence of neural IF (neurofilaments and GFAP) in teratomas. Detection of these IFPs in such testicular tumours can be useful in their diagnosis, subclassification and investigation of their histogenesis and potentials of differentiation.

Conclusions
Based on these studies we conclude that intermediate filament typing of testicular tumours provides a useful adjunct to routine histology and determination of serum markers in determining therapy and prognosis, especially in cases of anaplastic tumours.

Acknowledgements
We wish to thank Mr O. Moesker, Mrs A. Huijsmans, Mr G. Schaart, Mr B. Hendriks and Mr P. Peelen for excellent technical assistance and all members of the Departments of Urology and Pathology for providing the tumour material and for their help in tumour diagnosis. This study was supported by grants from The Netherlands Cancer Foundation.

References
Achtstaetter, T., Moll, R., Moore, B. & Franke, W. W. (1982) Cytokeratin polypeptide pattern of different epithelia of the human male urogenital tract: immunofluorescence and gel electrophoretic studies. *Journal of Histochemistry and Cytochemistry*, **33**, 415–426.
Battifora, H., Sheibani, K., Tubbs, R. R., Kopinski, M. I. & Sun, T. T. (1984) Antikeratin antibodies in tumor diagnosis. Distinction between seminoma and embryonal carcinoma. *Cancer*, **54**, 843–848.
Cooper, D., Schermer, A. & Sun, T. T. (1985) Classification of human epithelia and their neoplasms using monoclonal antibodies to keratins: strategies, applications, and limitations. *Laboratory Investigation*, **52**, 243–256.
Damjanov, I. & Andrews, P. W. (1983) Ultrastructural differentiation of a clonal human embryonal carcinoma cell line in vitro. *Cancer Research*, **43**, 2190–2198.
Haugen, O. A. & Taylor, C. R. (1984) Immunohistochemical studies of ovarian and testicular teratomas with antiserum to glial fibrillary acidic protein. *Acta Pathologica et Microbiologica Scandinavica* [A], **92**, 9–18.

Miettinen, M., Virtanen, I. & Talerman, A. (1985) Intermediate filament proteins in human testis and testicular germ-cell tumors. *American Journal of Pathology*, **120**, 402–410.

Moll, R., Franke, W. W., Schiller, D. L., Geiger, B. & Krepler, R. (1982) The catalog of human cytokeratins: patterns of expression in normal epithelia, tumors and cultured cells. *Cell*, **31**, 11–24.

Moll, R., Levy, R., Czernobilsky, B., Hohlweg-Majert, P., Dallenbach-Hellweg, G. & Franke, W. (1983) Cytokeratins of normal epithelia and some neoplasms of the female genital tract. *Laboratory Investigation*, **49**, 599–606.

Osborn, M. & Weber, K. (1983) Tumor diagnosis by intermediate filament typing: a novel tool for surgical pathology. *Laboratory Investigation*, **48**, 372–393.

Ramaekers, F. C. S., Puts, J. J. G., Moesker, O., Kant, A., Vooijs, G. P. & Jap, P. H. K. (1983) Intermediate filaments in malignant melanomas. Identification and use as marker in surgical pathology. *Journal of Clinical Investigation*, **71**, 635–643.

Ramaekers, F. C. S., Puts, J. J. G., Moesker, O., Kant, A., Huysmans, A., Haag, D., Jap, P. H. K., Herman, C. J. & Vooijs, G. P. (1983) Antibodies to intermediate filament proteins in the immunohistochemical identification of human tumours: an overview. *Histochemical Journal*, **15**, 691–731.

Ramaekers, F. C. S., Feitz, W. J. F., Moesker, O., Schaart, G., Herman, C. J., Debruyne, F. M. J. & Vooijs, G. P. (1986) Antibodies to cytokeratin and vimentin in testis tumor diagnosis. *Virchows Archiv* [A], **408**, 127-142.

Trojanowski, J. O. & Hickey, W. F. (1984) Human teratomas express differentiated neural antigens, an inumunohistochemical study with anti-neurofilament, anti-glial filament, and anti-myelin basic protein monoclonal antibodies. *American Journal of Pathology*, **115**, 383–392.

Virtanen, I., Badley, R. A., Paasivuo, R. & Letho, V. P. (1984) Distinct cytoskeletal domains revealed in sperm cells. *Journal of Cell Biology*, **99**, 1083–1092.

Discussion

Skakkebæk Have you compared seminiferous tubules containing CIS with tubules which are adjacent to testicular tumours and contain tumour cells? Both types of intratubular cells are morphologically similar but they may have functional differences and it is possible that differentiation from CIS cells into tumour cells starts intratubularly.

Debruyne We have not looked specifically at this.

Oliver Have you looked at mixed tumours and if so do you see zones of differing cytoskeletal antigen expression?

Debruyne Most of our seminoma tumours were classical seminomas except one, and we divided the nonseminomatous tumours into embryonal carcinoma and teratocarcinoma. We did not specifically look at the different seminomatous and nonseminomatous patterns. We were more interested to see what was the staining pattern of the nonseminomatous part of the tumour and especially to differentiate between the different monoclonal antibodies.

G. K. Jacobsen What were your criteria for using the term 'anaplastic' seminoma?

Debruyne Our pathologist called it an anaplastic seminoma because of a high mitotic index of greater than 3–5 mitoses per HPF. I have heard a suggestion that we should not use the term 'anaplastic' and should call it 'seminoma with a high mitotic index'.

Holstein I was not sure of the localization of vimentin in seminoma. Was the staining within the cells or around the cells?

Debruyne Vimentin was in the tumour cells, but not in the surrounding tissue.

Niemi I think that there is a place for the use of antibodies to intermediate filaments as tumour markers, but I do not agree with your criteria that they are such specific markers. There is overlapping in many tissues.

Debruyne There is of course a lot of overlap. I did not try to imply that they can be used as specific markers to differentiate the different types of tumour components in every tumour. But I think that they can be used in some difficult cases to give some additional objective information about the original composition of the tumour.

Oncogenes and germ cell tumours

K. SIKORA,* G. EVAN and J. WATSON   *Ludwig Institute for Cancer Research, M.R.C. Centre, Cambridge, and *Department of Clinical Oncology, Royal Postgraduate Medical School*

Summary

The central problem in cancer therapy is the poor selectivity of current systemic agents against the common solid tumours. The demonstration that unique segments of DNA, constant in location and conserved in evolution are involved in growth control opens new avenues for basic and clinical research. The function of the products of these genes needs to be elucidated. Examples of growth control functions include homology to growth factors, surface receptors, protein kinases and cell cycle control proteins. From DNA sequence data peptides predicted to be exposed within intact molecules can be constructed and used to produce monoclonal antibodies to oncogene products. Such antibodies have now been successfully used to demonstrate the intracellular localization of gene products as well as the cell cycle regulatory role of the *c-myc* protein. By having a battery of antibodies against the different gene products their direct clinical application for diagnosis and prognosis has become a reality. Immunohistology and flow cytometry permit the geographical and quantitative analysis of function in normal and neoplastic tissues. Furthermore, by purification and biochemical analysis the molecular basis for their action can be elucidated. It is likely that by the end of the decade new drugs that inhibit oncoprotein function will be available for clinical trial.

Key words.   Oncogenes, growth factors, monoclonal antibodies, germ cell tumours.

Introduction

Oncogenes are highly conserved regions of the normal genome and over twenty-five have now been identified, cloned and sequenced. Changes in either the coding or control regions of these genes have been implicated in the development of cancer. Several molecular mechanisms, resulting in the increased production of normal oncogene products or the development of aberrant proteins which subvert the normal growth control processes, have now been uncovered (Cooper & Lane, 1984; Hamlyn & Sikora, 1983). These include gene amplification, translocation, mutation translocation, insertion and re-arrangement. Such changes have been documented in fresh tumour biopsies from patients, as well as cultured cell lines (Slamon *et al.*, 1984; Spandidos & Kerr, 1984). The structure and function of oncogene protein products are now under investigation. Those of *c-sis* and *c-erb*B respectively code for a sub-unit of platelet derived growth factor (PDGF) and the internal domain of epidermal growth factor receptor (Waterfield *et al.*, 1983;

Correspondence: Karol Sikora, Department of Clinical Oncology, Royal Postgraduate Medical School, Hammersmith Hospital, DuCane Road, London W12 0HS.

Downward et al., 1984). Indeed, more recently, several others have been found to have a function related to cell growth control.

Tumours of the testis arise predominantly from cells of the germ cell lineage. Malignant teratoma tissue often contains a wide range of differentiated cells identifiable by light microscopy, in addition to the undifferentiated and replicating stem cells. It therefore provides an intriguing biological system in which to examine the role of oncogene product function in differentiation and neoplasia. Considerable interest has surrounded the *c-ras* and *c-myc* genes as marked variation has been found in the quantity of their transcripts in clinical biopsies at the RNA level (Thor et al., 1984). The *c-myc* gene product is a 62,000 molecular weight protein which is particularly intriguing, with regard to human cancer, as there is now evidence that this oncoprotein is involved in cell cycle control. The level of *c-myc* m-RNA increases as cells are stimulated into division. Both m-RNA transcripts and the protein itself have unusually short half lives of 20–30 min (Rabbitts et al., 1985). This is a prerequisite for their putative cell cycle control function. Furthermore, the protein binds to the nucleus, one of the most likely sites for such control.

DNA and RNA hybridization analysis is difficult to perform with many clinical samples. Low copy number genes and message cannot be detected with current methods. Hybridization techniques cannot normally be applied to fixed embedded material stored in pathology departments. Furthermore, they tell us nothing about the ultimate concentration and distribution in the cell of the final gene product: the oncoprotein.

In order to examine the relevance of *c-myc* in clinical samples, a set of mouse monoclonal antibodies were constructed against the *c-myc* protein (Evan et al., 1985). One of these antibodies (*Myc* 1-6E10) has been used to localize p62$^{c\text{-}myc}$ in formalin fixed histological sections from patients with testicular cancer. Furthermore, a quantitative flow cytometric assay for p62$^{c\text{-}myc}$, using the same monoclonal antibody was developed for nuclei extracted from paraffin embedded testicular cancer biopsies. Such studies can be applied to many other oncoproteins, when the appropriate reagents become available.

Materials and Methods

Peptide synthesis, the immunization protocol and screening procedures for deriving *Myc* 1-6E10 are described elsewhere and summarized in Fig. 1. Hybridoma cells were grown in the ascites fluid of female Balb/c mice. The antibody was purified by octanoic acid precipitation followed by ammonium sulphate concentration. Purified antibody was adjusted to a concentration of 2 mg ml^{-1} in PBS with 0.0001% sodium azide, aliquoted and stored at −20°C. A control mouse immunoglobulin of the same subclass (IgG1K) was obtained from ascites fluid of the mouse myeloma line X-63. It was similarly purified and adjusted to a concentration of mg ml^{-1}.

Immunohistology

Paraffin blocks containing surgical biopsies were obtained from the archives of the Department of Pathology. Sections (5 μm) were cut and placed on standard microscope slides previously immersed in a 0.5% gelatin solution which also contained 250 mg chrome alum and 30 mg sodium azide 100 ml^{-1} and air-dried

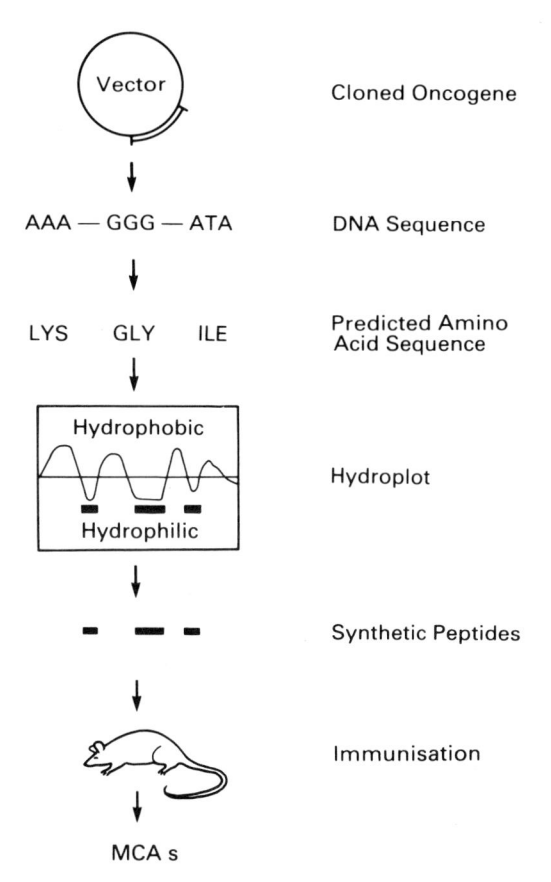

Fig. 1. Schema for the production of monoclonal antibodies from synthetic peptides (with permission of Sikora et al. and British Journal of Cancer, 1985).

overnight. An avidin–biotin technique was used to stain the sections (Vectorstain ABC Kit, Vector Labs). Sections were dewaxed and rehydrated using xylene and alcohol, incubated for 30 min with 0.5% hydrogen peroxide in methanol, washed and incubated for 20 min in diluted normal serum. Excess serum was blotted and the sections incubated for 60 min with 100 µl *Myc* 1-6E10 diluted 1/500 in PBS, 1% BSA and 0.25% Triton X-100 (pH 7.3). Sections were washed and then incubated with a biotinylated rabbit anti-mouse immunoglobulin. After a further wash, sections were incubated for 45 min with the Vector stain ABC reagent. A final incubation in diaminobenzidine (100 mg in 200 ml 0.5% hydrogen peroxide solution) was performed for 30 min and the sections washed with tap water and counterstained in Mayer's haemalum for 60 s.

Extraction of nuclei, staining and flow cytometry
The full technical details have been published (Watson, Sikora & Evan, 1985), but for convenience, the methodology is summarized in Fig. 2. Isolated nuclei were extracted from the archival material by pepsin digestion after dewaxing with xylene

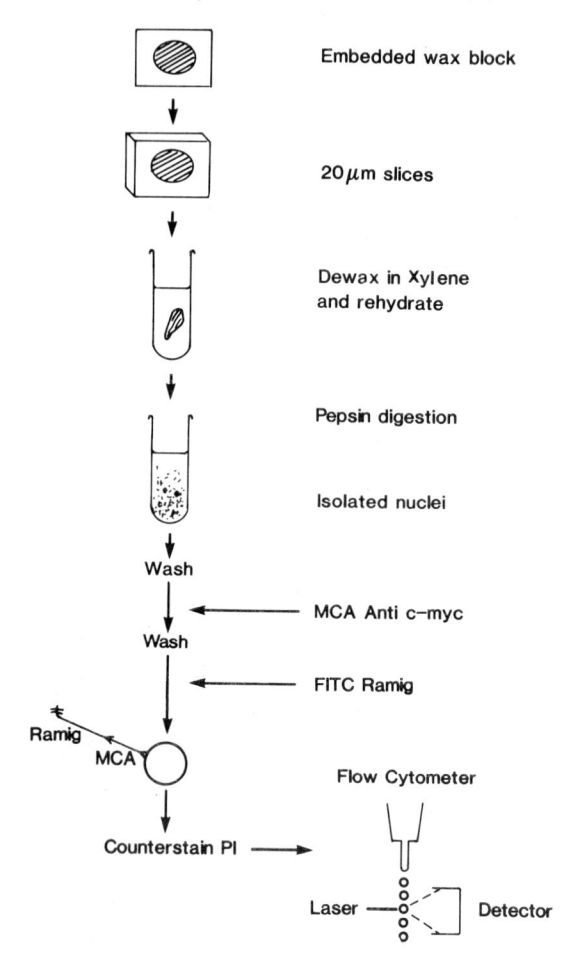

Fig. 2. Flow cytometric analysis of *c-myc* content of isolated nuclei.

and rehydration. The suspension containing isolated nuclei was filtered through a 35 μm nylon mesh to remove debris and clumps, centrifuged at 200 g and resuspended in phosphate buffered saline, pH 7.4 at a concentration of 10^6 nuclei ml^{-1}.

Aliquots of 1.0 ml of the nuclear suspension were then placed into 1.5 ml tubes and spun down in an Eppendorph centrifuge. The supernatants were carefully removed and the nuclear pellets were resuspended in dilutions of *Myc* 1-6E10. A fluorescein labelled rabbit anti-mouse immunoglobulin was added to probe the *Myc* 1-6E10 and the nuclei were counterstained with propidium iodide to assess DNA content.

The nuclei were analysed in the Cambridge M.R.C. custom-built flow cytometer using the argon laser tuned to 488 nm which simultaneously excites red (DNA) and green (oncoprotein) fluorescence from individual nuclei. The data were stored on computer disc and following collection were recalled and the median of the p62^{c-myc} fluorescence distribution associated with either the diploid or aneuploid peak (if present) was computed.

Results

Specificity controls

Most seminomas and teratomas showed considerable staining using *Myc* 1-6E10 when compared to normal testis. An irrelevant mouse monoclonal immunoglobulin (X63 IgG) of the same immunoglobulin subclass showed no binding. Staining by *Myc* 1-6E10 was blocked by the addition of 1 µg of the peptide used as the immunogen added to 100 µl of antibody prior to its addition to tumour sections.

Normal testis

Small amounts of p62$^{c\text{-}myc}$ were demonstrated in the cytoplasm and nuclei of the more peripheral spermatogonia of the normal seminiferous tubule (Fig. 3). The amounts decreased towards the lumen of the tubules. It was also present in the cytoplasm of the interstitial cells of Leydig. There was no variation between different areas of the same testis.

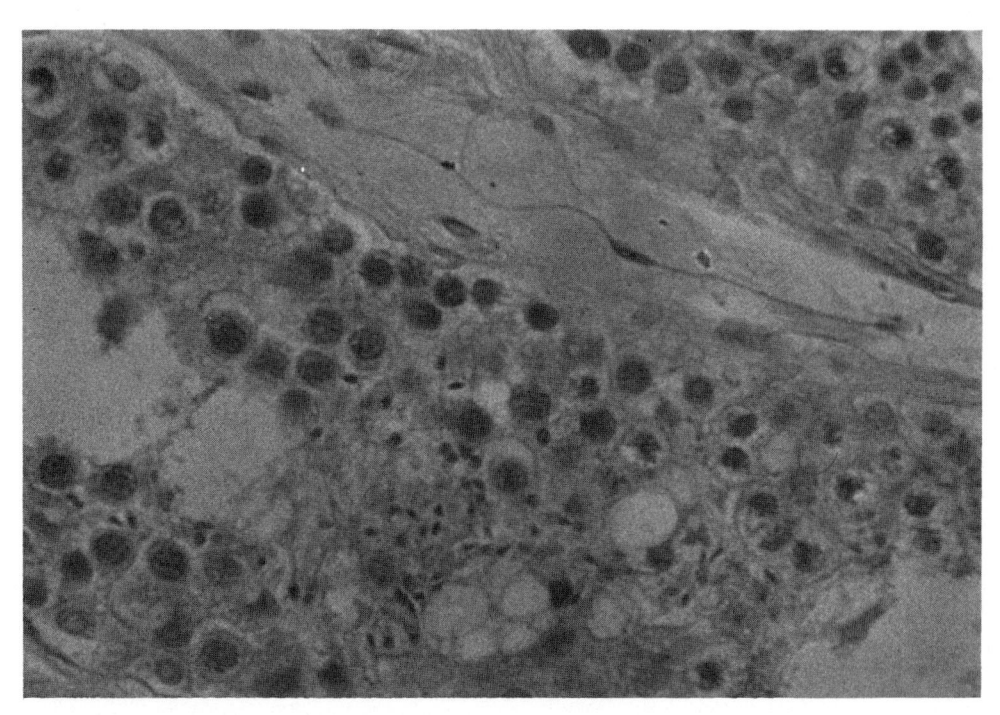

Fig. 3. Immunoperoxidase staining of p62$^{c\text{-}myc}$ in normal testis.

Seminoma

Eleven patients with seminoma were studied. All showed increased p62$^{c\text{-}myc}$ staining predominantly located in cell nuclei but with some cytoplasmic increase. There was considerable variation between different areas of the same tumour and between different tumours (Fig. 4). Infiltrating lymphocytes showed little or no staining.

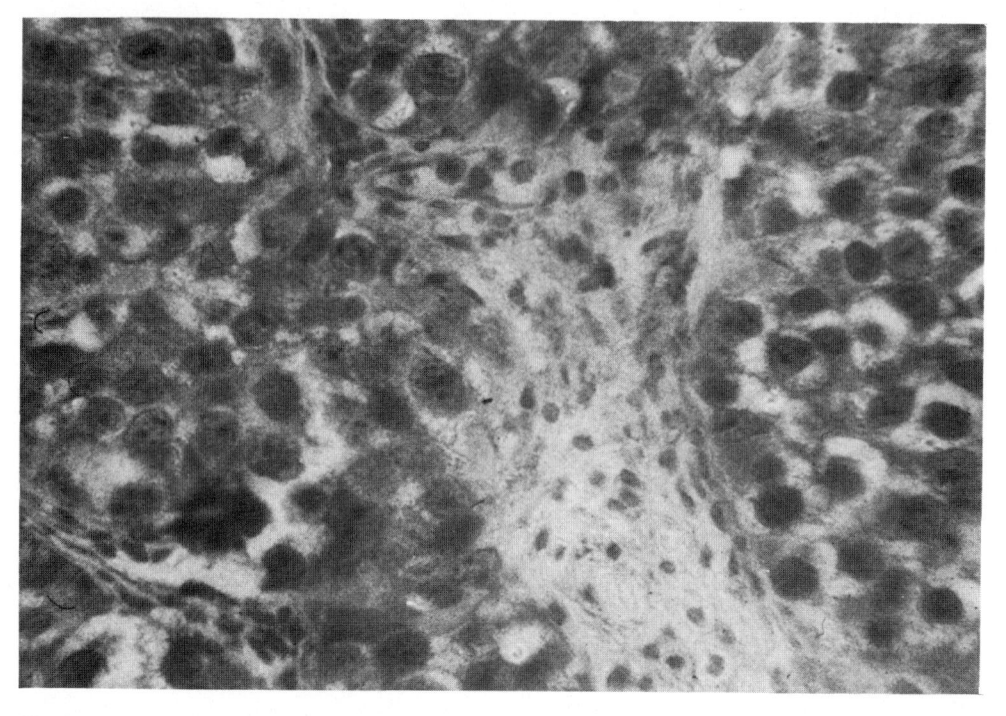

Fig. 4. p62^{c-myc} distribution in seminoma.

Malignant teratoma
There was considerable variation in staining intensity between different parts of the individual tumours in the twenty-one teratomas examined. Undifferentiated areas showed little p62^{c-myc} activity, often less than the basal spermatogonia of normal testes. Areas of greatest intensity were clustered at sites of outgrowth of differentiating structures (Fig. 5). Certain tumours, especially those with yolk sac differentiation, showed intense staining (Fig. 6). Little or no staining was seen in areas of trophoblastic differentiation.

No correlation of p62^{c-myc} staining was observed between the stage of the disease or the preoperative serum level of human chorionic gonadotrophin. Five patients who subsequently died from their disease, and one who is currently undergoing chemotherapy for a recurrence, all had small amounts of the p62^{c-myc} in their tumour.

An overall summary of p62^{c-myc} quantitation in testicular cancer versus clinical outcome is given in Fig. 7. The patients were divided into two groups, those who were alive and well with no recurrence at 3 years after diagnosis and those who developed recurrence within this interval. The mean oncoprotein levels, with their standard deviations, were 513 ± 275 and 155 ± 77 for the good and bad prognosis groups respectively. Student's *t*-test for comparison of the means with their variances was 3.4 with 36 degrees of freedom, $P < 0.001$. The good prognosis group contained eleven patients with seminoma all of whom are alive and well. When this subset was excluded the mean p62^{c-myc} level was 456 ± 305 for the teratoma patients

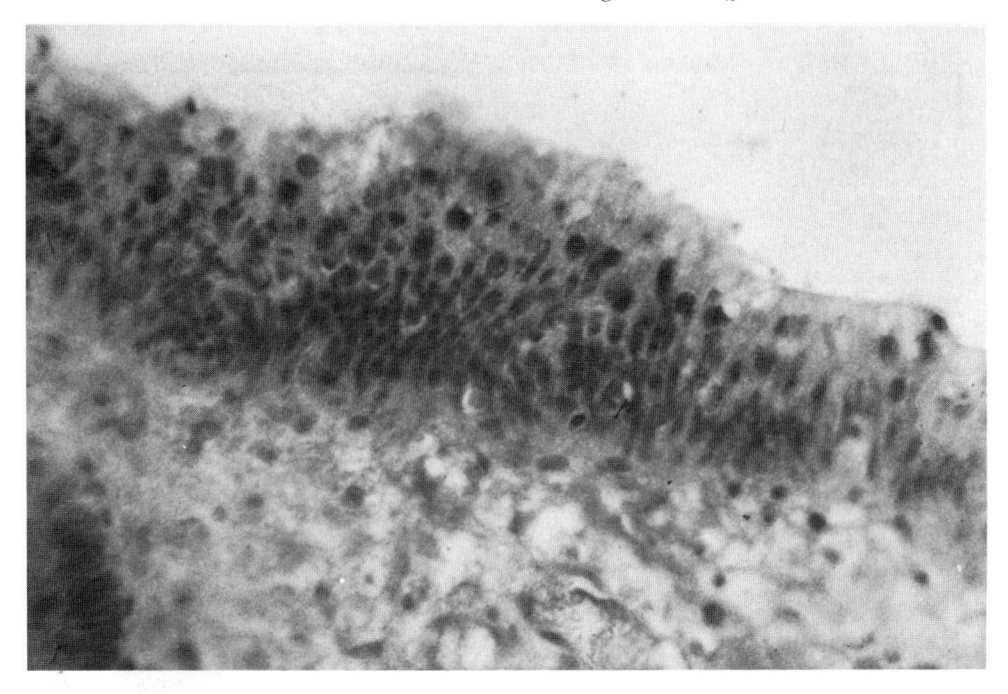

Fig. 5. p62$^{c\text{-}myc}$ distribution in differentiating area of malignant teratoma intermediate.

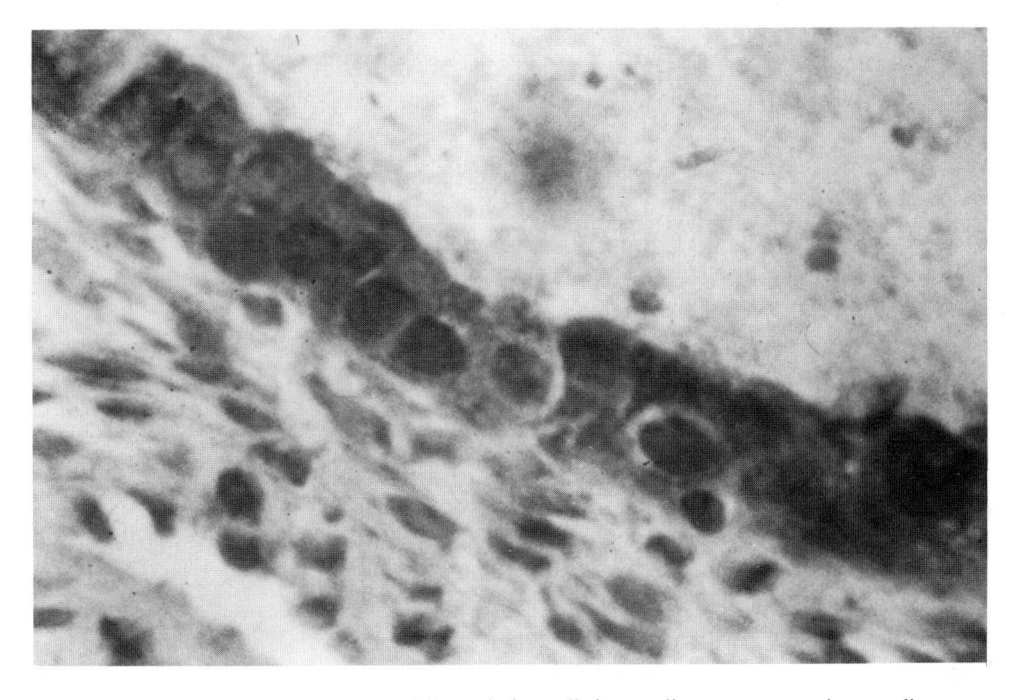

Fig. 6. p62$^{c\text{-}myc}$ distribution in yolk sac differentiating cells in a malignant teratoma intermediate.

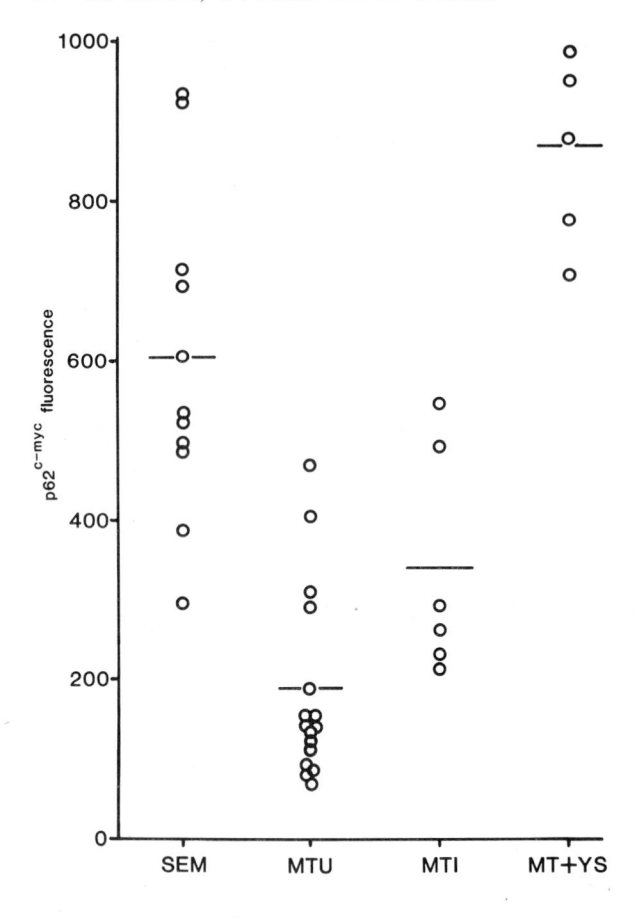

Fig. 7. p62$^{c\text{-}myc}$ content of isolated nuclei from seminomas; malignant teratoma undifferentiated; malignant teratoma intermediate; and teratomas with yolk sac elements.

who are alive and well. Comparison of this group with those who developed recurrence gave $t = 2.4$ with 25 degrees of freedom, $P < 0.02$.

There was no correlation between p62$^{c\text{-}myc}$ level and the age of the patients, stage of disease, or serum levels of human chorionic gonadotrophin. The pretreatment alpha fetoprotein levels were compared with p62$^{c\text{-}myc}$ and there was no correlation in MTU or MTI but a good correlation with tumours showing yolk sac differentiation.

Only three patients exhibited an aneuploid component on the DNA histogram. All were teratomas but the numbers are too small to make any useful observations.

Discussion

The development of monoclonal antibodies to oncogene products provides essential reagents for characterizing oncoprotein function and distribution in health and disease. The remarkable conservation of the DNA sequence of individual oncogenes across wide reaches of evolutionary time points to an essential role of their gene products in normal development. Testicular cancer produces a biologically as well as clinically relevant system for study.

The examination of *c-myc* m-RNA in the developing human placenta indicates that the peak of *myc* transcription occurs at 4–5 weeks after conception (Pfeifer-Ohlsson et al., 1984). Other oncogene RNA transcripts have been found to be elevated in differentiating systems. During liver regeneration the expression of *H-ras* and *c-myc* genes are increased (Goyette et al., 1983) and the *c-fos* gene product is specifically elevated in developing bone (Muller et al., 1982). In most cells the level of *c-myc* m-RNA has been found to be low but increases with the rate of cell division. In the normal dividing germ cells of the mouse testis very few *c-myc* m-RNA transcripts have been found. The drive to proliferate, at least for several divisions, may therefore come from other gene products. By partially purifying mouse testicular cells, it has been demonstrated that *c-myc* expression was greatest in spermatogonia during the process of their differentiation into spermatocytes (Stewart, Bellve & Leder, 1984). The results described here suggest a similar pattern in normal human testis.

The control of cell division and differentiation are complex requiring the interaction of many different molecular mechanisms. The *c-myc* gene product is probably involved in both processes. Normal differentiation of germ cells requires the transient expression of high quantities of p62^{c-myc}. Malignant cells can also arise with several differentiation characteristics and containing various amounts of p62^{c-myc}. The most undifferentiated and therefore clinically aggressive teratomas contain low levels of this protein as measured by our antibody. Tumours can differentiate so expressing elevated levels, especially those with yolk sac elements. Fully differentiated tissue reverts to lower *c-myc* expression (Fig. 8). This model

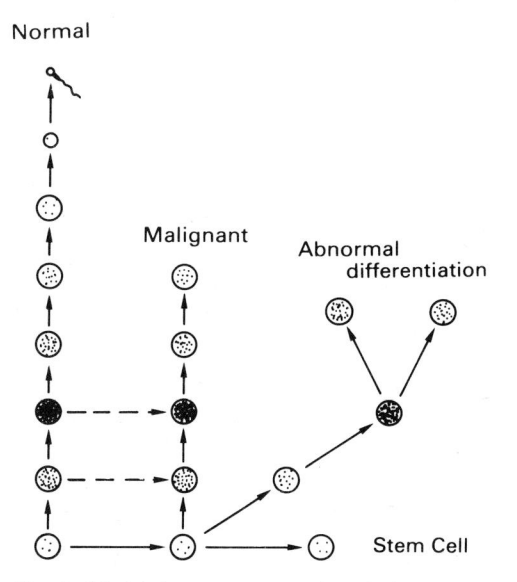

Fig. 8. Model for *c-myc* expression during normal spermatogenesis and the development of germ cell tumours. (Permission of Sikora et al., and *British Journal of Cancer*, 1985).

accounts for our observations in testicular cancer. Studying the expression of different gene products in histological material may result in greater precision of diagnosis and prognosis as well as opening new avenues for future therapy.

References

Cooper, G. M. & Lane, M. A. (1984) Cellular transforming genes and oncogenesis. *Biochimica et Biophysica Acta*, **738**, 9–12.

Downward, J., Morden, M., Mayes, E., et al. (1984) Close similarities of epidermal growth factor receptor and v-erb B oncogene protein sequences. *Nature*, **307**, 521–526.

Evan, G., Lewis, G. K., Ramsay, G., et al. (1985) Isolation of monoclonal antibodies specific for human and mouse proto-oncogene products. *Molecular and Cellular Biochemistry*, **5**, 3610–3618.

Goyette, M., Petropoonlos, C. J., Shank, P. R., et al. (1983) Expression of a cellular oncogene during liver regeneration. *Science*, **219**, 510–514.

Hamlyn, P. H. & Sikora, K. (1983) Oncogenes. *Lancet*, **ii**, 326–329.

Muller, R., Slamon, D. J., Tremblay, J. et al. (1982) Differential expression of cellular oncogenes during pre- and post-natal development of the mouse. *Nature*, **299**, 640–644.

Pfeifer-Ohlsson, S., Gronsten, A. S., Rydnert, J. et al. (1984) Spatial and temporal pattern of cellular *myc* oncogene expression in developing human placenta: Implications for embryonic cell proliferation. *Cell*, **38**, 585–591.

Rabbitts, P. H., Lamond, A., Watson, J. V. et al. (1985) Metabolism of *c-myc* gene products: *c-myc* mRNA and protein expression in the cell cycle. *EMBO Journal*, **4**, 2009–2014.

Sikora, K., Evan, G., Stewart, J. & Watson, J. V. (1985) Detection of the *c-myc* oncogene product in testicular cancer. *British Journal of Cancer*, **52**, 171–176.

Slamon, D. J., de Kernion, J. B., Verma, I. M. et al. (1984) Expression of cellular oncogenes in human malignancies. *Science*, **224**, 256–261.

Spandidos, D. A. & Kerr, I. B. (1984) Elevated expression of the human *ras* oncogene family in premalignant and malignant tumours of the colorectum. *British Journal of Cancer*, **49**, 681–686.

Stewart, T. A., Bellve, A. & Leder, P. (1984) Transcription and promotor usage of the *myc* gene in normal somatic and spermatogenic cells. *Science*, **226**, 707–712.

Thor, A., Hand, H., Wunderlich, D., Caruso, A., Mararo, R. & Schlom, J. (1984) Monoclonal antibodies define differential *ras* gene expression in malignant and benign colonic disease. *Nature*, **311**, 562–567.

Waterfield, M. D., Scrace, G. T., Whittle, N. et al. (1983) Platelet derived growth factor is structurally related to the putative transforming protein p28^{sis} of simian sarcoma virus. *Nature*, **304**, 35–39.

Watson, J. V., Sikora, K. E. & Evan, G. I. (1985) A simultaneous flow cytometric assay for *c-myc* oncoprotein and DNA in nuclei from paraffin embedded material. *Journal of Immunological Methods*, **83**, 179–186.

Discussion

Engström Your work indicates a fundamental difference between mice and men. Murine embryonal carcinoma cells induced to differentiate *in vitro* decrease their expression of *c-myc*, whereas human testicular neoplasms behave quite differently.

The high expression of *c-myc* in human trophoblastic tissue may indicate that the expression of this oncogene is related not only to the state of proliferation but perhaps also to invasiveness and metastatic potential. Would you care to speculate?

Sikora A good point: the trophoblast is indeed an invasive tissue. I believe that *c-myc* expression is related to a subsequent series of changes in gene expression. Some of the changes in gene expression result in the development of specific patterns which we recognize as differentiation. Other changes may be directly related to invasion.

Niemi I have doubts about the use of immunoperoxidase staining as a quantitative technique although I agree that flow cytometry is quantitative.

Sikora There is no doubt that immunohistochemical assessment is subjective, therefore we have developed a flow cytometric assay in parallel which is more objective and more precise.

Niemi You described $p62^{c-myc}$ as a peptide combining with nuclear lamins, but your preparations also showed strong cytoplasmic staining. Are you at present using monoclonal antibodies against nuclear lamins?

Sikora We do not have monoclonal antibodies to nuclear lamins. Cellular localization by immunohistochemistry is a different problem particularly as the pH of fixation alters the distribution of $p62^{c-myc}$ across the nuclear membrane.

Oosterhuis Have you compared *c-myc* expression in primary embryonal carcinoma with its expression in residual metastatic carcinoma of similar morphology but after having been treated with chemotherapy?

Sikora We have not been able to perform such a comparison because in every case biopsy of the residual tumour has shown a different degree of histological differentiation than that of the primary tumour.

Oosterhuis The NTERA-2 system may tell us if a higher level of somatic differentiation in embryonal carcinoma is associated with a higher level of *c-myc* expression.

Cytogenetic studies of human testicular germ cell tumours

CELIA D. DELOZIER-BLANCHET, H. WALT,*
E. ENGEL and P. VUAGNAT† *University Institute of Medical Genetics, Geneva, *Institute of Pathology, University of Zurich, Zurich, and †University Institute of Mathematics, Geneva, Switzerland*

Summary

In a search for consistent cytogenetic alterations in testicular germ cell cancers we have thus far studied some twenty surgical specimens of seminomas and nonseminomatous tumours. From the literature and our results it is now clear that such testicular tumours generally have a hyperdiploid to hypotriploid chromosomal content, and frequently possess a possibly site-specific chromosomal marker, an isochromosome 12p. A significant correlation between the presence of the i(12p) and advanced clinical stages has been revealed in our study. Several other chromosomal regions are consistently involved in cytogenetic changes: 1p and 1q, 6q, 7p, 9q, 12p, 17q, and 22q. Although there is little doubt that characteristic chromosomal lesions exist in testicular germ cell tumours, the impact which specific lesions may have on tumour progression is still unclear.

Key words. Testicular germ cell tumours, teratocarcinoma (human), cancer cytogenetics, chromosomes 1, 6, 12, 17.

Introduction

Consistent cytogenetic alterations have been shown to be correlated with diagnosis and prognosis for a growing number of haematological and solid tumour types (Berger, Bloomfield & Sutherland, 1985; Mitelman, 1985). A search for the cytogenetic changes significant in testicular cancer is thus of interest both to assess their potential clinical importance and to gain insight into tumour development and progression. The study of cytogenetic aberrations in human testicular tumours is, however, still in its infancy, for only a handful of banded chromosome analyses of such malignancies have been reported. Our ongoing study of human testicular germ cell tumours has as a major goal the establishment of karyotypes from surgical specimens. As initial and follow-up information is collected on the patients, it should be possible to evaluate the potential clinical utility of cytogenetic studies of testicular germ cell tumours.

Correspondence: Dr C. D. DeLozier-Blanchet, Institute of Medical Genetics, CMU, 9 avenue de Champel, CH-1211 Geneva 4, Switzerland.

Materials and Methods

We have thus far received some thirty specimens of testicular germ cell tumours, primarily teratocarcinomas, following surgery, or occasionally after their passage in nude mouse hosts. All specimens have served for cytogenetic study by direct techniques (see DeLozier-Blanchet, 1986), and most nonseminomatous tumours have been implanted *in vitro* and into nude mice. In addition to light microscopic histological analysis, some samples have been selected for electron microscopic study and/or DNA flow cytometry (Walt *et al.*, 1986). Baseline clinical data, including alphafetoprotein (AFP) and β-human chorionic gonadotrophin (β-hCG) values, are obtained from the patients' charts, and in some cases the constitutional karyotypes of the patients are established from peripheral blood or testicular tissues.

The tumours which can be passaged serially *in vitro* or as xenografted lines are similarly analysed for their histological, cytogenetic, and biochemical characteristics (Walt *et al.*, 1986).

We use primarily Giemsa-trypsin banding for chromosomal identification, but C-banding, quinacrine fluorescence and Ag-NOR staining are also helpful.

Results

Direct cytogenetic analyses allowing assessment of both chromosome number and structural alterations are, in our experience, possible from about two-thirds of surgical specimens. In some cases cytogenetic analyses can be performed on, or complemented by, the study of xenografted or cultured tumour material. Most early passage xenografts of human testicular tumours are remarkably similar both histologically and cytogenetically to their parent tumours (DeLozier-Blanchet, 1986; Walt *et al.*, 1986).

We have thus far studied the constitutional karyotype of twelve testicular tumours patients. In all cases it was 46,XY. Eight of the patients, however, showed two or more aneuploid cells, and a number of breaks and structural abnormalities have been observed. Although these might be metastatic cells on the basis of chromosomal number, the presence or absence of the marker chromosomes typical of their tumours could not be confirmed. An explanation in the case of several patients might be that the aberrations in peripheral blood were secondary to chemotherapy.

The following discussion of the cytogenetics of testicular germ cell tumours is thus drawn both from the literature and from our personal experience (DeLozier-Blanchet, Engel & Walt, 1985; DeLozier-Blanchet, 1986).

Discussion

CHROMOSOME NUMBER

Early cytogenetic studies of testicular tumours (Martineau, 1969; Atkin, 1973) described the generally hyperdiploid to hypotriploid chromosome complement of testicular germ cell tumours: only a small percentage have a diploid or near-diploid chromosomal constitution, although most aneuploid tumours contain some diploid cells. The modal chromosome number of seminomas, usually 60–69, was higher than that of teratomas, 50–59, and combined tumours had intermediate modes.

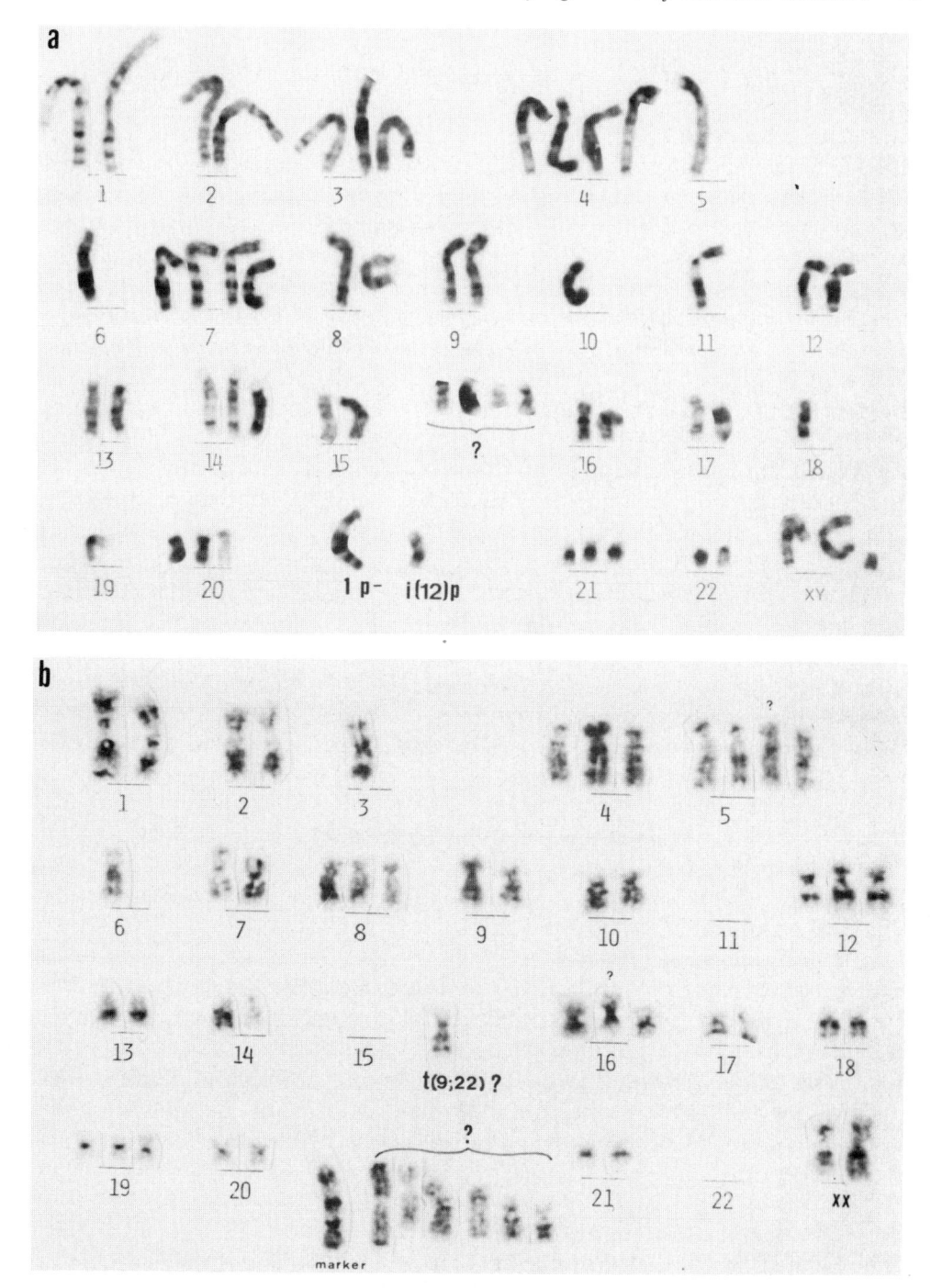

Fig. 1. Representative karyotypes from testicular germ cell tumours. (a) Giemsa-banded metaphase from an embryonal carcinoma, showing 55 chromosomes, several of which have unknown origins, and two consistent chromosomal markers: del(1)(p13) and i(12p). (b) Giemsa-banded metaphase from a seminoma, showing 53 chromosomes (the modal number was 66), including numerous unidentifiable chromosomes and a long acrocentric marker frequent in seminomas.

The distribution of extra chromosomes was found to be nonrandom, with a relative deficiency of B-group and an excess of C- and F-group-sized chromosomes.

Results from direct harvests of our first eighteen surgical testicular tumour specimens confirmed these observations (DeLozier-Blanchet, 1986) (Fig. 1). Although minor populations of near-diploid or diploid cells were observed, only two tumours had modal numbers of 46. When the aneuploid cell populations only are considered, the average modal number for seminomas was 69, in an embryonal carcinoma (EC) it was 54, and for tumours of mixed histology it was 59. The correlation of higher modal chromosome number with seminomatous, as compared to nonseminomatous histology, was significant at the 0.007 level. However, at variance with Atkin (1973), we found seminomas showed a wider range of chromosome number (often from 30 to over 100 in cells from the same tumour) than did nonseminomatous germ cell tumours (NSGCT). This higher chromosome content and variability of seminoma cells is consistent with the concept that these malignancies have a longer evolution prior to their detection. Seminomas, which are differentiated tumours probably lacking a pluripotent stem cell, have slower growth and less aggressive behaviour than NSGCT. In contrast to tumours containing EC or teratocarcinoma (TC) parts, we have not been able to propagate classical seminoma either *in vitro* or in the nude mouse, which again suggests a paucity of pluripotent stem cells.

TYPES OF CHROMOSOMAL CHANGES IN TUMOUR CELLS

Gross chromosomal changes are the rule in most solid tumours, an observation which led Bullerdiek *et al.* (1985) to suggest that cytogenetic alterations in carcinomas may fall into three major categories; this should be kept in mind during the discussion which follows:
1. *primary*, specific chromosomal changes that are characteristic of, or even unique to, a particular histological tumour type;
2. *secondary but nonrandom* alterations, leading for example to increased malignant change and metastatic potential; and
3. *random* chromosomal changes.

From our experience with testicular tumours, we agree with Bullerdiek *et al.* (1985) that few of the aberrations observed in highly aneuploid testicular tumours are primary. Many structural alterations, even when detected in multiple tumours, may be secondary although nonrandom alterations: nonrandom because these structural aberrations are common to other tumour types, and because some may be site-specific, secondary because they are associated with advanced clinical stages.

STRUCTURAL CHROMOSOMAL ALTERATIONS

Given the high and heterogeneous chromosome count of most testicular tumours, current studies focus on the identification of structurally altered chromosomes. Investigations prior to the banding era (Martineau, 1969; Atkin, 1973) had already shown that the majority of such cancers have 'marker' chromosomes; a large acrocentric or submetacentric marker was described in a number of specimens (Martineau, 1969). Our studies indicate multiple abnormal karyotype members in cells from almost all tumours, irrespective of histological type. Although in our experience, as in the literature (Wang et al., 1980; Atkin & Baker, 1985; Gibas et al., 1986), some of these alterations are both undefined and inconsistent from cell to cell, a certain number of recurring chromosomal deletions or rearrangements can be delineated.

1. *Potentially site-specific (primary?) chromosomal alterations*

(a) *Isochromosome 12p.* The most common structural anomaly in testicular germ cell tumours is probably the isochromosome 12p (Atkin & Baker, 1983; DeLozier-Blanchet et al., 1985) which may even be the sole structural abnormality detectable (Gibas, Prout & Sandberg, 1984). Its occurrence in the various histological types of testicular germ cell tumours points out their aetiological interrelationships and suggests that the i(12p) arises in a stem cell. The isochromosome 12p produces an amplification of genes on the short arm of this chromosome, often two to four copies of a normal 12 being present as well as one to four of the isochromosome. In our experience, which thus far differs from that of Atkin & Baker (1983), the isochromosome is found in duplicate or triplicate only in NSGCT.

The involvement of the short arm of chromosome 12 in nontesticular neoplasms (ovary, breast, colon) has also been reported (Mitelman, 1985), albeit only rarely.

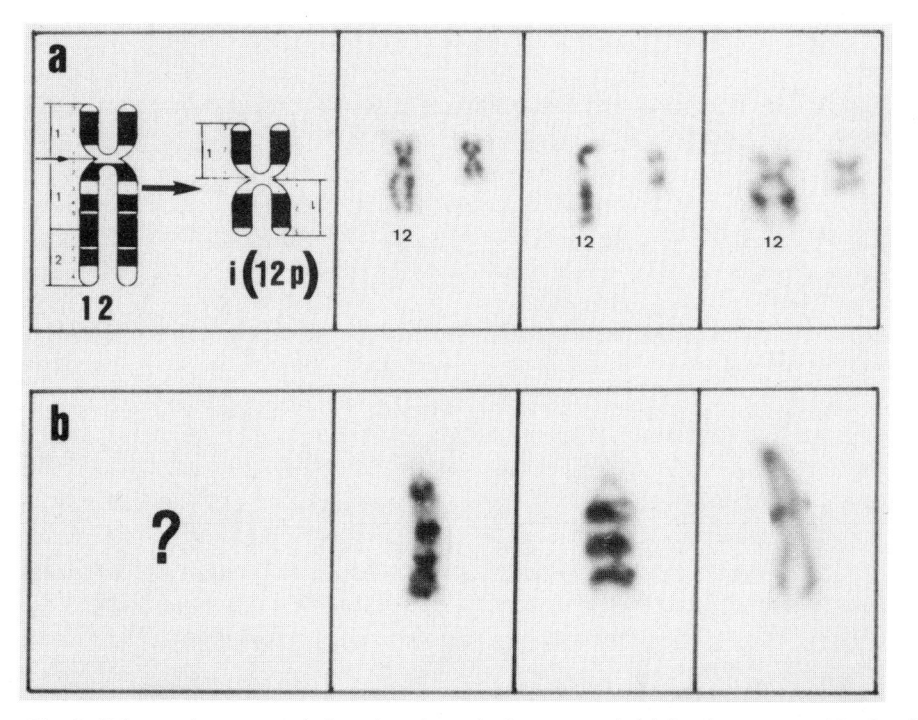

Fig. 2. Primary chromosomal alterations in testicular tumours? (a) Isochromosome 12p: in addition to a schematic diagram of isochromosome content, extracts from cells of two NSGCT and one seminoma are shown. The i(12p) in each case is represented next to a normal chromosome 12 from the same cell. (b) Long acrocentric marker: abstracts from cells of three seminomas demonstrate this long chromosome, larger than a number 1, which is of unknown identity. We have observed such a chromosome only in seminomas.

If the i(12p) itself is considered, however, we know of only a single report of its occurrence, in an adenocarcinoma of the colon (Riet-Fox, Retief & Niekerk, 1979). This aberration may thus prove to be a site-specific chromosomal anomaly, and as such a marker with clinical relevance. In our initial study (DeLozier-Blanchet, 1986) the presence of i(12p) was significantly correlated with evidence of metastatic disease. We think that this may be particularly true when multiple copies of i(12p) are present. Tumours with the isochromosome are also more likely in our experience to grow as xenografts in the nude mouse, thus attesting to their aggressive behaviour.

(b) *Long acrocentric marker*. We, as others, have found in a number of seminomas a long acrocentric chromosome (Fig. 2b) which corresponds to no normal member. In our initial study (DeLozier-Blanchet, 1986) this marker was found only in seminomas, so that the correlation with seminomatous histology (and early clinical stage) was significant. The possibility that such a marker represents a site-specific or even histology-specific anomaly will await knowledge of its origin. Although its content may be variable in different tumours, tandem duplication of large chromosomal regions was suggested by banding patterns.

2. *Chromosomal alterations also observed in tumours from other sites* (Fig. 3)

(a) *Aberrations of chromosome 1*. The frequent occurrence of chromosome 1 aberrations in cell lines derived from testicular germ cell tumours was pointed out by Wang *et al.* (1980). Atkin & Baker (1985) and Parrington, West & Povey (1986) confirmed these findings in surgical specimens or cultured cells, and the latter group observed breakage and loss of genetic material in the paracentromeric area of chromosome 1. We personally have observed chromosome 1 aberrations in at least seven tumours of various histological types: deletions of 1p are the most frequent but 1q anomalies may also be found (DeLozier-Blanchet, 1986).

Structural aberrations of chromosome 1 are frequent in haematological malignancies as well as in other solid tumours (Atkin & Brito-Babapulle, 1981; Mitelman, 1985), where they appear to occur late in tumour evolution. Such alterations may thus be related to tumour progression and enhanced invasiveness (Atkin & Brito-Babapulle, 1981). In the testicle we suspect that chromosome 1 anomalies signal enhanced metastatic potential: they are more frequent in established cell lines (Wang *et al.*, 1980) than in surgical specimens (DeLozier-Blanchet, 1986), and we have found the chromosome to be more often and more extensively affected in NSGCT than in seminomas.

(b) *Alterations involving 17q*. We have detected a translocation chromosome apparently containing 17q in at least nine testicular tumours. In tumours with EC or TC components such extra or modified 17q regions may be present in multiple-copy markers.

An isochromosome for 17q is a well known anomaly in haematological malignancies (Engel *et al.*, 1975; Fourth International Workshop on Chromosomes in Leukemia, 1984), where it is considered a late-appearing change in clonal evolution. 17q is also implicated in a number of solid tumour types (Mitelman, 1985).

(c) *Rearrangement of 6q*. 6q modifications are also found in a number of haematological and solid tumours (Mitelman, 1985), and we have so far observed

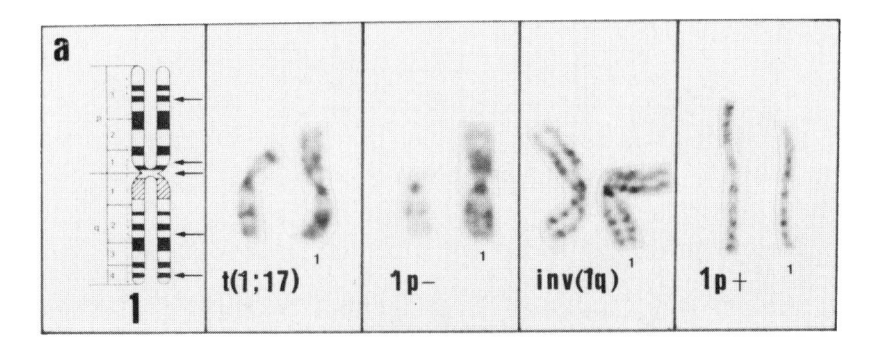

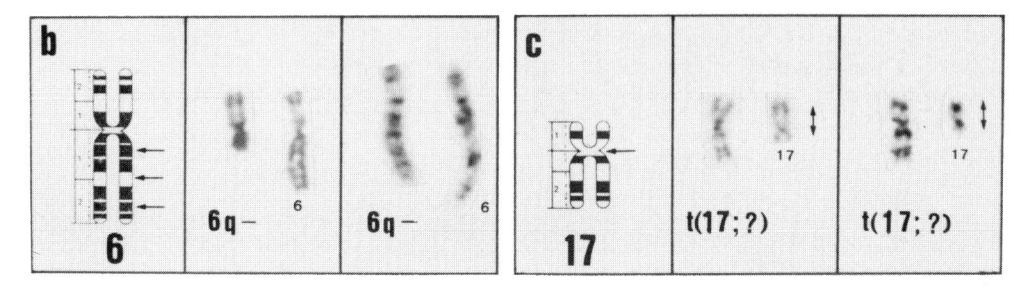

Fig. 3. Secondary chromosomal aberrations in testicular tumours? (a) Examples of chromosome 1 anomalies: Pictured on the left is a diagram of chromosome 1, on which the breakpoints from four NSGCT are indicated. The cytogenetic abstracts from cells of the four tumours show the altered number 1 next to a normal number 1 from the same cell. (b) Examples of aberrations involving 6q: A deleted chromosome 6 is shown next to a normal 6 from the same cell, in a tumour of combined histology (left) and a seminoma (right). (c) Examples of the involvement of 17q in structural alterations: A frequent marker chromosome in testicular tumours, apparently a translocation including 17q, is shown with a normal 17 from the same cell in each of two NSGCT. A translocation, t(1;17) appears in Fig. 3(a).

cells with a deletion or translocation involving 6q in three testicular tumours. To our knowledge, 6q aberrations have but rarely been described in testicular germ cell tumours, but four metastases from a mediastinal germ cell tumour presented an identical translocation involving chromosomes 6 and 11 (Oosterhuis et al., 1985).

A number of other chromosomal regions are less consistently modified in testicular germ cell tumours. In our initial study (DeLozier-Blanchet, 1986) the chromosomal regions affected most frequently by structural aberrations in testicular malignancies included 1p, 1q, 6q, 9q, 12p, 17q, 22q, and possibly 7p, 11p, and Xq. These apparently nonrandom chromosomal aberrations included deletions, translocations, and duplication by isochromosome formation, suggesting several different mechanisms through which chromosomal changes might qualitatively or quantitatively alter gene expression: gene dosage effects, gene amplification, position effects, gene activation or repression.

THE POTENTIAL ROLE OF ONCOGENES IN TESTICULAR CANCER (Fig. 4)
Initial reports from the literature have thus far suggested that the oncogenes *myc* (Sikora et al., 1985), *myb* (Oosterhuis et al., 1985) and *ras* (Tainsky et al., 1984)

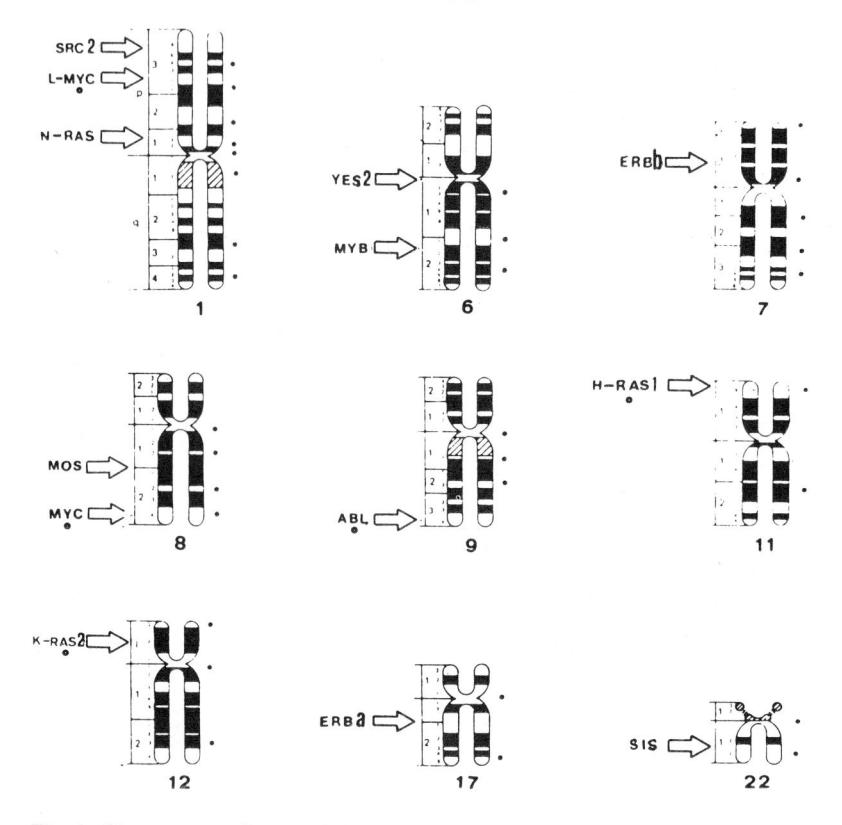

Fig. 4. Chromosomes frequently involved in structural rearrangements in testicular tumours, and their oncogene content. Those chromosomes most frequently involved in testicular tumours are shown with, on the right, what appear to be the most common breakpoints (*). To the left of each chromosome are indicated the oncogenes which have been mapped to them: (⇨) oncogenes localized to a specific band, and (⇨) those localized only to a chromosomal region.

may be activated or altered in testicular tumours. The characteristic cytogenetic alterations, on the other hand would suggest that genes on other chromosomal regions may play a role in either tumour initiation or evolution. Chromosome 1 contains the oncogenes *N-ras*, *l-myc*, and *src2*; 12p is the site of the *K-ras2* oncogene and 11p of the related *H-ras*. The *myb* oncogene has been mapped to 6q22–24 and *c-erb* is on 7p. Fig. 4 summarizes the correspondence between frequent chromosomal breakpoints in testicular tumours and the oncogenes located in the same regions. Our future studies will focus on these associations.

Note added in proof. An isochromosome 12p has recently been observed in an ovarian dysgerminoma (N.B. Atkin & M. C. Baker, in press) which might suggest that this chromosomal marker is characteristic of germ cell tumours in general rather than of testicular germ cell tumours in particular.

Acknowledgements
This work was supported in part by the Geneva (Geneva) Anticancer League and The Krebsliga des Kantons Zurich.

References

Atkin, N. B. (1973) High chromosome numbers of seminomata and malignant teratomata of the testis: A review of data on 103 tumors. *British Journal of Cancer*, **28**, 275–279.

Atkin, N. B. & Baker, M. C. (1983) i(12p): specific chromosomal marker in seminoma and malignant teratoma of the testis? *Cancer Genetics and Cytogenetics*, **10**, 199–204.

Atkin, N. B. & Baker, M. C. (1985) Chromosome analysis of three seminomas. *Cancer Genetics and Cytogenetics*, **17**, 315–323.

Atkin, N. B. & Brito-Babapulle, V. (1981) Heterochromatin polymorphism and human cancer. *Cancer Genetics and Cytogenetics*, **3**, 261–272.

Berger, R., Bloomfield, C. D. & Sutherland, G. R. (1985) Report of the Committee on chromosome rearrangements in neoplasia and on fragile sites. Human Gene Mapping 8, Helsinki. *Cancer Genetics and Cell Genetics*, **40**, 491–535.

Bullerdiek, J., Bartnitzke, S., Kahrs, E. & Schloot, W. (1985) Further evidence for nonrandom chromosome changes in carcinoma cells: A report of 28 cases. *Cancer Genetics and Cytogenetics*, **9**, 301–304.

DeLozier-Blanchet, C. D. (1986) Human testicular germ cell tumors: cytogenetic studies of surgical and xenografted specimens. Ph.D. thesis, Indiana University, Indianapolis, Indiana.

DeLozier-Blanchet, C. D., Engel, E. & Walt, H. (1985) Isochromosome 12p in human testicular tumors. *Cancer Genetics and Cytogenetics*, **15**, 375–376.

Engel, E., McKee, L. C., Flexner, J. M. & McGee, B. J. (1975) 17 long arm isochromosome. A common anomaly in malignant blood disorders. *Annals of Genetics*, **18**, 56–60.

Fourth International Workshop on Chromosomes in Leukemia (1984) *Cancer Genetics and Cytogenetics*, **11**, 249–360.

Gibas, A., Prout, G. R. & Sandberg, A. A. (1984) Malignant teratoma of the testis with an isochromosome No. 12, i(12p), as the sole structural cytogenetic abnormality. *Journal of Urology*, **131**, 762–763.

Gibas, A., Prout, G. R., Pontes, J. E. & Sandberg, A. A. (1986) Chromosome changes in germ cell tumors of the testis. *Cancer Genetics and Cytogenetics*, **19**, 245–252.

Martineau, M. (1969) Chromosomes in human testicular tumors. *Journal of Pathology*, **99**, 271–282.

Mitelman, F. (1985) *Catalog of Chromosome Aberrations in Cancer*. Second edition. Alan R. Liss, New York.

Oosterhuis, J. W., de Jong, B., van Dalen, I., van der Meer, I., Visser, M., de Leij, L., Mesander, G., Collard, J. G., Koops, H. S. & Sleijfer, D. T. (1985) Identical chromosome translocations involving the region of the c-myb oncogene in four metastases of mediastinal teratocarcinoma. *Cancer Genetics and Cytogenetics*, **15**, 99–107.

Parrington, J. M., West, L. F. & Povey, S. (1986) Chromosome changes in germ cell tumors. In *Germ Cell Tumours II* (ed. by W. C. Jones et al.), pp. 61–67. Pergamon Press, Oxford.

Riet-Fox, M. F., Retief, A. E. & Niekerk, W. A. (1979) Chromosome changes in 17 human neoplasms studied with banding. *Cancer*, **44**, 2108–2119.

Sikora, K., Evan, G., Stewart, J. & Watson, J. V. (1985) Detection of the c-myc oncogene product in testicular cancer. *British Journal of Cancer*, **52**, 171–176.

Tainsky, M. A., Cooper, C. S., Giovanella, B. C. & Vande Woude, G. F. (1984) An activated ras gene: Deteted in late but not early passage human PA1 teratocarcinoma cells. *Science*, **225**, 643–645.

Walt, H., Arrenbrecht, S., DeLozier-Blanchet, C. D., Keller, P. J., Nauer, R. & Hedinger, C. E. (1986) A human testicular germ cell tumor with borderline histology between seminoma and embryonal carcinoma secreted β-human gonadotropin and α-fetoprotein only as a xenograft. *Cancer*, **58**, 139–146.

Wang, N., Trend, B., Bronson, D. L. & Fraley, E. E. (1980) Nonrandom abnormalities in chromosome 1 in human testicular cancers. *Cancer Research*, **40**, 796–802.

Expression of growth regulatory genes in primary human testicular neoplasms

W. ENGSTRÖM, B. HOPKINS and P. SCHOFIELD
Department of Zoology, University of Oxford

Summary

Seven testicular tumours of different histological type—two seminomas, two teratomas/teratocarcinomas/embryonal carcinomas, one mixed seminoma/teratoma, one Leydig cell tumour and one testicular lymphoma—were examined for the expression of four potentially growth regulatory genes by Northern blotting. Seven out of seven testicular tumours contained transcripts that hybridized with a human insulin cDNA-probe whereas only four out of seven tumours contained IGF II transcripts. One tumour contained high levels of LDL-receptor transcript whereas all seven tumours contained significant quantities of HMG-CoA-reductase mRNA.

Key words. Germ cell tumours, insulin, insulin-like growth factors, cholesterol.

Introduction

Germ cell tumours, like other malignant neoplasms, are characterized by unrestricted proliferation *in vivo*. Despite recent improvements in therapeutic management, little is known about the cell biology of these tumours. Embryonal carcinoma stem cells can—in the mouse at least—participate in normal development after introduction into early embryo (Mintz & Illmensee, 1975). Conversely, it has been possible to derive embryonal carcinoma-like cells directly from early embryos (Evans & Kaufman, 1981, 1983). Therefore it has been suggested that germ cell tumour cells phenotypically resemble normal embryonic cells (Gardner, 1983).

Early embryonic development is characterized by a finely tuned interplay between growth and differentiation. It is conceivable that growth factors and hormones play an important role in controlling these processes (Engström & Heath, 1986). Recent studies which have analysed the growth phenotype of embryonal carcinoma cells *in vitro*, point at two classes of factors—transport proteins (transferrin, LDL, HDL) and members of the insulin family (insulin, IGF II)—as important determinants for embryonic stem cell proliferation (Heath, 1983; Engström, Rees & Heath, 1985; Engström & Heath, 1986; Heath & Shi, 1986). The present study was aimed at examining the expression of the insulin, IGF II, LDL-receptor and HMG-CoA-reductase genes in developmental tumours. We collected samples from human testicular tumours and examined the expression of the four genes by Northern blotting.

Correspondence: Dr W. Engström, Department of Zoology, University of Oxford, South Parks Road, Oxford OX1 3PS.

Materials and Methods

1. Isolation of RNA

Surgical specimens from eight human tumours were obtained from the John Radcliffe Hospital, Oxford. The histopathological type was determined for each tumour by light microscopy. RNA extraction from the tissue was started within 2 h after surgery.

The material was quickly dissolved by high-speed homogenization using an Ultra Turrax homogenizer in aqueous 4 M guanidiniumisothiocyanate (Fluka, F.R.G.) with 5 mM sodium citrate, 0.1 M beta-mercaptoethanol and 0.5% (v/v) Sarkosyl, and processed immediately. The dissolved samples were layered over a 2.2 ml 5.7 M CsCl 100 mM EDTA cushion in 12.6 ml capacity tubes (Beckman). They were centrifuged in a SW 40 Ti rotor at 33,000 rpm for 24 h at 15°C (Chirgwin et al., 1979).

The pellets of RNA were dissolved in 100 µl of aqueous 10 mM tris base (Sigma) with 1 mM EDTA at pH 7.4 (TE buffer). Next, they were ethanol precipitated twice, redissolved again in 100 µl TE buffer, and stored at −20°C. The concentration of RNA was measured by absorbance at 260 nm.

2. Labelling of the DNA probes with ^{32}P

The IGF II and insulin probes were in the form of cDNA sequences and were gifts from Dr J. Scott, MRC Clinical Research Centre, Harrow, U.K. The IGF II cDNA consisted of the Pst1 fragment containing a small amount of the 5′ non coding and the entire coding sequences cut from plasmid phigf2. The insulin probe consisted of the entire cDNA coding sequence cut from plasmid pcHI-1 with Pst1 (Bell et al., 1979).

The HMG-CoA-reductase and LDL-receptor probes were in the form of cDNA sequences and were a kind gift from Drs Kenneth Luskey, David Russel, Michael Brown and Joseph Goldstein, University of Texas, U.S.A. The hamster HMG-CoA-reductase cDNA probe (Chin et al., 1982) consisted of the 1200 bp Hind111-fragment which contains only a segment of the final peptide cut from plasmid pRED-10. The human LDL-receptor cDNA-probe (Yamamoto et al., 1984) consisted of a 1919 Bam H1 fragment which contains a part of the 5.3 kB coding sequence and was cut from a pSP64-vector.

The probes were cut from the vectors and isolated using low gelling temperature 1.5% (w/v) agarose gels (FMC Seakem) with 1 µg/ml ethidium-bromide (Sigma); and subsequently purified through NACS prepack columns (BRL) according to the manufacturer's instructions. The probes were labelled with ^{32}P-dATP by random hexanucleotide priming (Feinberg & Vogelstein, 1984) to a specific activity $> 4 \times 10^8$ cpm/µg DNA.

3. Northern blotting

Solutions of total extractable RNA (5–20 µg) were denatured for 15 min at 60°C. The 20 µl final reaction volume contained 20 mM MOPS (3-(N-morpholine) propanesulfonic acid), 5 mM Na acetate, 1 mM EDTA at pH 7.0 (1 × MOPS) with 50% (v/v) deionized formamide and 1.87% (v/v) formaldehyde. Before gel loading, 2 µl of 6× loading buffer was added. This contained aqueous 15% (w/v) Ficoll 400, 0.25% (w/v) bromophenol blue, and 0.25% (w/v) xylene cyanol. The samples were run on a 1.0% (w/v) denaturing agarose gel containing 1 × MOPS buffer and 0.23 M formaldehyde. Gels sized 11 × 14 cm were run at 60 mA, in 1 × MOPS with 8.79% (v/v) formaldehyde. An end-labelled Hind111 digest of DNA was used as a set of molecular weight markers.

The RNA was transferred to nitrocellulose filters (Schleicher & Schull BA 85, 0.45 μm pore size), by blotting overnight in 20 × SSC (1 × SSC = aqueous 0.15 M NaCl, 0.015 M Na citrate, pH 7.0). The blots were washed in 1 M EDTA pH 8, air dried and baked for 4 h at 80°C between two sheets of Whatman 3 mm chrome paper, then prehybridized overnight with 250 μg/ml of sonicated and denatured salmon sperm DNA in 5 × SSC, 50 mM phosphate buffer at pH 6.8, 5× Denhardt's solution (Denhardt, 1966), 0.1% (w/v) sodium dodecyl sulphate (SDS) and 50% (v/v) deionized formamide. They were hybridized with the labelled probes for at least 48 h at 42°C of a final radioactivity concentration of 3×10^6 cpm per ml. The hybridizing buffer contained 5 × SSC, 25 mM phosphate buffer at pH 6.8, 2.5× Denhardt's solution, 0.1% (w/v) SDS, 50% (v/v) deionized formamide and 250 μg sonicated and denatured salmon sperm DNA/ml. The probe was denatured before adding the buffer. The filters were washed at high stringency with a final wash at 55°C for 30 min in 0.2 × SSC. Radioactivity was detected with preflashed Kodak X-OMATS film (Laskey & Mills, 1977).

Results and Discussion

Seven testicular tumours of different histological type—two seminomas, two teratomas/teratocarcinomas/embryonal carcinomas, one mixed seminoma/teratocarcinoma, one Leydig cell tumour and one testicular lymphoma—were used as primary material for this study. One pancreatic insulin-producing islet cell tumour was used as a positive control for insulin.

Table 1 summarizes how the insulin, IGF II, HMG-CoA-reductase and LDL-receptor genes are expressed in these eight tumours. It was found that the human insulin cDNA probe hybridized with RNA from all seven testicular tumours. However, the probe mainly hybridized with a 6 kB size transcript instead of the expected 0.55 kB size transcript. This signal remained at high stringency washing up to 65°C at 0.2 × SSC.

In contrast, the insulinoma contained very high amounts of 0.55 kB insulin mRNA but no detectable levels of the 6 kB transcript as seen in the testicular tumours. When the testicular tumours were examined for IGF II expression, we found three tumours: one seminoma, one teratoma and one lymphoma, to be IGF II-negative. One teratocarcinoma (embryonal carcinoma) and one Leydig cell tumour displayed high levels of IGF II mRNA, whereas one seminoma and one mixed seminoma/teratocarcinoma were characterized by low levels of IGF II transcript. In all four cases, the cDNA probe hybridized with a 6.0 kB and a 1.9 kB band but only faintly with the additional 4.8 kB band as has been described in other developmental tumours (Scott et al., 1985). The ratio between the 6.0 and 1.9 kB band intensities remained constant although the absolute levels differed between the four tumours.

Thus, seven out of seven testicular tumours contain transcripts that hybridize with a human insulin cDNA-probe, whereas only four out of seven tumours contained IGF II transcripts. There was no correlation between expression of the two genes in the sense that any tumour contained high amounts of both transcripts.

Table 1. Presence of insulin IGF II, HMG-CoA-reductase and LDL-receptor transcripts in human primary tumours

Tumour number	Histological type	Insulin mRNA	IGFII mRNA	LDL-receptor mRNA	HMG-CoA-reductase mRNA
1	Seminoma	+++[1]	−	(+)[4]	++[5]
2	Seminoma	+[1]	+[2]	(+)[4]	++[5]
3	Seminoma/teratocarcinoma	+[1]	+[2]	+[4]	+++[6]
4	Teratoma	+[1]	−	+[4]	+++[6,3]
5	Embryonal carcinoma	+[1]	++++[2]	++++[4]	++[6]
6	Leydig cell tumour	+[1]	++[2]	(+)[4]	+[6]
7	Lymphoma	++[1]	−	(+)[4]	+++[6,3]
8	Insulinoma	+++++[3]	n.d.	(+)[4]	+++[6,3]

1 = 6 kB transcripts, 2 = 6 and 1.9 kB transcripts, 3 = 0.55 kB transcripts, 4 = 5.3 kB transcripts, 5 = 4.2, 3.1 and 1.1 kB transcripts, 6 = 4.2, 3.1, 1.1, 0.95 and 0.78 kB transcripts.
(−) = negative, n.d. = not determined.

The size of the transcripts which hybridized with the human IGF II probe were comparable to those reported elsewhere (Scott et al., 1985). However, we unexpectedly found that the insulin probe hybridized with a 6 kB band instead of the normal 0.55 kB band (Cordell et al., 1982). The insulin and IGF II genes are located on the short arm of chromosome 11 and are separated by a 12.6 kB stretch (Bell et al., 1985). It may be assumed that, if the known insulin promoter is used, the transcription in testicular tumours will terminate a long way in the intergenic region between the insulin and IGF II genes. The existence of 'large' insulin transcripts in testicular tumours is interesting in the light of Muglia & Lochers (1984) finding that the expression of the insulin gene in rat extrapancreatic tissues such as liver and the fetal yolk sack yielded two transcripts of 2.4 and 0.72 kB. In contrast, the corresponding pancreatic tissue only produced the expected 0.55 kB transcript. The significance of these findings is at present unclear, but the data suggests that in testicular tumours, as well as in normal extrapancreatic tissue, the insulin gene is transcribed actively but evidently not processed (Muglia & Locher, 1984; Rosenzweig et al., 1980).

It thereafter became of interest to examine how two genes that are involved in the regulation of the supply of cholesterol to cells are expressed in these tumours. Table 1 shows that only one tumour—an embryonal carcinoma—contained very high levels of LDL-receptor transcript. Northern blotting confirmed that our probe mainly hybridized with the expected 5.3 kB-transcript (Yamamoto et al., 1984). When the tumours were examined for HMG-CoA-reductase expression it was found that the hamster HMG-CoA-reductase probe hybridized with RNA from all eight tumours. The normal 4.2 kB band (Chin et al., 1982) was visible in all tumours. In addition, all tumours contained a weak 3.1 kB band, as well as a 1.1 kB size transcript. The latter band was prominent in five of the tumours, namely one embryonal carcinoma, one teratoma, one mixed teratoma/seminoma, one lymphoma and one insulinoma. These five tumours also contained large amounts of two 0.95 and 0.78 kB transcripts. Finally, three tumours, a teratoma, a lymphoma and an insulinoma produced a 0.55 kB transcript that hybridized with the HMG-CoA-reductase probe. Taken together, there appears to be a qualitative difference between Leydig cell tumours and the seminomas on the one hand, and the teratoma, embryonal carcinoma, insulinoma and lymphoma on the other. The Leydig cell tumours and seminomas only displayed the expected 4.2 kB transcript and low levels of 3.1 kB and 1.1 kB transcript. All other tumours contained at least two and sometimes three smaller transcripts.

The biological significance of this finding remains difficult to grasp, but it is possible that some malignant cells produce prematurely terminated or aberrantly spliced transcripts. Whether or not this finding can be used as a future diagnostic tool remains unclear.

Acknowledgements
The authors wish to express their gratitude to Professor C. F. Graham, F.R.S., Mr J. C. Smith, F.R.C.S. and Miss Amanda Lee, and to the Cancer Research Campaign for generous support.

References
Bell, G. I., Gerhard, D. S., Fong, M. M., Sanchez Pescador, R. & Rall, L. B. (1985) Isolation of the human insulin-like growth factor genes: Insulin-like growth factor II and insulin genes are contiguous. *Proceedings of the National Academy of Sciences of the United States of America*, **82**, 6450–6454.

Bell, G. I., Swain, W. F., Pictet, R., Cordell, R., Cordell, B., Goodman, H. M. & Rutter, W. J. (1979) Nucleotide sequence of a cDNA clone encoding human preproinsulin. *Nature*, **282**, 525–527.

Brown, M. S. & Goldstein, I. L. (1980) Multivalent feedback regulation of HMG-CoA-redusctase. A control mechanism corrdinating isoprenoid synthesis and cell growth. *Journal of Lipid Research*, **21**, 505–517.

Chin, D. J., Luskey, K. L., Faust, I. R., MacDonald, R. J., Brown, M. S. & Goldstein, I. L. (1982) Molecular cloning of 3-hydroxy-3-methylglutarylcoenzyme A reductase and evidence for regulation of its RNA in UT-1 cells. *Proceedings of the National Academy of Sciences of the United States of America*, **79**, 7704–7708.

Chirgwin, J. M., Przbyla, A. E., MacDonald, R. J. & Rutter, W. J. (1979) Isolation of biologically active ribonucleic acid from sources enriched in ribonuclease. *Biochemistry*, **18**, 5294–5299.

Cordell, B., Diamond, D., Smith, S., Punder, I., Schöne, H. H. & Goodman, H. (1982) Disproportionate expression of the two non-allelic rat insulin genes in a pancreatic tumour is due to translational control. *Cell*, **32**, 531–542.

Denhardt, D. T. (1966) A membrane-filter technique for the detection of complementary DNA. *Biochemical and Biophysical Research Communications*, **23**, 641–646.

Engström, W., Rees, A. R. & Heath, J. K. (1985) Proliferation of a human embryonal carcinoma derived cell like in a defined serum-free medium. Interrelationship between growth factor requirement and membrane receptor expression. *Journal of Cell Science*, **73**, 361–373.

Engström, W. & Heath, J. K. (1986) Growth factors in early embryonic development. *Perinatal Medicine*, **9**, 1–24.

Evans, M. J. & Kaufman, M. H. (1981) Establishment in culture of pluripotential cells from mouse embryos. *Nature*, **292**, 154-156.

Evans, M. J. & Kaufman, M. H. (1983) Pluripotential cells grown directly from normal mouse embryos. *Cancer Surveys*, **2**, 185–207.

Gardner, R. L. (1983) Teratomas in perspective. *Cancer Surveys*, **2**, 1–19

Heath, J. K. (1983) Regulation of murine embryonal carcinoma cell proliferation and differentiation. *Cancer Surveys*, **2**, 141–164.

Heath, J. K. & Shi, W. K. (1986) Developmentally regulated expression of insulin like growth factors by differentiated murine teratocarcinomas and extraembryonic mesoderm *Journal of Embryology and Experimental Morphology*, **95**, 193–212.

Laskey, R. & Mills, A. D. (1977) Enhanced autoradiographic detection of ^{32}P and ^{125}P using intensifying screens and hypersensitized films. *Federation of European Biochemical Societies Letters*, **82**, 314–316.

Mintz, B. & Illmensee, K. (1975) Normal genetically mosaic mice produced from malignant teratocarcinoma cells. *Proceedings of the National Academy of Sciences of the United States of America*, **72**, 3585–3589.

Muglia, L. & Locker, J. (1984) Extrapancreatic insulin gene expression in the fetal rat. *Proceedings of the National Academy of Sciences of the United States of America*, **81**, 3635–3639.

Rosenzweig, I. C., Havrankova, J., Lesniak, M., Brownstein, M. & Roth, J. (1980) Insulin is ubiquitous in extrapancreatic tissues of rats and humans. *Proceedings of the National Academy of Sciences of the United States of America*, **77**, 572–576.

Scott, J., Cowell, J., Robertson, M. E., Priestley, C. M., Wadey, R., Hopkins, B., Bell, G. I., Pritchard, J., Rall, C. B., Graham, C. F. & Knott, T. (1985) Insulin like growth factor II gene expression in Wilms tumour and embryonic tissues. *Nature*, **317**, 260–262.

Yamamoto, T., Davis, C. G., Brown, M. S., Schneider, W. J., Casey, M. L., Goldstein, J. L. & Russel, D. W. (1984) The human LDL-receptor; A cysteine rich protein with multiple Alu sequences in its mRNA. *Cell*, **38**, 27–38.

Discussion

Sikora How did you collect your material and why did you have so much degradation of DNA in your tissue?

Engström The samples were collected directly from the operating theatre in the hospital and homogenized in 4 M guadinium isothiocyanate to stop RNA degradation. To examine if the background on the blots is due to RNA from degraded tissue, we rehybridized the filters with a c-DNA probe for glyceraldehyde-3-phosphate dehydrogenase. The autoradiographs showed a clean 1.6 kB band in all samples.

Walt Did you analyse metastatic tumour cells?

Engström All the tumours included in this survey were primary tumours, although I do not know if any of them had metastasized.

Niemi Can your probes be used for *in-situ* hydridization?

Have you any evidence that insulin or insulin-like growth factors are actually produced by the tumours and not just the transcripts?

Engström All probes can be used for *in-situ* hydridization experiments, but we have not yet tried this technique.

We have not actually looked for insulin or the IGF II protein product in the testicular tumours. However, the existence of an unprocessed insulin mRNA transcript makes it less likely that insulin itself would be found.

HLA phenotype and clinicopathological behaviour of germ cell tumours: possible evidence for clonal evolution from seminomas to nonseminomas

R. T. D. OLIVER *The London and St Bartholomew's Hospital Medical Colleges and The Institute of Urology*

Summary

Analysis of 101 patients with germ cell tumours of the testis who have been typed for HLA DR antigens has provided confirmatory evidence for an association of DR5 with the development of seminoma and demonstrated an association of DR7 with metastases. These observations taken with the suggestion of HLA linkage in the small numbers of familial cases reviewed, does suggest that there is an HLA linked gene involved in the clinicopathological behaviour of germ cell tumours. Though of only theoretical interest at present these observations may be of considerable importance in the future given the observation in mice that transfection of missing MHC genes into a malignant tumour can produce a vaccine that enables previously unexposed animals to resist the original malignant tumour (Hui *et al.*, 1984).

Key words. HLA, germ cell tumours, clonal evolution.

Introduction

Little is known about what, apart from age at diagnosis, determines whether a germ cell tumour will be a seminoma or nonseminoma.

As both are associated with *in-situ* carcinoma, there is debate as to whether seminomas develop as an entirely separate entity from nonseminomas or is an integral stage in their development (Fig. 1).

The most convincing evidence that study of genetic factors may be relevant to understanding the factors determining the occurrence of seminomas or nonseminomas comes from study of familial germ cell tumours.

Despite incomplete enquiry the incidence of familial tumours is higher than the one in 450 life-time risk amongst unrelated individuals of that age. Pugh (1976) reported six patients in his series of 2763 while Oliver *et al.* (1986) recorded three familial cases in a series of 493 patients treated at The London Hospital. As this data is retrospective, a formal prospective follow-up of a large series with correction for the number of years follow-up and the number of males at risk in each family would be necessary to define the precise risk. Such a study is currently in progress through the auspices of The Imperial Cancer Research Fund

Correspondence: R. T. D. Oliver, Department of Medical Oncology, The London Hospital, Whitechapel, London E1 1BB.

Table 2. DR locus antigen frequency (%) in different pathological and clinical staging in subgroups

	Controls (n = 390)	Seminoma (n = 31)	MTI & TD (n = 29)	MTU & MTT & YS (n = 41)	Stage II & III (n = 31)	Stage IV (n = 42)	(n = 28)
DR1	16	29	34†	15	36‡	24	14
DR2	29	13	24	29	16	26	25
DR3	23	13	17	29	23	19	21
DR4	31	32	38	22	32	29	29
DR5	19	36*	7	20	16	19	29
DRW6	19	13	17	24	16	29	7
DR7	26	29	41	32	23	29	54§
DRW8	7	0	3	2	3	0	4
DRW9	2	0	0	0	0	0	0

MTI = Malignant teratoma intermediate = teratocarcinoma.
TD = Teratoma differentiated = mature teratoma.
MTU = Malignant teratoma undifferentiated = embryonal carcinoma.
MTT = Malignant teratoma trophoblastic = choriocarcinoma.
YS = Yolk sac tumour.
*vs control $\chi^2 = 3.9$, $P = 0.04$ uncorrected.
†vs control $\chi^2 = 5.4$, $P = 0.22$ corrected.
‡vs control $\chi^2 = 6.4$, $P = 0.09$ corrected.
§vs control $\chi^2 = 8.9$, $P = 0.045$ corrected.

Table 3. DR3/DR5 frequency in seminoma patients

		Seminoma		Control	
		Number	Frequency (%)	Number	Frequency (%)
Oliver et al. (1985)	DR5	31	36[a]	390	19
Pollack et al. (1983)	DR5	15	54[b]	176	25
Total	DR5	46	41[c]	566	21
Oliver et al. (1985)	DR3	31	13	390	23
Pollack et al. (1983)	DR3	15	0[d]	176	22
Total	DR3	46	9[e]	566	23

(a) vs control $P < 0.04$, RR = 2.38.
(b) vs control $P < 0.05$, RR = 3.38.
(c) vs control $P < 0.01$, RR = 2.60.
(d) vs control $P < 0.05$, RR = 0.11.
(e) vs control $P < 0.05$, RR = 0.32.

Table 4. DR7/DW7 frequency in published series of testicular germ cell tumours

	Patients		Controls	
	Number	Frequency (%)	Number	Frequency (%)
Oliver et al. (1986)*	101	34	390	26
Pollack et al. (1982)*	103	32	176	28
DeWolf et al. (1979)†	53	28	150	9
Aiginger et al. (1983)*	69	29	160	28
Total	328	32[a]	862	24[b]

(a) vs (b) $\chi^2 = 3.9$ ($P < 0.05$).
*DR7.
†DW7.

DR antigens themselves. Alternatively if a cofactor in the initiation process were an endemic virus, in different parts of the world it might have evolved to infect a different group of susceptible individuals.

HLA studies in familial germ cell tumour

Evidence in favour of the linked gene hypothesis comes from HLA studies of familial testis tumour. Although only seven families have been studied (Table 5), 100% of the affected pairs share one or more HLA haplotype compared to 75% expected. If confirmed in a larger series this would suggest that the association of HLA DR in unrelated individuals is not due to the HLA genes themselves but an as yet undefined linked gene. This is similar to the situation in Hodgkin's disease, which also shows minor but consistent HLA associations amongst non-relatives (Walford, 1972), but strong HLA linkage in families (Hors et al., 1984).

The relative rarity of familial testicular tumours means that to collect sufficient informative families will require international collaboration. In an attempt to do this the Medical Research Council Working Party on Testicular Tumours in

Table 5. HLA genotype of family members with germ cell tumour

Family no.	Relationship	Genotype
1	Patient	A1 B8/AX, BX
	Uncle	A1, B8/A2, B7
2	Patient	A3 BW44/AW30, B70
	Nephew	A3, BW44/AW26, BW57
3	Patient	A32, B27/A2, B12
	Brother	A32, B27/A29, B7
	Brother	A32, B27/A2, B12
4	Patient	A2, B12/A28, B12
	Non-identical twin brother	A2, B12/A28, B12
5	Patient	A3, B7/A2, B17
	Brother	A3, B7/A28, B14
6	Patient	A3, BW35/A24, B7
	Brother	A3, BW35/A28, B44
7	Patient	A3, B7/A28, B44
	Brother	A3, B7/A2, B40

1, 2, 3 = Oliver *et al.* (1986).
4, 5, 6 = Pollack *et al.* (1982).
7 = E. R. Heise (1985), personal communication.

collaboration with The Imperial Cancer Research Fund Epidemiology and Clinical Trials Unit in Oxford is currently registering all familial cases including twins and arranging for pathological review and HLA typing if this cannot be arranged locally.

An additional approach to study the significance of this observation would be to transfect different MHC genes into germ cell tumour lines and study their morphology in immune deficient mice as this may shed light on the controversy of the relationship of seminoma and nonseminoma (Fig. 1).

According to Mostofi and coworkers (Mostofi, 1984; Sesterhenn, 1986), the tumours are polyclonal and each cell type is a separate monoclonal proliferation from a separate premalignant germ cell precursor. The second theory favoured by Raghavan *et al.* (1982) and the author of this paper, suggests that the tumours are monoclonal with seminomas as a stage after *in-situ* carcinoma through which all germ cell tumours progress. The variable cell morphology seen is a reflection of the host genetic make up and which gene set has been activated during the serial mutagenic oncogenic process. Support for this latter hypothesis comes from the results of the HLA studies reviewed in this paper and study of DNA content of germ cell tumours. The average DNA ploidy value of seminomas (3.6N) is intermediate between that of the premalignant *in-situ* carcinoma cell (4.2N) and the average ploidy value of nonseminomas (2.7N) which is still higher than the ploidy values of the normal spermatogonium which is 2.0N (Atkin & Kay, 1979; Müller & Skakkebæk, 1981).

References

Aiginger, P., Schwartz, H. P., Kuzmits, R., Kuhback, J., Schemper, M., Mayr, W. R. & Karrer, K. (1983) HLA-A, B, C and Dr-antigens and testicular cancer: a prospective study. *Proceedings of the American Association for Cancer Research*, **24**, 190.

Atkin, N. B. & Kay, R. (1979) Prognostic significance of modal DNA value and other factors in malignant tumours, based on 1465 cases. *British Journal of Cancer*, **40**, 210.

DeWolf, W. C., Lange, P. H., Einaison, M. E. & Yunus, E. J. (1979) HLA and testicular cancer. *Nature*, **277**, 216–217.

Hart, I. R. (1985) Molecular basis of tumour spread. *Nature*, **315**, 274–275.

Hors, J., Bonaiti-Perrie, C., D'Agacy, M. F., Rappaport, M., Andrieux, J. M., deWaal, L. P., de Lange, G. G. & Feingold, N. (1984) *Hodgkin's Disease, Histocompatibility Testing*, pp. 411–414. Springer-Verlag, Berlin.

Hui, K., Grosveld, F. & Festenstein, H. (1984) Rejection of transplantable AKR leukaemia cells following MHC DNA-mediated cell transformation. *Nature*, **311**, 750–752.

Lancet Editorial (1985) New views on HLA and disease. *Lancet*, **i**, 559–561.

Lilly, F. & Pincus, T. (1973) Genetic control of murine leukemogenesis. *Advances in Cancer Research*, **17**, 231–277.

Mostofi, F. K. (1984) Tumour markers and pathology of testicular tumours. *Progress and Controversies in Oncological Urology*, pp. 69–87. Alan R. Liss, New York.

Müller, J. & Skakkebæk, N. E. (1981) Microspectrophotometric DNA measurements of carcinoma-*in-situ* germ cells in the testis. *International Journal of Andrology*, Suppl. 4, 211–221.

Oliver, R. T. D. (1982) Biology of host/tumour cell interactions. *Scientific Basis of Urology* (ed. by Chisholm, G. S. & Innes Williams, D.), pp. 624–631. Wm. Heinemann, London.

Oliver, R. T. D., Stephenson, C. A., Parkinson, M. C., Forman, D., Atkinson, A., Bodmer, J. & Bodmer, W. F. (1986) Germ cell tumours of the testicle as a model of MHC influence on human malignancy. *Lancet*, **i**, 1506.

Oliver, R. T. D., Ward, J. & Bodmer, K. (1986) In preparation.

Pollack, M. S., Vugrin, D., Hennessy, W., Herr, H. W., Dupont, B. & Whitmore, W. (1982) HLA antigens in patients with germ cell cancers of the testis. *Cancer Research*, **42**, 2470–2473.

Pugh, R. C. B. (1976) Testicular tumours. *Pathology of the Testis* (ed. Pugh, R. C. B.), pp. 139–159. Blackwell Scientific Publications, Oxford.

Raghavan, D., Sullivan, A. L., Peckham, M. J. & Neville, M. (1982) Elevated serum alphafetoprotein and seminoma: clinical evidence for a histological continuum. *Cancer*, **50**, 982–989.

Sesterhenn, I. A. (1986) The role of intratubular malignant germ cells in the histogenesis of germ cell tumours. In: *Germ Cell Tumours II* (ed. by Jones, W. G., Milford Ward, A. & Anderson, C. K.). Pergamon Press, Oxford.

Walford, R. L. (1972) Histocompatibility systems and disease states with particular reference to cancer. *Transplantation Reviews*, **8**, 1–15

Weissbach, L. & Widman, T. (1986) Familial tumour of the testis. *European Journal of Urology*, **12**, 104–108.

Discussion

Dieckmann In our series of 180 patients with testicular cancer we found three pairs of brothers. One pair had nonidentical histology and two pairs had identical histology. Cryptorchidism was not present in any of these related cases.

Oliver Such an incidence of testicular tumours within families is much higher than reported from previous registry data and fits in with our preliminary data from the prospective study.

Bannwart There are some instances of familial testicular cancer in the Swiss experience, the latest example being in identical twins. The first twin had a unilateral orchidectomy for palpable tumour and this showed teratocarcinoma. Biopsy of the contralateral testis showed seminoma-in-situ. A few weeks later, a testicular biopsy from the second twin showed seminoma-in-situ in one testis and he will be receiving therapy.

Skakkebæk I think that your findings give further evidence for our theory that all germ cell tumours except spermatocytic seminoma have their origin from the CIS

pathologists commonly fall into the nullipotent category, and many cell lines derived from them similarly possess little capacity for differentiation (Damjanov, 1983; Andrews, 1983). This rarity of pluripotency, together with the apparent differences from their murine counterparts (discussed below) and the pleomorphism of cells labelled EC by pathologists, have all contributed to the difficulties of defining objective criteria for human EC cells, and of studying their differentiation into the other components of human germ cell tumours. For these reasons we have concentrated our studies on clonal derivatives of two human cell lines isolated from different testicular germ cell tumours, 2102Ep and TERA-2: in nude mice 2102Ep forms tumours consistent with pure human embryonal carcinoma, and we have regarded 2102Ep cells as prototypical human EC cells (Andrews *et al.*, 1982). Although some cell lines described as human EC cells differ from this prototype, the properties of the 2102Ep cells are generally shared by a substantial subset of histologically identified human EC-like cells (e.g. Damjanov *et al.*, 1982). Moreover, stem cell clones isolated from TERA-2 exhibit similar properties to the 2102Ep cells but are also capable of differentiating into a variety of somatic cell types (Andrews *et al.*, 1984b; Andrews, 1984). Thus we have been able to define criteria for a group of human teratocarcinoma stem cells that appear to form a counterpart to the murine EC cells. Nevertheless, variation in the expression of several markers, including the globo-series carbohydrate antigens SSEA-3 and SSEA-4, and the class I MHC antigens, has been observed even amongst different clones of TERA-2-derived human stem cells (Thompson *et al.*, 1984; Andrews *et al.*, 1985). Here we review the characteristics of 2102Ep and TERA-2 human EC cells, the changes that accompany their differentiation, and some of the variations in EC cell properties that occur.

Properties of 2102Ep and TERA-2 EC cells
For our studies of the 2102Ep and TERA-2 cell lines, we used clonally derived sublines grown from isolated single cells (Andrews *et al.*, 1982, 1984b). In the case of TERA-2, most of these clones were from a subline, NTERA-2, that was rederived from a nude mouse tumour of TERA-2. When maintained at a high cell density ($>7 \times 10^4/\text{cm}^2$), 2102Ep and NTERA-2 cultures consist mostly of densely packed cells with little cytoplasm, which contains few organelles other than free ribosomes, and nuclei with prominent nucleoli, features common to murine EC cells. However, unlike murine EC cells, which contain vimentin intermediate filaments, both human lines express cytokeratin (40, 45 and 52 kD polypeptides) (Damjanov, Clark & Andrews, 1984).

The cells from high-density cultures of 2102Ep and NTERA-2 express several monoclonal antibody-defined surface antigens, SSEA-3, SSEA-4, TRA-1-60 and TRA-1-81, which are commonly expressed by EC-like cells in other specimens of human germ cell tumours, but by few other cell types (Damjanov *et al.*, 1982; Shevinsky *et al.*, 1982; Andrews *et al.*, 1984a). SSEA-4 and -3 are epitopes comprising the terminal and subterminal region, respectively, of an extended globo-series ganglioside (Table 1); these antigens are also expressed by human erythrocytes and correspond to the 'Luke' and 'P' blood group antigens (Tippett *et al.*, 1986). Murine EC cells do not express either SSEA-3 or -4 (Shevinsky *et al.*, 1982), but do express SSEA-1, a carbohydrate epitope composed of fucose($\alpha1\rightarrow3$)N-acetylglucosamine carried on a type 2 polylactosamine chain (Solter & Knowles, 1978; Kannagi *et al.*,

Table 1. Glycolipid structures identified in TERA-2-derived EC cells or their differentiated derivatives

Glycolipid structure	Glycolipid/antigen	Reference
Galβ1→3GalNAcβ1→3Galα1→4Galβ1→4Glcβ1→Cer*	Gb$_5$, SSEA-3[†]	Kannagi et al., 1983
NeuNAcα2→3Galβ1→3GalNAcβ1→3Galα1→4Galβ1→4Glcβ1→Cer	Gl$_7$, SSEA-3, SSEA-4[†]	Fenderson et al., 1986
Fucα1→2Galβ1→3GalNAcβ1→3Galα1→4Galβ1→4Glcβ1→Cer	Globo H	
GalNAcα1→3Galβ1→3GalNAcβ1→3Galα1→4Galβ1→4Glcβ1→Cer	Globo A	
↑ 2 Fucα1		

1. Globo-series

2. Lacto-series

Galβ1→4GlcNAcβ1→3Galβ1→4Glcβ1→Cer*
         ↑ 3
       Fucα1

| | Le^x, SSEA-1 | Kannagi et al., 1982 |

3. Ganglio-series[‡]

(9-0-acetyl)NeuNAcα2→8NeuNAcα2→3Galβ1→4Glcβ1→Cer*
NeuNAcα2→8NeuNAcα2→3Galβ1→4Glcβ1→Cer

| | 9-0-AcGD$_3$, ME311 | Thurin et al., 1985 |
| | GT$_3$, A2B5 | Fenderson et al., 1986 |

*Key control points in switching between synthesis of globo-series, lacto-series and ganglio-series core structures.
[†]SSEA-3 corresponds to the P blood group antigen and SSEA-4 to the Luke blood group antigen.
[‡]Other ganglio-series structures identified in TERA-2-derived cells include GM$_3$, GM$_2$ and GD$_3$ and GD$_2$.

1982). The 2102Ep and NTERA-2 EC cells lack SSEA-1, although it appears on some of their differentiated derivatives. The structures of the TRA-1-60 and TRA-1-81 epitopes, carried by high molecular weight polypeptides, are currently unknown, but they appear to be human-specific. Other surface markers expressed by the 2102Ep and NTERA-2 cells include high levels of alkaline phosphatase (ALP), low levels of epidermal growth factor receptor (Carlin & Andrews, 1985), and low levels of MHC class I (HLA-A,B,C) antigens. Most of the ALP is composed of the liver isozyme, but a form of resembling placental ALP is also detectable (Benham et al., 1981).

Variations in the expression of SSEA-3 and -4
Several EC-like clones isolated from the original TERA-2 line by Graham and colleagues (Thompson et al., 1984), and by ourselves (Andrews et al., 1985), do not express cell surface-reactive SSEA-3 or -4, although they express TRA-1-60 and TRA-1-81, and resemble NTERA-2 EC cells in other ways, including ability to differentiate. The distinction between the TERA-2 and NTERA-2 clones is not merely due to passage of the latter in a nude mouse, since of the two TERA-2 clones we studied (cl.w1 and cl.w2), cl.w1 EC cells do not express SSEA-3 and -4 while cl.w2 EC cells do (Andrews et al., 1985). Nevertheless, passage through a nude mouse does induce SSEA-3 and -4 in some cl.w1 cells. This suggests a relationship between EC cell tumour growth and expression of these antigens, and in turn raises the question of whether P-blood group genotype influences the behaviour of germ cell tumours in human patients.

Differentiation of 2102Ep and NTERA-2 EC cells
The growth of 2102Ep cells at a low cell density (1.5×10^3 cells/cm^2) results in morphological and biochemical changes, including a reduction in SSEA-3 and -4 expression, and the appearance of SSEA-1-positive cells synthesizing fibronectin (Andrews, 1982) and a few cells containing immunoreactive cytoplasmic hCG (Damjanov & Andrews, 1983). The latter suggests limited differentiation along a trophoblastic lineage. However, many cells retain an EC phenotype, and more extensive differentiation is not induced by chemical agents such as retinoic acid. By contrast, NTERA-2 cells differentiate extensively in response to retinoic acid, forming a variety of cell types such as neurons expresssing tetanus toxin receptors and all three neurofilament polypeptides (Andrews, 1984; Lee & Andrews, 1986). Unlike 2102Ep EC cells, NTERA-2 EC cells also differentiate, forming glandular structures and smooth muscle, in addition to neurectodermal elements, when grown as xenograft tumours.

Glycolipids of TERA-2 EC cells and their changes during differentiation
Undifferentiated NTERA-2 (cl.D1) cells express predominantly globo-series glycolipids including Gb$_3$, Gb$_5$ (SSEA-3), sialosyl Gb$_5$ (SSEA-4), fucosyl Gb$_5$ (globo-H), and globo-A (Fenderson et al., 1986) (Fig. 1). When these cells are induced to differentiate by retinoic acid, a shift from globo-series to lacto- and ganglio-series glycolipids occurs: globo-series structures declining, particularly during the period 7–20 days after first exposure to retinoic acid, while lacto-series structures, including sialosyl type 2 chain and fucosyl type 2 chain (SSEA-1), and ganglio-series structures

A. Sialosyl Glycolipids (Gangliosides)

B. Upper Neutral Glycolipids

Fig. 1. TLC immunostaining analysis of glycolipids from TERA-2 EC cells and their differentiated derivatives. Upper phase sialosyl (A) and neutral (B) glycolipids were obtained from NTERA-2 cells cultured in the presence of 10^{-5} M retinoic acid for 0–9 days (lanes 0 and 9), and from undifferentiated cultures of TERA-2 cl.w1 and w2 cells (lanes W1 and W2). Each lane contains glycolipid from approximately 2×10^7 cells. Upper phase neutral glycolipids obtained from human type A or type O whole blood cells are included on the right side of each panel in part B for reference; other glycolipid standards include GL_7 and Le^x pentasaccharide. Plates were developed using chloroform/methanol/water (50:40:10) containing 0.05% $CaCl_2$ and either stained for carbohydrate by the orcinol/sulphuric acid reaction (orcinol) or labelled with monoclonal antibody to SSEA-3, SSEA-4, globo-A, or SSEA-1 and ^{125}I-protein A. Note that SSEA-3 and -4-reactive glycolipids GL_7 and GL_9 and globo-A-reactive glycolipid are readily detectable in NTERA-2 stem cells (0 days) but are much reduced in the differentiated cells (9 days). Conversely, SSEA-1-reactive Le^x-reactive glycolipids appear by 9 days. Like NTERA-2 EC cells, cl.w2 cells express SSEA-3 and -4-reactive GL_7 and GL_9, but GL_7 is absent from cl.w1 cells which do not exhibit cell surface reactivity for either anti-SSEA-3 or -4. Thus GL_7 is probably the immunodominant globo-series glycolipid on the surface of human EC cells.

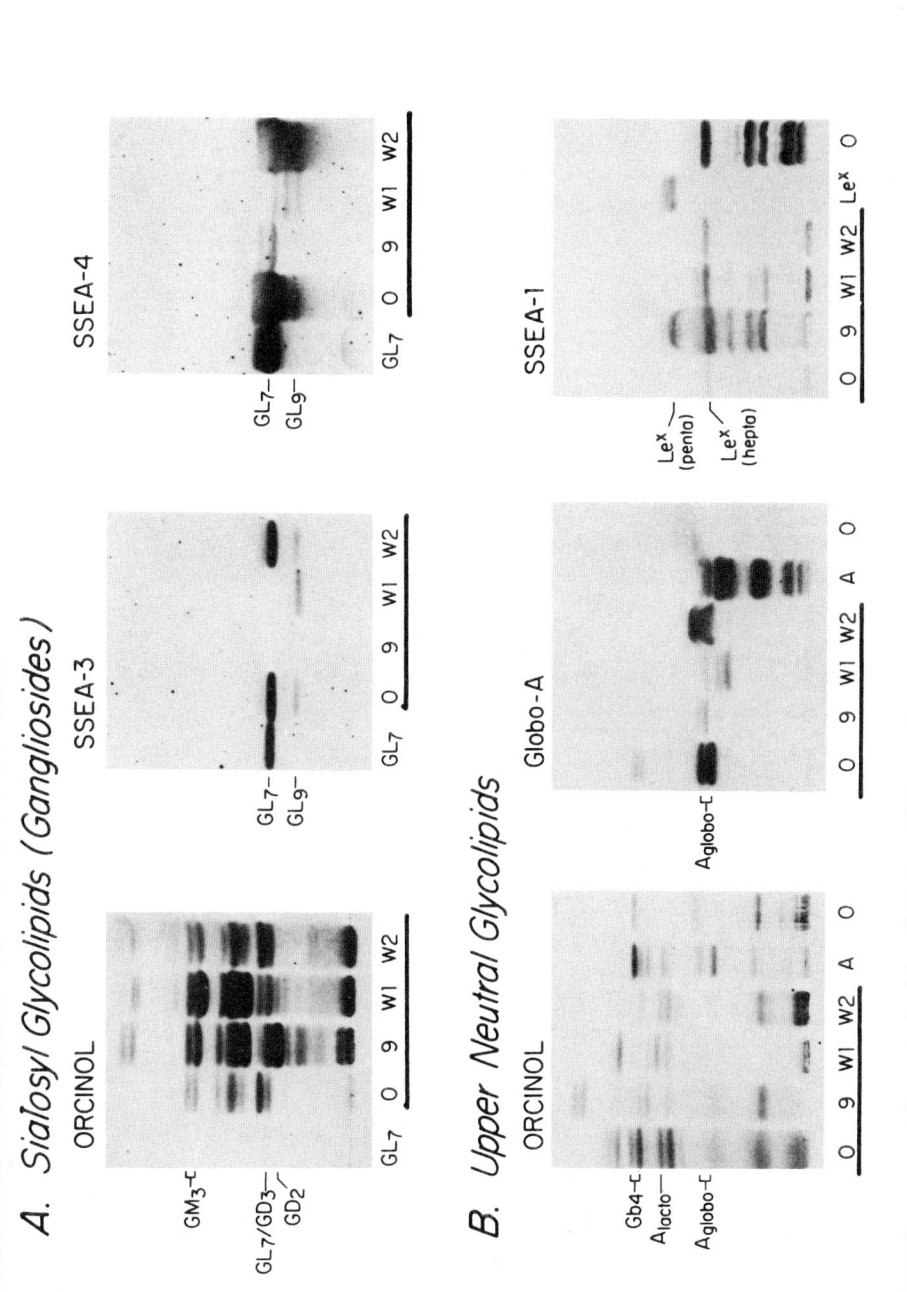

including GM$_3$, GD$_3$, 9-0-acetyl-GD$_3$, GM$_2$, GD$_2$ and GT$_3$, increase. The lacto-series structures later decline, and the overall changes in glycolipid expression may be represented as shown in Fig. 2. This scheme, however, masks the fact that NTERA-2 differentiation leads to multiple cell types, in which these various glycolipid antigens are differentially expressed. For example, GT$_3$ (A2B5) is strongly expressed by the neuronal derivatives, and a subset of other cells, while 9-0-acetyl GD$_3$ (ME311) is only expressed by a subset of non-neuronal cells.

In contrast to the NTERA-2 EC cells, the TERA-2 cl.w1 and w2 cells co-express globo-, lacto- and ganglio-series glycolipids (Fig. 1), suggesting that these EC lines have initiated a developmental programme of core structure switching but that other changes associated with the complete loss of an EC phenotype have not occurred. Curiously, although cl.w1 cells lack reactivity with antibodies to SSEA-3 and -4, they clearly contain the glycolipids carrying these epitopes. Thus cell surface reactivity is dependent upon the organization of these glycolipids in the plasma membrane and not merely upon their presence or absence.

The presence of globo-A antigens in undifferentiated NTERA-2 cells (Fig. 1, panel B) raises the question of whether globo-series ABH antigens are stage-specific embryonic antigens, whose expression is not correlated with adult ABH blood group status. To explore this we compared two additional EC cell lines, derived from patients of B and O blood types, with TERA-2 cells which came from a blood type A patient. The globo-H antigen was identified in EC cells irrespective of the host's blood group status, but the globo-A antigen was clearly detected only in the TERA-2 EC cells. Thus, globo-series ABH expression in human EC cells appears to be determined by adult ABH genotype.

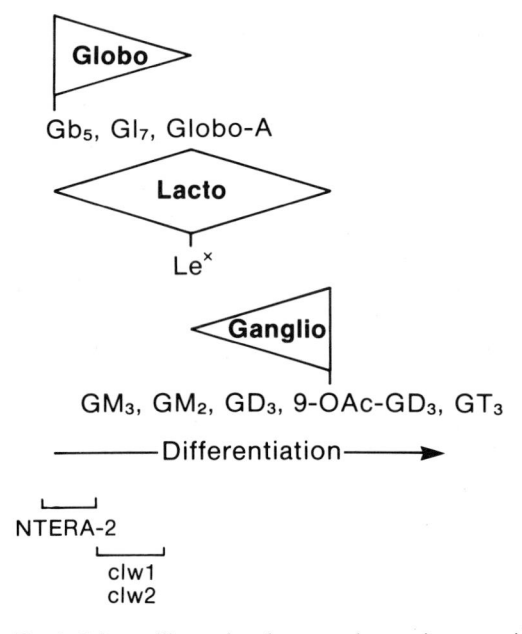

Fig. 2. Scheme illustrating the gross changes in expression of glycolipid antigens during TERA-2 EC cell differentiation. The differences in expression between NTERA-2 EC cells and TERA-2 cl.w1 and cl.w2 EC cells may indicate that the latter have already initiated some of the changes associated with differentiation.

Our results suggest that glycosyltransferases, particularly those involved in controlling glycoconjugate core structure assembly, are key enzymes that are regulated during the differentiation of human EC cells and, by implication, during human embryogenesis. These enzymes may include $\alpha 1 \rightarrow 4$ galactosyltransferase (globo-core), $\alpha 1 \rightarrow 3$ N-acetylglucosaminyltransferase (lacto-core), and $\alpha 2 \rightarrow 3$ sialyltransferase (ganglio-core) (see Table 1). However, the differential expression of some antigens (e.g. A2B5 and ME311) by different subsets of NTERA-2 cells suggests that some of the chain modification enzymes may also be regulated.

Variation in the expression of MHC antigens—induction by interferon
MHC class I antigens (HLA-A,B,C) and β_2-microglobulin (β_2m) are usually detectable in the 2102Ep and NTERA-2 EC cells (Andrews et al., 1982, 1984), in contrast to the absence of the homologous H-2 antigens in murine EC cells. However, expression of HLA-A,B,C and β_2m is weak and variable, especially in the case of NTERA-2; in a few experiments we have not observed them at all, while Thompson et al. (1984) never detected these antigens in their TERA-2 clones. We investigated whether MHC antigens are induced in human and mouse EC cells by interferon (IFN), since this antiviral agent induces MHC antigen expression in other cell types. In murine EC cells, IFN is known to produce only a partial response, inducing certain enzymes usually associated with the development of an antiviral state (e.g. 2'-5'oligo(A) synthetase), but without inducing complete virus resistance. We have now found that, similarly, neither 2102Ep nor NTERA-2 respond to IFN-α, -β or -γ by becoming resistant to vesicular stomatitis virus or, in this case, even by expressing 2'-5'oligo(A) synthetase (Andrews et al., 1986). On the other hand, both human EC cells express much higher levels of HLA-A,B,C and β_2m when exposed to IFN, especially IFN-γ, without any evidence of differentiation. Even in NTERA-2 cultures that did not express detectable HLA-A,B,C and β_2m, expression was detectable 1 day after exposure to 100 U/ml IFN-γ. However, class II antigens were not induced. We also found that murine IFN-γ induces MHC class I (H-2D^b), but not class II (Ia^b), antigens in at least one murine EC cell line: in one subline of PCC4aza^R, H-2D^b was strongly induced, while in another subline a low level of expression was detectable following exposure to 500 U/ml IFN-γ. On the other hand, expression of H-2D^b was not inducible in F9 EC cells. Despite their expression of MHC antigens, the PCC4aza^R cells retained a typical murine EC phenotype in the presence of IFN-γ without evidence of differentiation. Thus, under certain circumstances, class I MHC antigens may be expressed by both human and mouse EC cells, raising the question of whether other agents or growth conditions might also induce these antigens without inducing differentiation. Variations in the low level expression of MHC antigens between different human EC cell lines, or between human and mouse EC cell lines, may then reflect a 'leaky' control system.

Conclusion
Our studies have focused on two cell lines derived from human germ cell tumours. These cell lines are identified as human EC cell lines on the basis of the histology of their tumours in nude mice (especially in the case of 2102Ep) and their ability to differentiate into distinct cell types (especially in the case of NTERA-2). These two

EC cell lines exhibit similar phenotypes and examination of their properties has provided objective criteria for defining at least a subgroup of human EC cells. Extensive comparative studies of other human germ cell tumours, and the isolation of new pluripotent human stem cell lines, is now necessary to determine the generality of these criteria. Meanwhile, the differentiation of TERA-2 EC cells in culture provides a model for studying cellular differentiation in a way relating to human early embryogenesis, as murine EC cell lines have provided a model for murine early embryogenesis.

Acknowledgements
This work was supported by USPHS grants CA29894 and HD18704 from the NIH. We thank Mr M. Dignazio, Mr G. O'Malley and Ms S. Judkins for excellent technical assistance.

References

Andrews, P. W. (1982) Human embryonal carcinoma cells in culture do not synthesize fibronectin until they differentiate. *International Journal of Cancer*, **30**, 567–571.

Andrews, P. W. (1983) The characteristics of cell lines derived from human germ-cell tumours. *The Human Teratomas; Experimental and Clinical Biology* (ed. by I. Damjanov, B. B. Knowles and D. Solter), pp. 285– 311. Humana Press, Clifton, N.J.

Andrews, P. W. (1984) Retinoic acid induces neuronal differentiation of a cloned human embryonal carcinoma cell line *in vitro*. *Developmental Biology*, **103**, 285–293.

Andrews, P. W., Banting, G. S., Damjanov, I., Arnaud, D. & Anver, P. (1984a) Three monoclonal antibodies defining distinct differentiation antigens associated with different high molecular weight polypeptides on the surface of human embryonal carcinoma cells. *Hybridoma*, **3**, 347–361.

Andrews, P. W., Damjanov, I., Simon, D., Banting, G., Carlin, C., Dracopoli, N. C. & Fogh, J. (1984b) Pluripotent embryonal carcinoma clones derived from the human teratocarcinoma cell line TERA-2: Differentiation *in vivo* and *in vitro*. *Laboratory Investigation*, **50**, 147–162.

Andrews, P. W., Damjanov, I., Simon, D. & Dignazio, M. (1985) A pluripotent human stem-cell clone isolated from the TERA-2 teratocarcinoma line lacks antigens SSEA-3 and SSEA-4 *in vitro*, but expresses these antigens when grown as a xenograft tumor. *Differentiation*, **29**, 127–135.

Andrews, P. W., Goodfellow, P. N., Shevinsky, L., Bronson, D. L. & Knowles, B. B. (1982) Cell surface antigens of a clonal human embryonal carcinoma cell line: Morphological and antigenic differentiation in culture. *International Journal of Cancer*, **29**, 523–531.

Andrews, P. W., Trinchieri, G., Perussia, B. & Baglioni, C. (1986) Interferon induces class I MHC antigens in human teratocarcinoma cells without inducing differentiation, growth inhibition or resistance to viral infection. (Manuscript in preparation.)

Benham, F. J., Andrews, P. W., Bronson, D. L., Knowles, B. B. & Harris, H. (1981) Alkaline phosphatase isozymes as possible markers of differentiation in human teratocarcinoma cell lines. *Developmental Biology*, **88**, 279–287.

Carlin, C. R. & Andrews, P. W. (1985) Human embryonal carcinoma cells express low levels of functional receptor for epidermal growth factor. *Experimental Cell Research*, **159**, 17–26.

Damjanov, I. (1983) The pathology of human teratomas. *The Human Teratomas; Experimental and Clinical Biology* (ed. by I. Damjanov, B. B. Knowles and D. Solter), pp. 23–66. Humana Press, Clifton, N.J.

Damjanov, I. & Andrews, P. W. (1983) Ultrastructural differentiation of a clonal human embryonal carcinoma cell line *in vitro*. *Cancer Research*, **43**, 2190–2198.

Damjanov, I., Clark, C. K. & Andrews, P. W. (1984) Cytoskeleton of human embryonal carcinoma cells. *Cell Differentiation*, **15**, 133–139.

Damjanov, I., Fox, N., Knowles, B. B., Solter, D., Lange, P. H. & Fraley, E. E. (1982) Immunohistochemical localization of murine stage-specific embryonic antigens in human testicular germ cell tumours. *American Journal of Pathology*, **108**, 225–230.

Fenderson, B. A., Andrews, P. W., Nudelman, E., Clausen, H. & Hakomori, S.-i. (1986) Core structure switching of glycolipids from globo- to lacto- and ganglio-series during retinoic acid-induced differentiation of TERA-2-derived human embryonal carcinoma cells. (Manuscript in preparation.)

Kannagi, R., Cochran, N. A., Ishigami, F., Hakomori, S.-i., Andrews, P. W., Knowles, B. B. & Solter, D. (1983) Stage-specific embryonic antigens (SSEA-3 and -4) are epitopes of a unique globo-series ganglioside isolated from human teratocarcinoma cells. *The EMBO Journal*, **2**, 2355–2361.

Kannagi, R., Nudelman, E., Levery, S. B. & Hakomori, S.-i. (1982) A series of human erythrocyte glycosphingolipids reacting to the monoclonal antibody directed to a developmentally regulated antigen, SSEA-1. *Journal of Biological Chemistry*, **257**, 14865–14874.

Kleinsmith, L. J. & Pierce, G. B. (1964) Multipotentiality of single embryonal carcinoma cells. *Cancer Research*, **24**, 1544–1551.

Lee, V. M.-Y. & Andrews, P. W. (1986) Differentiation of NTERA-2 clonal human embryonal carcinoma cells into neurons involves the induction of all three neurofilament proteins. *Journal of Neuroscience Research*, **6**, (2), 514–521.

Martin, G. R. (1980) Teratocarcinoma and mammalian embryogenesis. *Science*, **209**, 768–776.

Shevinsky, L. H., Knowles, B. B., Damjanov, I. & Solter, D. (1982) Monoclonal antibody to murine embryos defines a stage-specific embryonic antigen expressed on mouse embryos and human teratocarcinoma cells. *Cell*, **30**, 697–705.

Solter, D. & Damjanov, I. (1979) Teratocarcinoma and the expression of oncodevelopmental genes. *Methods in Cancer Research*, **18**, 277–332.

Solter, D. & Knowles, B. B. (1978) Monoclonal antibody defining a stage-specific mouse embryonic antigen (SSEA-1). *Proceedings of the National Academy of Science of the United States of America*, **75**, 5565–5569.

Thompson, S., Stern, P. L., Webb, M., Walsh, F. S., Engstrom, W., Evans, E. P., Shi, W.-K., Hopkins, B. & Graham, C. F. (1984) Cloned human teratoma cells differentiate into neuron-like cells and other cell types in retinoic acid. *Journal of Cell Science*, **72**, 37–64.

Thurin, J., Herlyn, M., Hindsgaul, O., Strömberg, N., Karlsson, K.-A., Elder, D., Steplewski, Z. & Koprowski, H. (1985) Proton NMR and fast atom bombardment mass spectrometry analysis of the melanoma-associated ganglioside 9-0-acetyl-GD$_3$. *Journal of Biological Chemistry*, **260**, 14556–14563.

Tippett, P., Andrews, P. W., Knowles, B. B., Solter, D. & Goodfellow, P. N. (1986) Red cell antigens P (globoside) and Luke: identification by monoclonal antibodies defining the murine stage-specific embyronic antigens -3 and -4 (SSEA-3 and -4). *Vox Sanguinis* (in press).

Discussion

Holstein I would like to ask you for a description of the histological appearance of cultured cells. We tried to culture testicular tumour cells but only obtained cultures of macrophages.

Andrews When grown at high cell density, the TERA-2 and 2102Ep embryonal carcinoma cells exhibit a similar morphology. They form tightly packed islands of round cells with a large nucleus containing one or few prominent nucleoli, and surrounded by a thin rim of cytoplasm. When grown at low cell density, the cells flatten out and appear to acquire more cytoplasm: within the nuclei, the nucleoli became greater in number and less distinct.

I should point out that it is often difficult to establish tumour cell lines in culture from testicular tumours and in many instances only a culture of fibroblasts is obtained.

Safirstein Is there a difference in drug sensitivity between the different cells based on their expression of surface antigens?

Andrews Together with Dr Oosterhuis we have examined the sensitivity of human EC cells, and also the differentiated derivatives of NTERA-2 cells, in culture to cisplatin. We have compared EC cells with the whole population of differentiated cells but have no information of the differential sensitivity of the various subsets of cells derived from NTERA-2 embryonal carcinoma cells. Our results do show the high sensitivity of EC cells to cisplatin and some changes in sensitivity as they differentiate.

Oosterhuis In general, human and murine embryonal carcinoma cells are more sensitive to cisplatin *in vitro* than their somatically differentiated derivatives by a factor of ×2 to ×4.

Walt What is the origin of the TERA-2 line and what was the histological classification of the primary tumour? Also, what is the DNA content of the cells of the TERA-2 culture?

Andrews TERA-2 was originally derived by Dr Jørgen Fogh from a lung metastasis of a testicular germ cell tumour. The report provided by Dr Fogh states that the histology of the explanted tumour was consistent with embryonal carcinoma; no information was provided concerning the histology of the primary tumour.

We have not measured DNA content directly but have made detailed studies of the karyotype of the TERA-2 cells. The cells are all aneuploid having 57–64 chromosomes, including a number of duplications and translocations; they possess a single X and Y chromosome. Different clones of TERA-2 have similar, but not identical, karyotypes to one another. Among the chromosome abnormalities is a chromosome 12 with a deletion of the tip of the long arm [del(12) (q^{13})].

Niemi Have you stained sections of human testicular tumours with SSEA-antibodies?

Andrews This has been done by Drs Damjanov and Oosterhuis. There is clear evidence that EC cells in clinical material are commonly SSEA-3 and -4 positive and SSEA-1 negative.

Vogelzang Do the clones of 2102E cells also exhibit the chromosomal abnormality on the short arm of the isochromosome 12 (i12p)?

Andrews The TERA-2 clones all contain what we have described as a deletion of the tip of the long arm of chromosome 12 [del(12) (q^{13})], rather than the isochromosome of the short arm (i12p) suggested by others. We have seen a similar chromosome in 2102Ep. The distinction between i(12p) and del(12)(q^{13}) is difficult in chromosome 12, but in any case, either involves loss of some genes from the long arm of 12.

Vogelzang Do the other cell lines in your laboratory contain the i12p marker?

Andrews We have not made a detailed study of the karyotypes of the other cell lines which we maintain.

Cell lines of human germinal cancer

J. CASPER,[1] H.-J. SCHMOLL,[1] U. SCHNAIDT[2] and
C. FONATSCH[3] [1]*Medical University of Hannover, Department of Hematology/Oncology, Konstanty-Gutschowstr., D-3000 Hannover 61, West Germany,* [2]*Pathologisches Institut, Caritas Klinik Rastpfuhl, Rheinstr. 2, D-6600 Saarbrücken, West Germany, and* [3]*Medical University of Lübeck, Institut für Humangenetik, Ratzeburger Allee 160, D-2400 Lübeck, West Germany*

Summary

Three new established human germ cell tumour lines, H 12.1, H 12.5 and H 12.7, are described. Cytogenetic and growth characteristics, morphology, histology, and tumour marker and steroid hormone production *in vitro* and/or *in vivo* revealed properties commonly found in other germ cell tumour lines and in patients with these tumours. *In vitro* oestrone and oestradiol were produced by the H 12 lines and four other lines (833 KE, 1156 Q, 1428 A and 2102 EP) under high and low density (differentiation inducing) conditions. AFP was produced by one line and β-hCG by six of seven lines under low density conditions. The pattern of oestrogen production suggests that these hormones could be useful in AFP and β-hCG negative patients. Differentiated elements of somatic and extraembryonic character, observed in tumours of H 12.1 and H 12.7, underline the value of these lines in the study of differentiation and other germ cell tumour related questions.

Key words. Germ cell tumours, nude mice, tumour marker, steroid hormones.

Introduction

Established cell lines, which provide a continuous source of otherwise limited or unavailable cancer cells, have contributed significantly to our knowledge about cancer. Since the first testicular germ cell tumour lines were described (Fogh & Trempe, 1975), considerable information has been gathered about their properties and behaviour and their similarities to, and differences from, the well-studied mouse teratocarcinoma system (Bronson, Bronson & Fraley, 1983). In this report we describe three new human testicular tumour lines and compare them with other lines, concentrating on tumour marker and steroid hormone production *in vitro* and properties of these lines *in vivo* (nude mouse). Because the role and prognostic significance of gynaecomastia and oestrogen elevations in patients with germ cell tumours is still controversial (Von Eyben, 1978; Tseng *et al.*, 1985) we studied the production of two oestrogenic substances by the cell lines under maintenance and differentiation-inducing culture conditions.

Correspondence: Dr J. Casper, Southwest Foundation for Biomedical Research, P. O. Box 28147, San Antonio, Texas 78284, U.S.A.

Materials and Methods

The lines H 12.1, H 12.5 and H 12.7 were established from a primary testicular germ cell tumour from a 19-year-old patient that was classified histologically as seminoma, embryonal carcinoma, mature teratoma and choriocarcinoma. Elevated levels of AFP, β-hCG, oestrone (E_1) and 17-β oestradiol (E_2) had been measured in serum samples from the patient, but no gynaecomastia was apparent. The tumour specimen was minced, and fragments (H 12.1 and H 12.5) and floating cells (H 12.7) were seeded in 25 cm^2 flasks. Cell lines 833 KE, 1156 Q, 1428 A and 2102 EP were a gift from Drs David L. Bronson and Elwin E. Fraley of the University of Minnesota Medical School, Minneapolis, U.S.A. The properties of these lines were described earlier (Bronson et al., 1980, 1983; Andrews et al., 1980; Wang et al., 1980). All cell lines were maintained and subcultured as described by Bronson et al. (1980). Population doubling times in cultures seeded at different cell densities (split ratios of 1:2 or 1:20) were calculated from growth curves in the exponential phase. For cytogenetic studies, colchicine-treated cultures were prepared and Giemsa banded as described by Fonatsch et al. (1980). For marker measurements in culture supernatant fluids and sera of tumour-bearing mice, an enzyme immunoassay (EIA) for AFP (Enzygnost AFP Behringwerke) and a radioimmunoassay (RIA) for β-hCG (Serono) were used. RIAs for E_1 and E_2 (reagents obtained from BioMérieux, NEN, Steranti and Organon) and an EIA for progesterone (BioLab) were used for culture fluids only. Medium blanks incubated in parallel or serum of non-tumour bearing mice were used as controls. Nude mice (BALBc nu/nu or NMRI nu/nu), obtained from the Institut für Versuchstierzucht of the Medical University of Hannover, were inoculated subcutaneously with 1×10^7 viable cells/mouse. Tumour diameters were measured twice weekly and the tumour volume calculated using the formula of Attia, De Ome & Weiss (1965). Semilogarithmic growth curves were used to determine the tumour-volume doubling time in the exponential growth phase. Tumours were removed after ether anaesthesia and blood was collected from the retroorbital veneplexus. Formalin-fixed tumours were Paraplast-embedded and stained with haematoxylin and eosin.

Results

Three lines, H 12.1, H 12.5 and H 12.7, were established from the same primary germ cell tumour and were maintained in tissue culture for more than 200 passages. Chromosomal analyses in passage 12 (H 12.5) and passage 20 (H 12.1 and H 12.7) revealed a modal number of 55 (range 52–57) for all three lines. Structural and numerical aberrations included changes in chromosome 1 (2×1, 1×1p abnormal) and 7 (2×7/2×7, 1×7p+) and an isochromosome of the short arm of chromosome 12 (i(12p)). A second Y chromosome was found in metaphases of H 12.7.

High-density cultures

When cultured at high density (split ratio 1:2), cells in all H 12 lines displayed the morphology characteristics of embryonal carcinoma cells (Fig. 1; Bronson et al., 1980, 1983; Andrews et al., 1980; Cotte et al., 1982). The median doubling time was 19±7 h (range 12–28 h). Increased levels of E_1 and E_2 were observed in the H 12 lines as well as in 833 KE, 1156 Q, 1428 A and 2102 EP (Table 1). In addition,

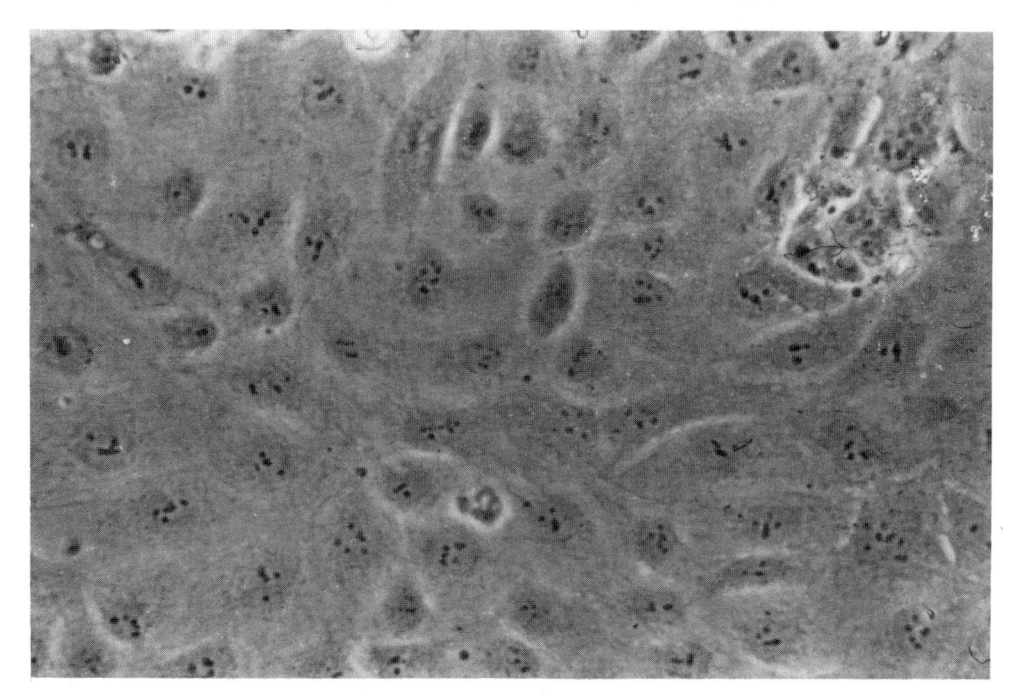

Fig. 1. Embryonal carcinoma cells *in vitro* (H 12.1; ×760).

Table 1. Hormone production of germ cell tumour lines *in vitro*

Line	E$_1$ (pg/ml)	E$_2$ (pg/ml)	Progesterone (ng/ml)	β-hCG (mIU/ml)	AFP (ng/ml)
High density cultures					
833 KE	36 (13–48)*	3 (2–8)	–†	—	—
1156 Q	43 (25–70)	13 (2–19)	–	–	–
1428 A	21 (0–69)	12 (8–15)	–	13 (6–19)	–
2102 EP	6 (0–9)	7 (4–11)	–	–	–
H 12.1	22 (0–55)	16 (0–39)	–	10 (6–12)	–
H 12.5	40 (25–52)	18 (5–32)	–	16 (11–23)	–
H 12.7	14 (0–35)	12 (4–21)	–	16 (9–41)	–
Low-density cultures					
833 KE	355 (221–503)	61 (13–119)	–	–	–
1156 Q	157 (33–324)	150 (17–368)	4 (0–11)	68 (53–85)	18 (7–28)
1428 A	163 (25–391)	379 (61–800)	3 (1–5)	16 (7–20)	–
2102 EP	75 (4–151)	59 (0–202)	1 (0–2)	16 (7–25)	–
H 12.1	148 (62–248)	307 (58–600)	2 (0–5)	161 (17–537)	–
H 12.5	198 (5–396)	315 (7–>800)	2 (0–4)	25 (6–41)	–
H 12.7	514 (53–1041)	849 (50–1803)	18 (2–28)	628 (14–1889)	–

*Median levels and in () range of hormone levels.
†No elevated hormone levels measured.

1428 A and the H 12 lines produced low levels of β-hCG (range 6–41 mIU/ml). No significant levels (Andrews *et al.*, 1980) of AFP or progesterone were detected.

Low-density cultures

At low cell density (split ratio 1:20), a condition that induces differentiation in some human germ cell tumour lines (Bronson et al., 1983; Bronson, Vessella & Fraley, 1984), a variety of cell types were observed. Besides enlarged cells, there were syncytial formations (Fig. 2), fibroblastoid cell types and spindle-shaped cells. These irreversible changes in cell morphology were most obvious in cultures of H 12.7. Tumour-cell doubling time decreased slightly during the first low-density passage of all three H 12 lines (18±4 h, range 14–24 h) and in subsequent passages at the same split ratio, a partial (H 12.1 and H 12.5) or total (H 12.7) growth stoppage was observed. E_1 and E_2 levels increased in cultures of all seven cell lines, reaching the highest levels in H 12.7 (Table 1) with 1041 ng/ml of E_1 (normal <10 ng/ml) and 1803 ng/ml of E_2 (normal <10 ng/ml). Low levels of β-hCG (<100 mIU/ml) were found in culture fluids from 1156 Q, 1428 A, 2102 EP and H 12.5 and high levels in H 12.1 and H 12.7 cultures, reaching a maximum of 1889 mIU/ml (normal <5 mIU/ml). Elevated progesterone levels (>0.5 ng/ml) were measured in cultures of 1156 Q, 1428 A, 2102 EP, H 12.1, H 12.5 and H 12.7, whereas AFP could be detected only in 1156 Q cultures.

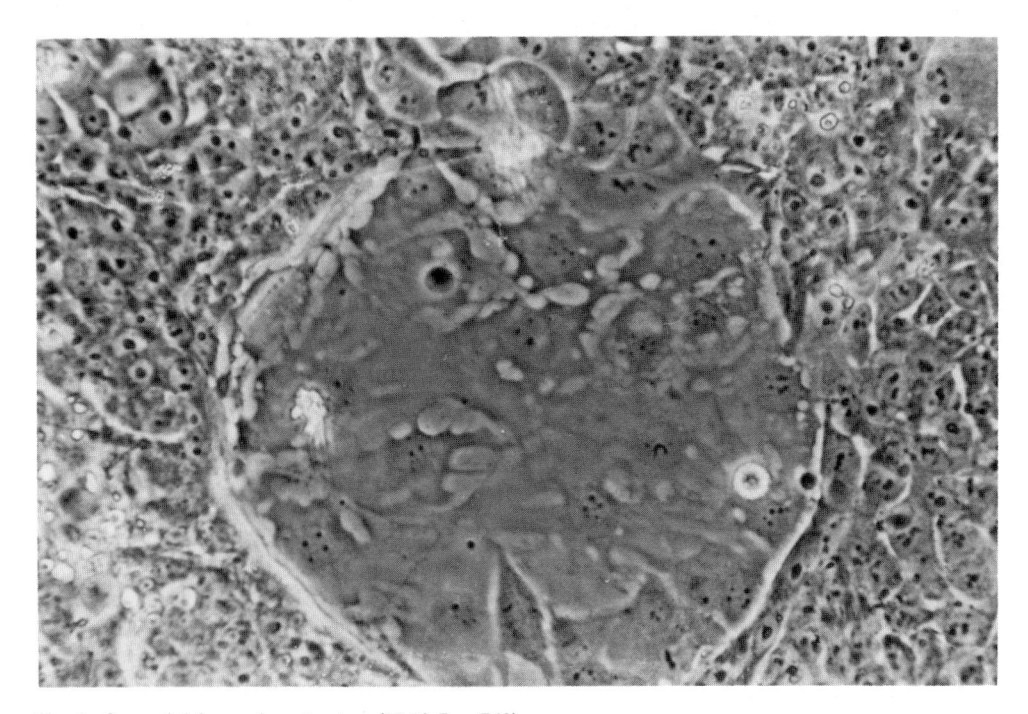

Fig. 2. Syncytial formations *in vitro* (H 12.7; ×760).

Cell lines in nude mice

Tumour take-rates ranged from 0 in 1156 Q to 63% (12/19 animals) in H 12.1. In the exponential growth phase, the mean tumour volume doubling time was 9±4 days (range 4–17 days). Differentiation in tumours (Table 2, Fig. 3) ranged from

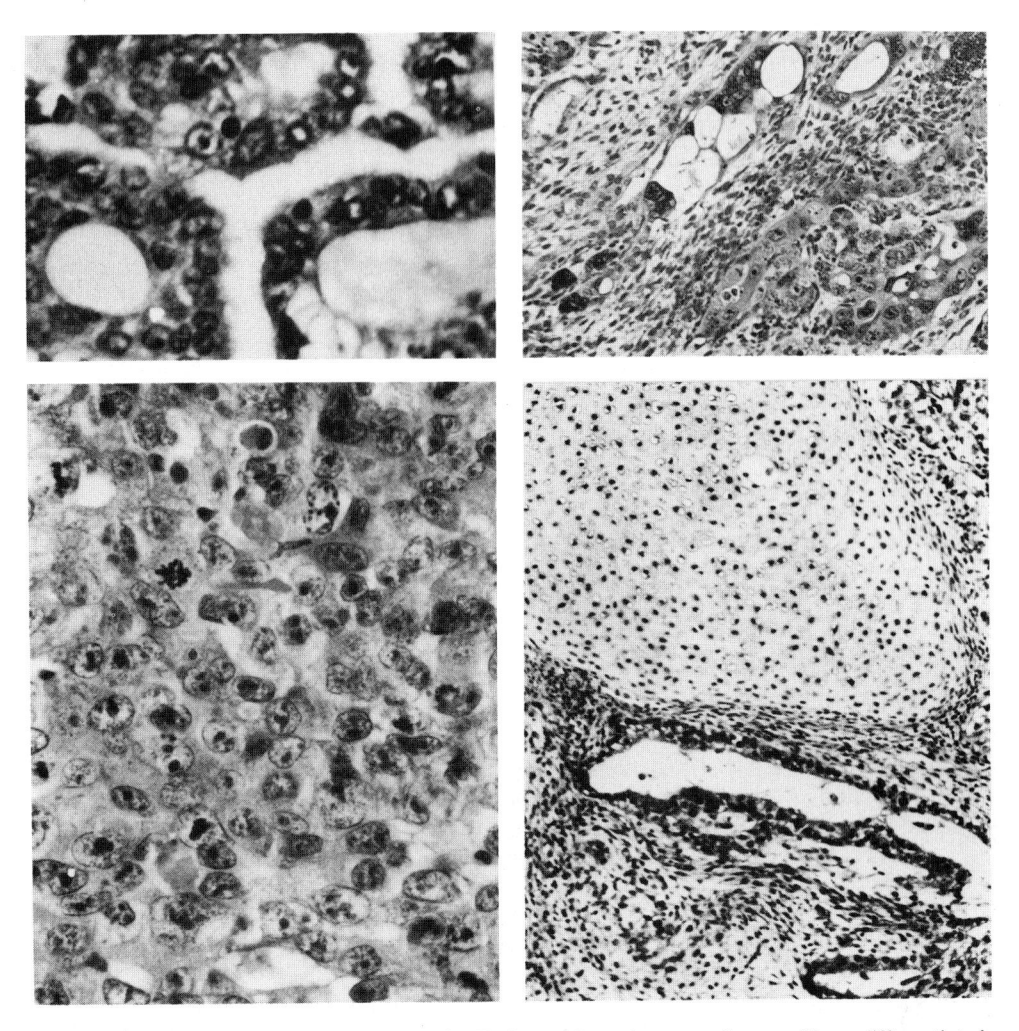

Fig. 3. Tumours in nude mice. Upper left: Embryonal carcinoma, adenopapillary differentiated. H & E, ×230. Lower left: Embryonal carcinoma, undifferentiated. The cells form a solid pattern. H & E, ×230. Upper right: Embryonal carcinoma and syncytiotrophoblastic giant cells. H & E, ×110. Lower right: Embryonal carcinoma and immature teratoma. In the upper section immature cartilage can be seen. H & E, ×110.

undifferentiated embryonal carcinoma (833 KE, 2102 EP and H 12.5) to embryonal carcinoma with teratoma and yolk sac tumour (H 12.7). In addition some tumours of 1428 A, H 12.1 and H 12.7 were accompanied by syncytiotrophoblastic giant cells (STGC). Elevated levels of β-hCG were found in sera of mice bearing all lines except 833 KE at a frequency ranging from 38% (2102 EP) to 100% (1428 A, H 12.7). The lowest levels of β-hCG were produced by 2102 EP cells (maximum 302 mIU/ml) and the highest levels by 1428 A, H 12.1 and H 12.7 cells (maximum 7550 mIU/ml). AFP could be detected in sera of 71–100% of mice bearing all cell lines, reaching 23,230 ng/ml in H 12.7-bearing mice. Only 2102 EP and H 12.1 did not produce elevated AFP levels in all tumour-bearing animals.

Table 2. Germ cell tumour lines in nude mice

Line	Take rate* (%)	Histology†	AFP (ng/ml)	hCG (mIU/ml)
833 KE	1/9 (11)	EC	64	–
1156 Q	0/3	–	–	–
1428 A	6/10 (60)	EC + STGC	1428–3345	>400
2102 EP	20/53 (38)	EC	0–276	0–302
H 12.1	12/19 (63)	EC + STGC + IT	0–>4000	0–6905
H 12.5	1/9 (11)	EC	12	13
H 12.7	19/44 (43)	EC + STGC + IT + YS	340–23230	343–7550

*Number of tumours/number of animals injected.
†EC = embryonal carcinoma; STGC = syncytiotrophoblastic giant cells; YS = yolk sac carcinoma; IT = immature teratoma.

Discussion

The seven lines investigated showed properties commonly found in other germ cell tumour lines and in patients with these tumours, including cytogenetic abnormalities (Wang et al., 1980; Atkin & Baker, 1983), marker production (Bronson et al., 1983, 1984; Vogelzang et al., 1985), growth characteristics (Cotte et al., 1982), and morphology and histology (Bronson et al., 1983, 1984; Andrews et al., 1980). In addition chromosome 7 changes, oestrogen production in vitro and formation of teratoma, STGC and β-hCG and/or AFP in vivo were found. It may be of prognostic significance that E_1 and E_2 are produced in high-density cultures of embryonal carcinoma lines and, in the absence of β-hCG and progesterone elevations, in low-density cultures. This pattern suggests that E_1 and E_2 could serve as markers of elements other than trophoblastic cells (embryonal carcinoma cells?) in AFP- and β-hCG-negative tumours. Progesterone should be ascribed to trophoblastic elements, as suspected by O'Hare et al. (1981), since we have shown production of high levels of both β-hCG and progesterone by our lines, which is similar to the pattern of production of these hormones by a gestational choriocarcinoma line (O'Hare et al., 1981). In the leukaemias seen in patients previously treated for germ cell tumours, changes in chromosome 7 have been a major finding (van Imhoff et al., 1986). The existence of chromosome 7 changes in the H 12 and some other germ cell tumour lines (Fonatsch, personal communication) is an argument for the chemotherapy-independent, teratomatous origin of these malignancies (reviewed by Loehrer, Sledge & Einhorn, 1985). Extensive differentiation of germ-cell tumour lines in vitro has already been shown (Bronson et al., 1984), and in the future we might learn how to direct such differentiation as a new approach for cancer treatment.

Acknowledgements

We thank Mrs E. Seyfert and her team, Department of Endocrinology, Medical University of Hannover, for tumour marker and hormone determinations and Mrs D. Reile and Mrs S. Schumacher for excellent technical assistance.

References

Andrews, P. W., Bronson, D. L., Benham, F., Strickland, S. & Knowles, B. B. (1980) A comparative study of eight cell lines derived from a human testicular teratocarcinoma. *International Journal of Cancer*, **26**, 269–280.

Atkin, N. B. & Baker, M. C. (1983) i(12p): specific chromosomal marker in the seminoma and malignant teratoma of the testis? *Cancer Genetics and Cytogenetics*, **10**, 199–204.

Attia, M. A., De Ome, K. B. & Weiss, D. W. (1965) Immunology of spontaneous mammary carcinomas in mice. II. Resistance to a rapidly and a slowly developing tumor. *Cancer Research*, **25**, 451–457.

Bronson, D. L., Andrews, P. W., Solter, D., Cervenka, J., Lange, P. H. & Fraley, E. E. (1980) Cell line derived from a metastasis of a human testicular germ cell tumor. *Cancer Research*, **40**, 2500–2506.

Bronson, D. L., Bronson, J. G. & Fraley, E. E. (1983) Germ cell tumors of mice and men: The teratocarcinoma models and their clinical implications. *Testis Tumors*, pp. 77–91. Williams & Wilkins, Baltimore.

Bronson, D. L., Vessella, R. L. & Fraley, E. E. (1984) Differentiation potential of human embryonal carcinoma cell lines. *Cell Differentiation*, **15**, 129–132.

Cotte, C., Raghavan, D., McIlhinney, R. A. & Monaghan, P. (1982) Characterization of a new human cell line derived from a xenografted embryonal carcinoma. *In Vitro*, **18**, 739–749.

Edler von Eyben, F. (1978) Biochemical markers in advanced testicular tumors: Serum lactate dehydrogenase, urinary chorionic gonadotropin and total urinary estrogens. *Cancer*, **41**, 648–652.

Fogh, J. & Trempe, G. (1975) New human tumor cell lines. *Human Tumor Cells In Vitro*, pp. 115–159. Plenum Press, New York.

Fonatsch, C., Schaadt, M., Kirchner, H. & Diehl, V. (1980) A possible correlation between the degree of karyotype aberrations and the rate of sister chromatid exchanges in lymphoma lines. *International Journal of Cancer*, **26**, 749–756.

Loehrer, P. J., Sledge, G. W. & Einhorn, L. W. (1985) Heterogeneity among germ cell tumors of the testis. *Seminars in Oncology*, **12**, 304–316.

O'Hare, M. J., Nice, E. C., McIlhinney, R. A. & Capp, M. (1981) Progesterone synthesis, secretion and metabolism by human teratoma-derived cell-lines. *Steroids*, **38**, 719–737.

Tseng, A., Horning, S. J., Freika, F. S., Resser, K. J., Hannigan, J. F. & Torti, F. M. (1985) Gynecomastia in testicular cancer patients. *Cancer*, **56**, 2534–2538.

Van Imhoff, G. W., Sleijfer, D. Th., Breunning, M. H., Anders, G. J. P. A., Mulder, N. H. & Halie, M. R. (1986) Acute nonlymphatic leukemia 5 years after treatment with cisplatin, vinblastine, and bleomycin for disseminated testicular cancer. *Cancer*, **57**, 984–987.

Vogelzang, N. J., Bronson, D. L., Savino, D., Vessella, R. L. & Fraley, E. F. (1985) A human embryonal-yolk sac carcinoma model system in athymic mice. *Cancer*, **55**, 2584–2593.

Wang, N., Trend, B., Bronson, D. L. & Fraley, E. E. (1980) Nonrandom abnormalities in chromosome 1 in human testicular cancers. *Cancer Research*, **40**, 769–802.

Discussion

Niemi You have succeeded well in establishing several permanent cell lines from one human germ cell tumour. Others have been less successful. Did you have any unsuccessful trials as well? Have you tried to culture many tumours and is this the only one with which you have had success? What are the optimal culture conditions for a successful transfer of malignant germ cell to grow in tissue culture?

Casper We have had several unsuccessful trials to establish cell lines in the beginning and now follow the procedures described by Bronson, Clayman & Fraley (in Damjanov, Solter & Knowles (eds) *The Human Teratocarcinomas: Experimental and Clinical Biology*. Humana Press, Clifton, New Jersey, pp. 267–284, 1983) who have established many germ cell tumour lines. They initially cultured tumours directly, but are now using a layer of feeder cells with a success rate of approximately 75% (Bronson *et al.*, 1983). We did not use feeder cells in establishing our lines. Feeder cells, as described by Bronson et al. (1983) are treated with mitomycin C so that the cells themselves may not be as important as perhaps a substance which is provided by these cells.

G. K. Jacobsen Have you been able to establish cell lines from seminoma, or do you know anyone who has?

Casper We have tried to culture several seminomas but at present no seminoma cell lines have been established in our studies, and I do not know of any other group who has successfully established seminoma cell lines *in vitro*.

Niemi Has anybody in the audience managed to culture seminoma cells?

Walt We have tried to culture seminomas in nude mice and in tissue culture, but without success.

Oosterhuis Does anyone have experience with culturing testicular germ cell tumours at a low temperature?

Walt We used a lower temperature of 30°C for the tissue culture studies. This did not appear to help.

Niemi There is no suggestion from the audience that germ cell tumour cultures might survive better if cultured at temperatures lower than 37°C. In my experience, the temperature does not play an essential role in the success of the *in vitro* growth and survival of the germ cell cultures.

Vogelzang Do the lines of H 12 lose the ability to produce AFP and hCG with tissue culture passage number.

In my work in Dr Bronson's Laboratory with cell line 1618 K the production of AFP and hCG declined with cell passage number. Also, nude mice tumours of 1618 K produced higher levels of AFP and hCG in mouse sera than in tissue culture media.

Casper The H12 lines did not lose the ability to produce β-hCG in culture up to passage number 100. Cell line H12.7 may represent an exception because it could not be induced to produce β-hCG by seeding cells at low density in passage numbers greater than 100 although these cells still produce oestrogens. Animals bearing H 12.7 tumour still had elevated serum β-hCG even after passage 100. This finding may direct future attention to the question of what controls tumour marker production.

Oliver You mentioned oestrogen production, but have you looked at human placental lactogen (hPL) production in the hCG-negative tumours? We have had experience with one patient who had gynaecomastia in association with extensive multiple small volume lung metastases involving the whole of both lung fields. This clinical picture is characteristic of choriocarcinoma but there was no measurable hCG although his tumour was hPL-positive.

Casper We have not measured hPL production *in vitro*, but this might be a promising investigation considering that quite a few placental substances are produced by germ cell tumours. You did not measure oestrogen production in your patient, and I wonder if he had elevated serum levels. Perhaps oestrogen should be measured as a tumour marker in testicular tumour patients.

Flow cytometry derived DNA content of the primary lesions of advanced germ cell tumours

G. W. SLEDGE, Jr, J. N. EBLE, B. J. ROTH, B. P. WUHRMAN *and* L. H. EINHORN   *Departments of Medicine and Pathology, Indiana University School of Medicine, and the Richard L. Roudebush VA Medical Center, Indianapolis, Indiana, U.S.A.*

Summary

We currently lack good prognostic indicators for patients with advanced disseminated germ cell tumours (GCT). An analysis of archival tumour samples of forty-nine patients with advanced GCT for flow cytometry derived DNA content suggests an inverse relationship between tumour proliferative activity and patient survival. The great majority of patients with advanced GCT have aneuploid tumour subpopulations. This analysis suggests that the survival of patients with advanced GCT may depend in part on kinetic variables present in the primary tumour.

Key words.   DNA flow cytometry, advanced germ cell tumours of the testis.

Introduction

The past decade has seen remarkable advances in the treatment of patients with disseminated germ cell tumours (GCT) of the testis. Prognosis in these patients depends in large part on the stage of the disease at the time of initial presentation. Patients with minimal to moderate disease in the Indiana University staging system achieved disease free status with cisplatin based chemotherapy in more than 90% of cases (Birch *et al.*, 1986). Patients with advanced disease (defined as advanced pulmonary metastases, palpable abdominal mass plus pulmonary metastases, or hepatic, osseous, or central nervous system metastases) belong to a less favourable prognostic group, with only 58% of patients surviving for more than 3 years (Birch *et al.*, 1986).

Among patients with advanced disease, there are few useful prognostic indices. A sophisticated multivariate analysis performed by the Southeastern Cancer Study Group (Birch *et al.*, 1986) suggested that only the number of elevated tumour markers had any statistical significance as a predictor of outcome in patients with advanced disease.

Recent studies in several human tumours have suggested that flow cytometry derived DNA content may prove useful as a prognostic indicator. Using a relatively new procedure (Hedley *et al.*, 1983) that allows the performance of flow cytometry for DNA content on archival tumour samples, we have evaluated the impact of

---

Correspondence: Dr George W. Sledge, Jr, Department of Medicine, V.A. Medical Center (111 H/O), 1481 W. 10th St., Indianapolis, IN 46202, U.S.A.

DNA content on survival in advanced GCT. Our data suggest that tumour proliferative index correlates with survival in patients with advanced disease.

Materials and Methods

We used a modification of the technique of Hedley *et al.* (1983) to examine the archival tumour samples of patients with advanced GCT. Tumour samples were derived from patients treated with cisplatin based chemotherapy at Indiana University on Southeastern Cancer Study Group trials 78 GU 240 or 82 GU 332. The former study evaluated the role of maintenance therapy in disseminated GCT (Einhorn *et al.*, 1981). The latter compared the use of cisplatin plus bleomycin plus either vinblastine or VP-16 (Williams *et al.*, 1985). Wherever possible, flow cytometry was performed on primary tumour samples (either testis or mediastinum): in two cases where no primary tissue had been obtained analysis was performed on lymph node metastases. Multiple blocks from individual patients were processed for flow cytometric analysis when available.

Multiple 50 micron thick sections were cut from paraffin blocks, deparaffinized, rehydrated through graded alcohol, and enzymatically digested with pepsin. Following digestion, suspensions were centrifuged over a 1 M sucrose solution, then resuspended in Tris HCl buffer containing propidium iodide and ribonuclease. Single cell suspensions were then analysed for DNA content on a Coulter 753 tunable dye laser flow cytometer with excitation at 488 nM.

We looked at the following flow cytometric measurements: ploidy status, DNA index, and proliferative index. DNA index was defined as equalling the peak channel of the aneuploid G_0/G_1 peak divided by the peak channel of the euploid (2N) G_0/G_1 peak. Proliferative indices were calculated in the manner of Naus, Dietch & deVere White (1985), by summing the counts in seven consecutive channels beginning with the third channel before the modal channel of the G_1 peak and in seven consecutive channels beginning with the third channel before the modal channel of the G_2+M peak. The ratio of the latter to the former was then expressed as a decimal fraction. Tumour sections adjacent to the sections cut for flow cytometry were stained with haematoxylin and eosin and reviewed histopathologically.

Results

We analysed the DNA content of forty-nine patients with advanced GCT. As mentioned above, in two of these cases only metastases to lymph nodes were available for analysis. The histopathology of these tumours is described in Table 1. A preliminary analysis revealed no relationship between tumour histopathology and either survival or DNA-related measurements.

We were able to analyse forty-five of forty-nine cases for DNA index and ploidy. All but seven of the tumours analysed contained an aneuploid subpopulation in at least one tumour block. Our experience has been that our ability to detect aneuploidy increased with the number of tumour samples (tissue blocks) analysed for each patient. This suggests both the presence of considerable intratumoral heterogeneity for aneuploidy, and the risk of selection bias if only a single block is analysed. The median DNA index was 1.47 (see Fig. 1). Survival appeared to be independent of ploidy and DNA index in our patients. Though six of seven patients with solely euploid peaks survived for more than 2 years, compared to twenty-one of thirty-eight patients with tumours containing aneuploid peaks, this difference was not statistically significant ($\chi^2 = 1.19$, $P = $ N.S.).

Table 1. Histopathology of patients with advanced GCT

Histological type	Number of patients
Mixed GCT	27
Embryonal carcinoma	9
Seminoma	8
Teratoma (immature)	2
Choriocarcinoma	1
Yolk sac tumour	1
Unclassified	1
Total	49

GCT = germ cell tumour.

We were able to calculate proliferative indices (PI) in forty-three patients. When more than one sample was analysed for PI, we calculated the average PI of the tumour for that patient. Calculations of proliferative indices (PI) suggested an inverse relationship between PI and overall survival (see Fig. 2). With a minimum follow-up period of over 2 years, fifteen of the eighteen patients dying had a PI greater than the mean PI for the entire group. Similarly, nineteen of twenty-five surviving patients had a PI less than the calculated group mean. Comparison of the

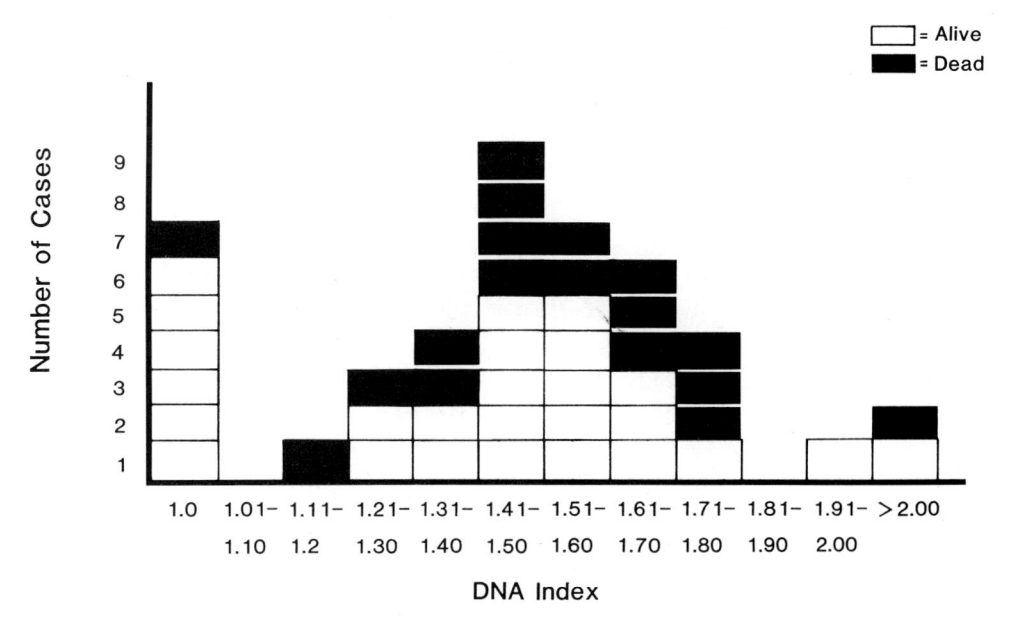

Fig. 1. DNA index and survival status.

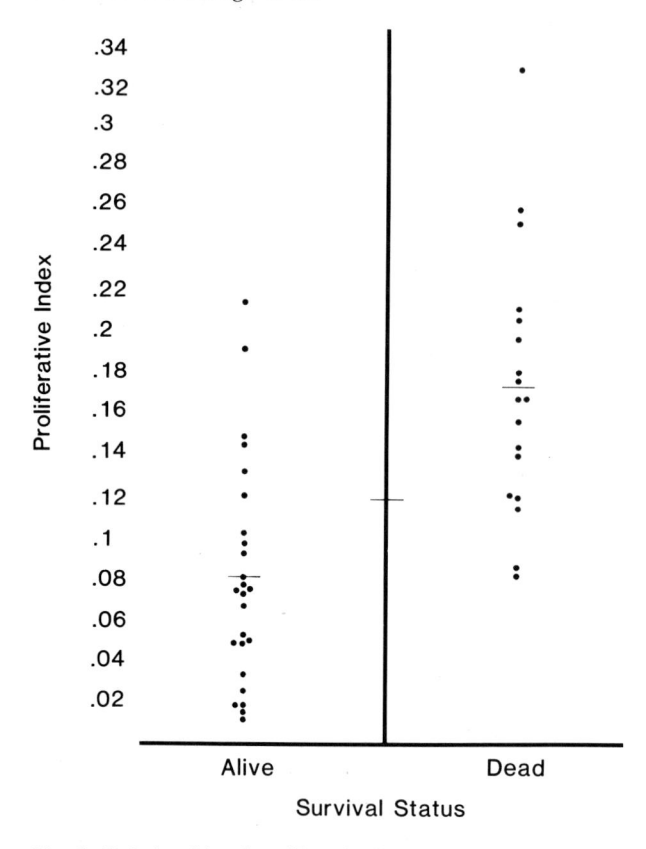

Fig. 2. Relationship of proliferative index to survival.

PI of surviving and dying patients using Student's t-test suggested a highly statistically significant difference ($t = 5.173$, $P < 0.0005$) between the two groups. These data suggest that patients with rapidly dividing tumours (as demonstrated by an increased proliferative index) appear to have impaired overall survival.

Discussion

Our retrospective study of forty-nine patients with advanced GCT suggests that the biology of the primary tumour sample may help determine the outcome of the patient's disease. The great majority (thirty-eight of forty-five) of the advanced GCT analysed contained aneuploid subpopulations. Given the high fraction of aneuploid tumours, aneuploidy is not a useful way to distinguish survivors from nonsurvivors. Similarly, DNA index does not appear to have any prognostic importance.

While our population size is too small to perform a sophisticated multivariate analysis, univariate analysis suggests that patients whose primary tumours contain a rapidly dividing subset (as indicated by an elevated proliferative index) have impaired survival.

This observation might have useful clinical implications. The volume of metastatic disease in patients with disseminated germ cell tumours clearly is prognostically important. However, 'advanced' disease is quite heterogenous both clinically and pathologically. The ability to segregate patients with 'advanced' disease from patients with less biologically aggressive disease, if confirmed in prospective studies, might allow the latter to be spared overly aggressive chemotherapy.

References

Birch, R., Williams, S., Cone, A., Einhorn, L., Roark, P., Turner, S. & Greco, E. A. (1986) Prognostic factors for favorable outcome in disseminated germ cell tumors. *Journal of Clinical Oncology*, **4**, 400–407.

Einhorn, L. H., Wiliams, S. D., Troner, M., *et al.* (1981) The role of maintenance therapy in disseminated testicular cancer. *New England Journal of Medicine*, **305**, 727–731.

Hedley, D. W., Friedlander, M. I., Taylor, J. W., Rugg, G. A. & Musgrove, E. A. (1983) Methods for analysis of cellular DNA content of paraffin-embedded pathological material using flow cytometry. *Journal of Histochemistry and Cytochemistry*, **31**, 1333–1338.

Naus, G. J., Deitch, A. D. & DeVere White, R. (1985) Predictive value of flow cytometric DNA content analysis of paraffin-embedded tissue in renal cell carcinoma. *Laboratory Investigation*, **52**, 47A.

Williams, S., Einhorn, L., Greco, A., Birch, R. & Irwin, L. (1985) Disseminated germ cell tumors: a comparison of cisplatin plus bleomycin plus either vinblastine (PVB) or VP-16 (BEP). *Proceedings of the American Society of Clinical Oncology*, **4**, 100.

Discussion

Oosterhuis In our material, we found no seminoma nor nonseminoma which was purely diploid among approximately 40 adult patients. However, among the nine infantile yolk sac tumours (orchidoblastomas) we found three diploid tumours. The details of these tumours and the median DNA indices are shown in the table:

Tumour histology	Number of patients	Mean age (years)	Clinical stage I	Clinical stage II	Clinical stage III	Median DNA indices
Orchidoblastoma	9	1.2	8	0	1	1.92
Seminoma	14	31	10	2	2	1.67
nonseminoma (adult)	23	28.7	8	4	11	1.39*

* The DNA index was not influenced by stage of tumour.

Sledge It is likely that the seven tumours which we called euploid in our analysis were not euploid in a strict cytogenetic sense for several reasons.

1 The resolving capacity of flow cytometry at its best is probably not adequate to pick up tumours that vary only minimally from a normal karyotype. For example, if the only karyotypic alteration was the presence of isochromosome 12p, I strongly suspect that no standard flow cytometer would have the requisite sensitivity to determine its presence.

2 We arbitrarily called any tumour with a single G 0/1 peak a euploid tumour. It is possible that a tumour containing entirely aneuploid cells and no (or very few) euploid cells may have a single G 0/1 peak and erroneously be called euploid. Investigations in other tumour systems such as breast and ovarian cancers have suggested that this is uncommon because nearly all tumours contain euploid host vascular and stromal tissue. All our material is archival and therefore our tissues do not contain an internal euploid standard which would allow us to distinguish an

aneuploid peak. Fresh tumour samples analysed for DNA content frequently have normal tissue available for a standard euploid peak.

3 Finally, our experience with the Hedley technique is that the proportion of tumours which we would label as being aneuploid increases with the number of tumour blocks analysed. This suggests the real possibility of selection bias in our 'euploid' tumours. Had we analysed more blocks from these tumours, we might have found more aneuploidy.

In my opinion the critical point that we should deduce from this analysis is that aneuploidy is common and euploidy (however defined) is rare whether analysed by flow cytometry or cytogenetically.

Oosterhuis I think that it is possible for seminoma to progress to nonseminoma in association with loss of chromosomes, because the DNA index of nonseminomas is significantly lower than the DNA index of seminomas.

Niemi The paper showed that ploidy does not correlate with prognosis and our discussion indicates that diploid seminoma cells do not exist. I feel that from a prognostic point of view it does not matter whether or not true diploid seminoma cells exist.

Rustin Could the difference in survival between patients who have tumours of low and high proliferative index be due to a greater proportion of the high proliferative index patients dying very early from bleeding brain metastases, respiratory failure, etc., rather than later from drug resistance? What is the cause of death in your high proliferative index patients?

Sledge I do not think your suggestion is the best explanation for our findings. The great majority of patients dying in our study do so some time after the time of initial presentation to our centre. Our clinical experience with brain metastases is that the prognosis in this group is determined by the response of the systemic disease to chemotherapy. Furthermore, a patient dying with respiratory failure may be said to have *de facto* resistance to cisplatin-based chemotherapy because most germ cell tumours respond rapidly to chemotherapy. The group of patients we studied experienced no obvious drug-related deaths.

Ultrastructure of syncytiotrophoblast-like cells in seminomas of the testis

M. SEHESTED[1] and GRETE K. JACOBSEN[2]
Departments of Pathology, [1]Herlev and [2]Gentofte Hospitals, Denmark

Summary

An ultrastructural examination of five syncytiotrophoblast-like cells (STLC) from three otherwise pure seminomas was performed. All five STLC demonstrated ultrastructural features identical to those of normal syncytiotrophoblastic cells. The STLC were surrounded by sinusoidal spaces and cells whose ultrastructure was compatible with that of seminoma cells, though the presence of cytotrophoblastic cells cannot be excluded with certainty. We conclude that (1) STLC in seminomas are indeed syncytiotrophoblastic and (2) their genesis remains an enigma.

Key words. Ultrastructure, syncytiotrophoblast-like cells, seminoma.

Introduction

Syncytiotrophoblast-like cells (STLC) have been reported to occur in 7–20% of otherwise pure seminomas of the testis (Bosman *et al.*, 1980; Jacobsen & Jacobsen, 1983; von Hochstetter *et al.*, 1985). In addition to a light microscopical (LM) similarity to normal syncytiotrophoblast, STLC also share functional properties with normal syncytiotrophoblast as STLC produce placental proteins such as hCG, SP1 and hPL (Bosman *et al.*, 1980; Heyderman & Neville, 1976; Heyderman, 1978; Jacobsen, Jacobsen & Clausen, 1981). Normal syncytiotrophoblast is considered to be derived from cytotrophoblast. However, cytotrophoblast has not been observed by LM in connection with STLC. The ultrastructure of STLC in seminomas has not, to our knowledge, previously been reported and the aim of the present study was therefore to investigate the ultrastructure of STLC together with the surrounding cells in order to answer the following questions: (1) is the ultrastructure of STLC compatible with syncytiotrophoblast? and (2) do the cells surrounding STLC resemble cytotrophoblast or seminoma cells?

Materials and Methods

During the period 1979–83 fresh tumour tissue was obtained for electron microscopy (EM) from all testicular tumours operated on at Herlev Hospital. The material included eighteen pure seminomas. The tumour tissue was immediately

Correspondence: Maxwell Sehested, Department of Pathology, KAS Herlev, DK-2730 Herlev, Denmark.

Grigor Some of your giant cells look as if they may be showing early embryogenesis as if they had been derived from totipotential cells. Do you think these giant cells are derived from seminoma and may be potential precursors of nonseminoma? In other words, do these cells represent a transition between seminoma and nonseminoma?

Sehested It is not possible to decide whether STLCs are derived from cytotrophoblast which has since disappeared, or directly from seminoma cells. I would expect that STLCs are end-stage cells.

Walt Do you know where the β-hCG is localized within the hCG-positive STLC?

Sehested A definitive answer would require immunocytochemistry at the electron microscopic level. However, I would expect β-hCG cells to be located in the numerous dilated rER cisternae.

Proliferation of human testicular tumours

H. M. RABES *Institute of Pathology, University of Munich, Munich, Federal Republic of Germany*

Summary

Whole tumour perfusion with radioactive DNA precursors reveals that proliferation of human testicular tumours differs widely depending on type and stage of development. In seminomas a homogeneous distribution of proliferating cells at early stages is followed by a shift of the growth fraction to the periphery at advanced stage. Embryonal carcinomas show a chessboard-like pattern of proliferating fractions with high ^{3}H-thymidine labelling indices and short t_{pot}. In mature teratomas proliferation is low. It increases in immature teratocarcinomas. Lack of proliferation is observed in β-hCG-positive syncytiotrophoblastic cells of choriocarcinomas, the growth fraction being limited to the cytotrophoblastic compartment.

Key words. Cell proliferation, DNA synthesis, heterogeneity, autoradiography, growth compartments, testicular tumour.

Introduction

Malignant transformation and tumour development go along with aberrations from the normal pattern of cell proliferation. Attempts have been made to analyse proliferation kinetics in a large variety of human tumours (Malaise, Chavaudra & Tubiana, 1973; Steel, 1977; Rabes, 1984). However, not much is known about the proliferation kinetics of human testicular tumours. Mitotic counts have been performed aimed at differentiating anaplastic and classical seminomas (von Hochstetter, 1981), but the modern quantitative techniques to determine cell proliferation

Table 1. ^{3}H-thymidine labelling indices in small fragments of human testicular tumours incubated for 1 h in ^{3}H-thymidine-containing medium (data from Silvestrini *et al.*, 1985)

Tumour type	No.	^{3}H-TdR labelling index (%)	Range
Seminoma	34	13.9	0.8–31.5
Embryonal carcinoma	46	42.0	1.6–77.3
Endodermal sinus tumour	4	29.6	17.0–30.5
Teratoma immature	5	8.5	0.1–25.0
Teratoma mature	7	1.4	0.01–7.0

Correspondence: Prof. Dr. med. H. M. Rabes, Institute of Pathology, University of Munich, Thalkirchner Str. 36, D-8000 Munich 2, F.R.G.

by means of tritiated thymidine-autoradiography have rarely been applied to testicular tumours. The only relevant study was published recently by Silvestrini et al. (1981, 1985) who determined the ^{3}H-thymidine (^{3}H-TdR) labelling index after incubation in vitro of small pieces of tumours from a total of 108 patients. Depending on the tumour type striking differences were observed (Table 1). Mature teratomas showed a very low labelling index which increased with the loss of differentiated function. The highest rate of proliferation was reported for embryonal carcinomas, seminomas showing a medium fraction of ^{3}H-TdR-labelled cells. Information on the changing rate of cell proliferation during tumour development, correlations between differentiation and cell kinetics, potential population doubling time and intratumoural heterogeneity of the proliferative pattern is still lacking.

The present study deals with some of these questions. To avoid artefactual estimation of growth rates from small and possibly non-representative pieces of tumour tissue, a new method was applied which takes advantage of the fact that an orchidectomy specimen can be perfused via the testicular artery under simulated physiological conditions (Rattenhuber et al., 1978; Rabes et al., 1985).

Methods

During surgery, a cannula is inserted into the testicular artery and, after the tumour-bearing testis has been resected, the specimen is connected via this vessel with a perfusion apparatus and perfused with dextran-diluted oxygenated blood in an open-perfusion system under controlled temperature and pressure. The details have been reported elsewhere (Rabes et al., 1985). After an equilibration period, tritiated thymidine is added to the perfusate for 20–30 min, followed by a 60–90 min isotope-free perfusion and a subsequent labelling with ^{14}C-TdR for 45 min. By this procedure it was possible to determine in autoradiographs not only the TdR labelling index, but also to calculate the duration of DNA synthesis (t_s) (Hilscher & Maurer, 1962; Wimber & Quastler, 1963) and to derive the potential population doubling time (t_{pot}) (Steel, 1977). Furthermore, ^{14}C-TdR labelled whole tumour autoradiographs of the perfused orchidectomy preparations provided a unique opportunity to get an insight into the heterogeneity of proliferating versus quiescent compartments in tumours as already shown for renal adenocarcinomas (Rabes et al., 1979).

Results

The kinetic analysis of clinically manifest seminomas of twelve patients revealed a mean TdR labelling index of 11.6 ± 1.4 and a DNA synthesis time of 15.9 ± 2.0 h. The calculated potential population doubling time t_{pot} was 4.7 ± 0.7 days (Table 2). It is remarkable that the variation of the labelling indices and of the calculated values for t_s and t_{pot} is high. For subpopulations of extreme labelling indices and short t_s values, doubling times of less than 1 day can be derived. This suggests that the human seminoma is a rapidly proliferating tumour, but it does not develop homogeneously in all subcompartments. In early stages of development, in the seminoma-in-situ, atypical spermatogonia with a high ^{3}H-TdR labelling index are found in the tubular lumina (Fig. 1). This homogeneity of proliferation is preserved

Table 2. Kinetics of perfused human seminomas (data from Rabes et al., 1985)

Patient's age (yr)	Tumour type	Diameter (cm)	Labelling index (%) Mean	Labelling index (%) Maximum	DNA synthesis time (t_s) (h)	Population doubling time (t_{pot}) (days) Mean	Population doubling time (t_{pot}) (days) Minimum
29	Typical seminoma	2.5	14.5	34.2	–	–	–
23	Typical seminoma	2.0	15.2	41.4	–	–	–
38	Seminoma and embryonal carcinoma	2.5	10.0	16.1	–	–	–
29	Typical seminoma	1.5	3.2	18.0	–	–	–
31	Typical seminoma	3.3	20.2	25.1	16.6	2.6	2.1
34	Typical seminoma	2.5	8.9	36.3	8.8	3.1	0.8
38	Typical seminoma	3.0	15.3	38.1	22.4	4.6	1.9
39	Typical seminoma	3.0	7.1	29.6	18.3	8.1	1.9
29	Anaplastic seminoma	2.5	16.6	41.9	10.0	1.9	0.8
26	Typical seminoma	3.5	6.6	21.9	10.1	4.8	1.4
34	Typical seminoma	5.0	11.2	36.4	21.3	5.9	1.8
37	Seminoma and teratoma	5.0	10.0	20.6	20.0	6.3	3.0
Mean ± SE			11.6 ± 1.4	30.0 ± 2.7	15.9 ± 2.0	4.7 ± 0.7	1.7 ± 0.3

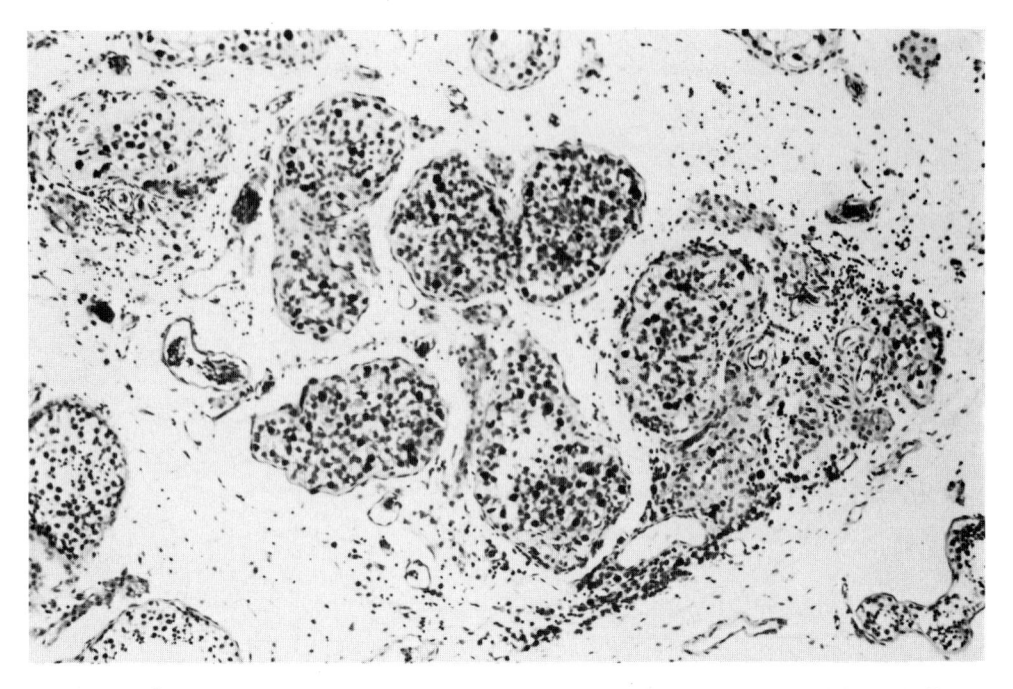

Fig. 1. High ^{3}H-TdR labelling index of atypical spermatogonia irregularly arranged in seminiferous tubules, 'seminoma-in-situ'. Autoradiograph, H & E, ×125. (From Rabes et al., 1985; reprinted by permission of Cancer, Philadelphia.)

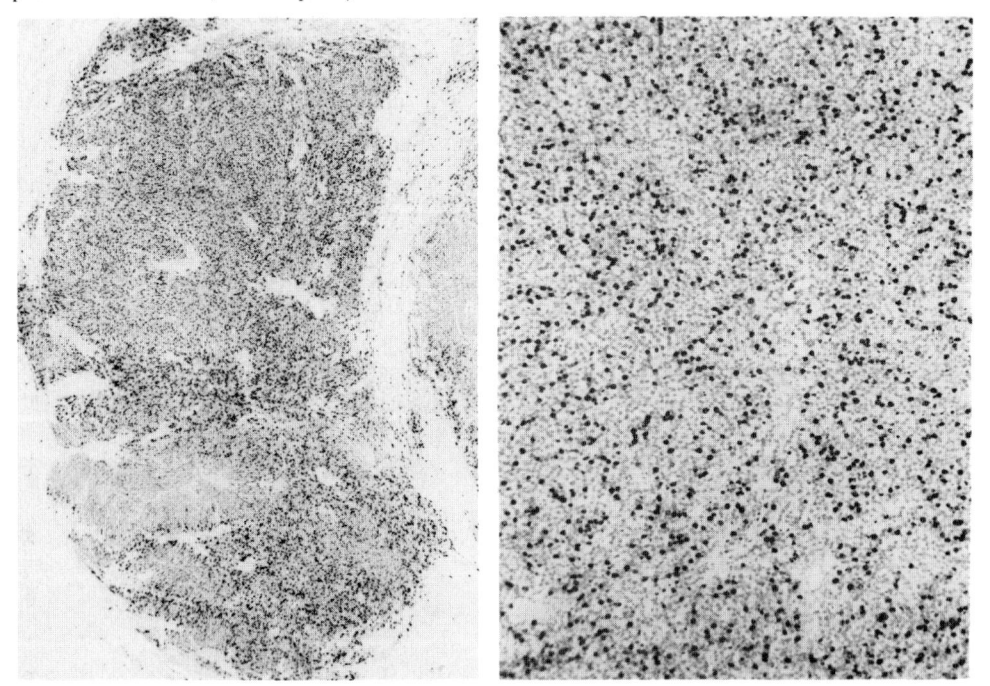

Fig. 2. Autoradiographs of rapidly proliferating subpopulations of a human seminoma after perfusion with tritiated thymidine. H & E. left, ×20; right, ×95. (From Rabes et al., 1985; reprinted by permission of Cancer, Philadelphia.)

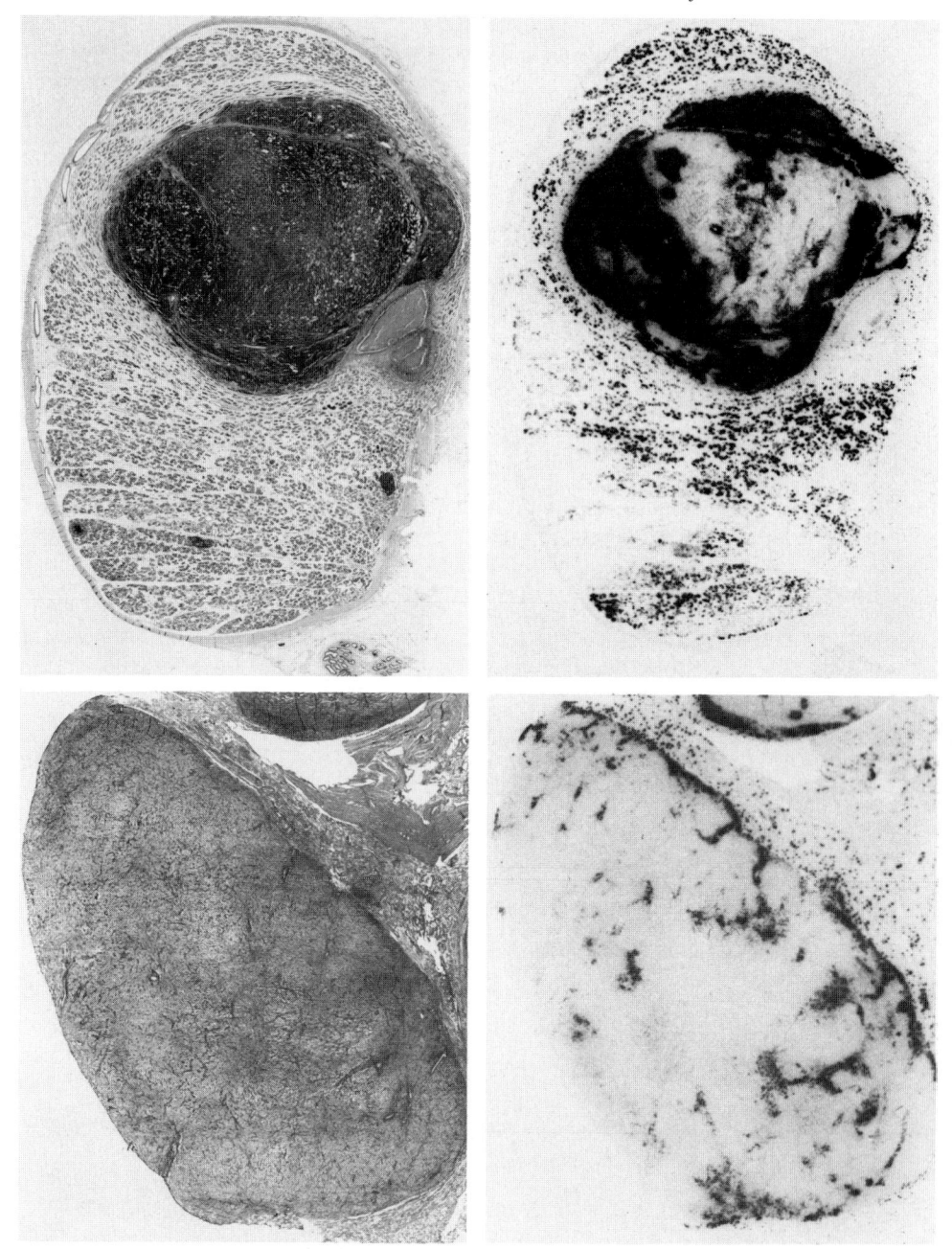

Fig. 3(a, b). Sections of seminoma-bearing testes after vascular perfusion with tritiated and ^{14}C-thymidine. Left, H & E stained sections; right, X-ray film autoradiographs after an exposure for 3 months. (a) Top, large seminoma with actively proliferating subpopulations at the tumour periphery; lack of DNA synthesizing cells in central parts of the tumour. In normal testicular tissue the majority of tubules contains labelled cells (×8). (b) Bottom, advanced stage of seminoma development. The proliferative fraction is limited to the boundary of the tumour and to small patches of tumour tissue immediately adjacent to the vascularization (×12). (From Rabes *et al.*, 1985; reprinted by permission of *Cancer*, Philadelphia.)

for a short time with an almost even distribution of DNA synthesizing cells in small seminoma foci. However, with increasing nodule size, the proliferative compartments become focally spread in the developing tumour, the invasive boundary showing the most pronounced rate of proliferation with labelling indices exceeding 40%. This ranks the human seminoma among the most rapidly proliferating human tumours (Fig. 2). However, this appears to be a typical transit stage, and large fractions of the tumour proceed into a stage of proliferative quiescence as the tumour enlarges, located mainly in the central parts of the tumour nodule. In the macroautoradiographs of a typical seminoma of this stage the central part contains a nonproliferative section with a broad frame of most rapidly proliferated tumour cells (Fig. 3a). Autoradiographs of ^{14}C-TdR-perfused whole tumours reveal that at a more advanced stage the growth compartment is confined to the peripheral parts of the tumour and to those intratumoural populations which are located immediately adjacent to the vascular tree (Fig. 3b). There is a steep decrease of labelling indices with increasing distance from the vascular pole. Finally, in big seminoma nodules an approximate steady-state develops, when the growing compartment becomes limited to the boundary at the well-vascularized normal testicular tissue, and to the vicinity of blood vessels. The other parts of the nodule are in G_o, but morphologically mostly intact. The rapidly proliferating and invasive fractions of this tumour may take the lead in the development of additional tumour nodules, and, in particular, in metastatic spread of tumour cells.

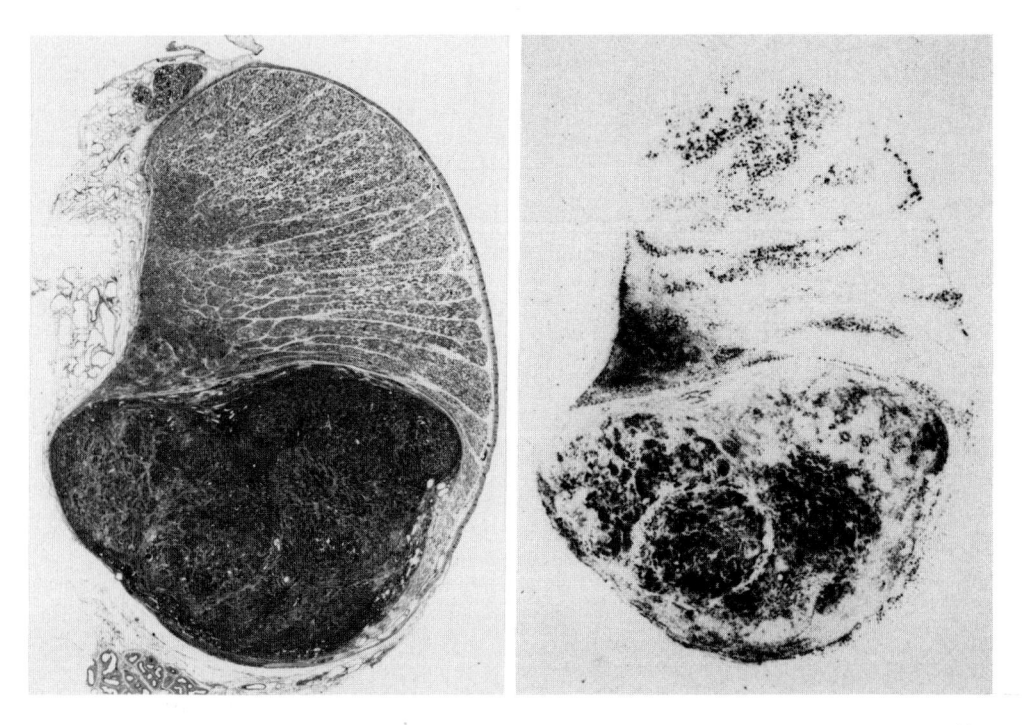

Fig. 4. Section of an embryonal carcinoma of the testis after vascular perfusion with tritiated and ^{14}C-thymidine. Left, H & E stained section; right, unstained autoradiograph on X-ray film after contact exposure for 3 months. (×8).

The relative homogeneous growth pattern and the changes from proliferating into quiescent compartments with increasing tumour size is in contrast to the embryonal carcinoma of the testis. The macroautoradiograph of an embryonal carcinoma at an advanced stage reveals that the growing compartments are spread over the entire tumour mass comprising not only the invasive boundary, but also the centre of the tumour (Fig. 4). The chessboard-like pattern of TdR-labelling evolves from the close association of highly proliferating and necrotic areas of the tumour (Rabes et al., 1978). A quantitative evaluation of the labelling indices in a cross-section of an embryonal carcinoma gives an impression of the extreme rates of proliferation with labelling indices of more than 80% surrounded by tumour necrosis (Fig. 5). With a DNA synthesis time of 16.9 h, the potential doubling time in the areas of maximum proliferation is about 0.6 days. As the clinical doubling time of this tumour is longer, an extremely high cell loss factor has to be assumed (Steel, 1967).

Much less impressive is the proliferation rate in the human mature teratoma. The whole-tumour autoradiograph shows only a few patches of ^{14}C-TdR labelling. The ^{3}H-TdR indices in a cross-section of this tumour are low, scattered irregularly depending on differentiation and histological structure (Fig. 6). They increase in immature teratomas (Fig. 6).

Choriocarcinomas perfused *in vitro* for the determination of the growth compartments release β-hCG in a considerable amount during the perfusion indicating

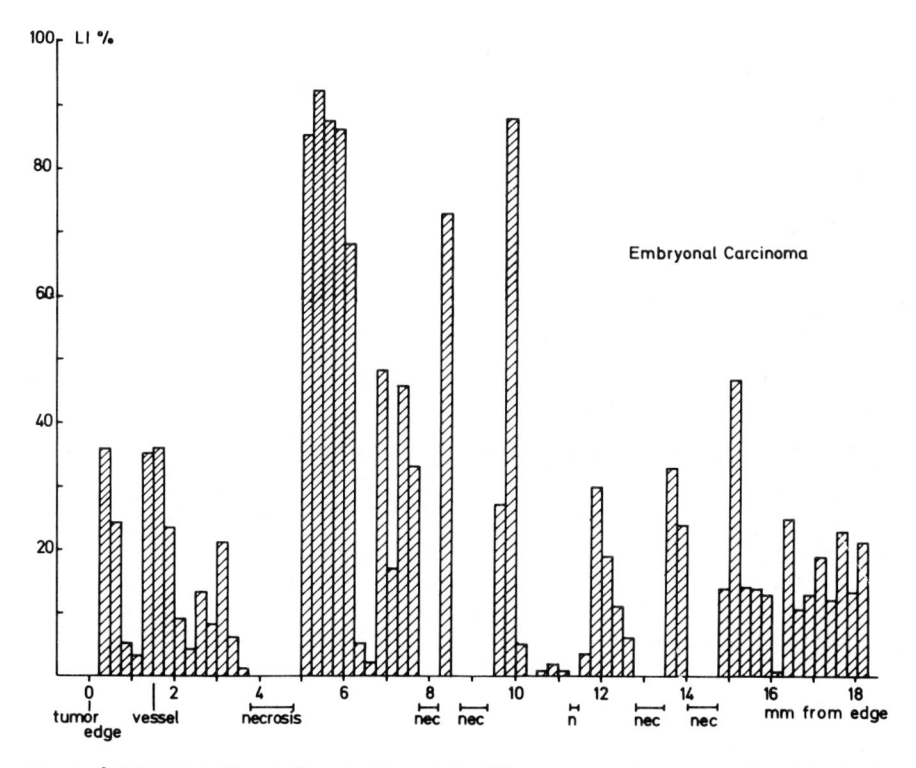

Fig. 5. ^{3}H-TdR labelling indices (ordinates) in different parts of a cross-section (abscissa) of a human embryonal carcinoma after vascular perfusion with tritiated thymidine.

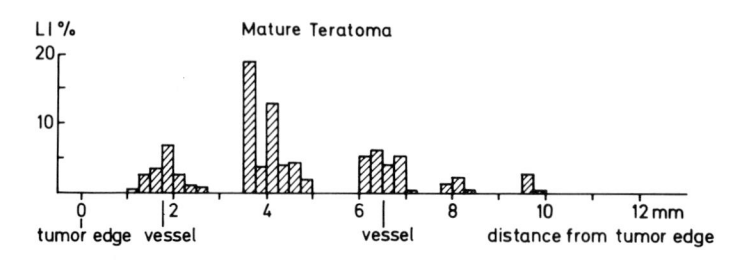

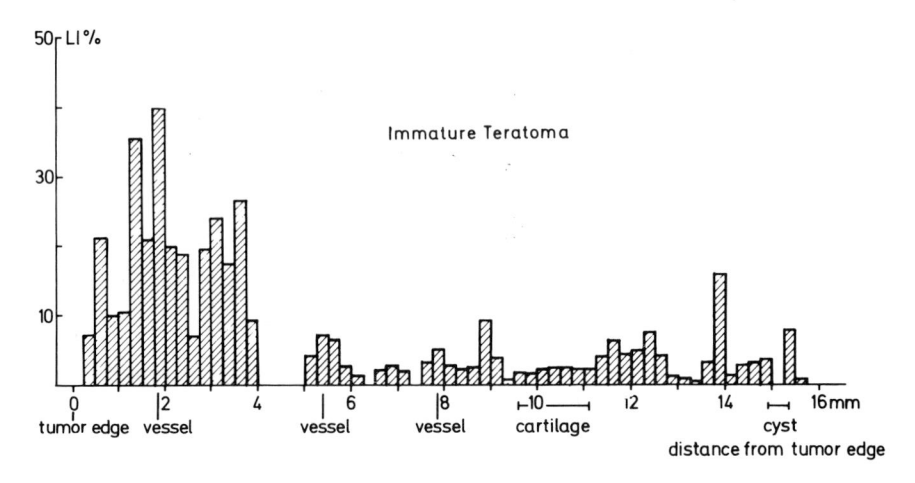

Fig. 6. ^{3}H-TdR labelling indices (ordinates) in a cross-section (abscissa) of a mature (top) and an immature teratoma (bottom) after vascular perfusion with tritiated thymidine.

a preserved physiological state under the conditions of perfusion after orchidectomy (Rattenhuber et al., 1978). The whole-tumour autoradiograph after ^{14}C-TdR exposure is characterized by large areas of necrosis which occupy most of the tumour mass.

However, the preserved tumour tissue located mainly at the periphery shows a burst of proliferative activity (Fig. 7). A closer view reveals an interesting distinction of three compartments. DNA labelling is almost exclusively seen in the cytotrophoblastic cell compartment. In contrast, β-hCG positive syncytiotrophoblastic cell nuclei remain unlabelled suggesting that the highly functionally active cell syncytium is not capable of any more proliferation. The third compartment, the necrotic areas, represents the final destiny of these actively proliferating and β-hCG producing cells. Again in this tumour the potential doubling time of the proliferating fraction is very short, but because of the high cell loss, the clinical doubling time is much larger.

By combination of immunohistochemical alphafetoprotein staining and thymidine autoradiography the proliferation pattern of AFP-positive endodermal sinus tumours can also be evaluated. In contrast to the β-hCG-positive syncytiotrophoblastic cells, AFP-positive functionally active cells were found to be labelled suggesting that in this tumour there is no strict separation into a functional and a proliferating compartment.

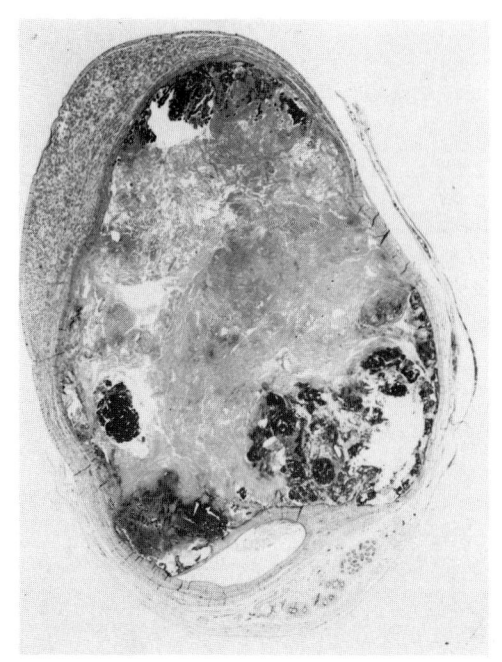

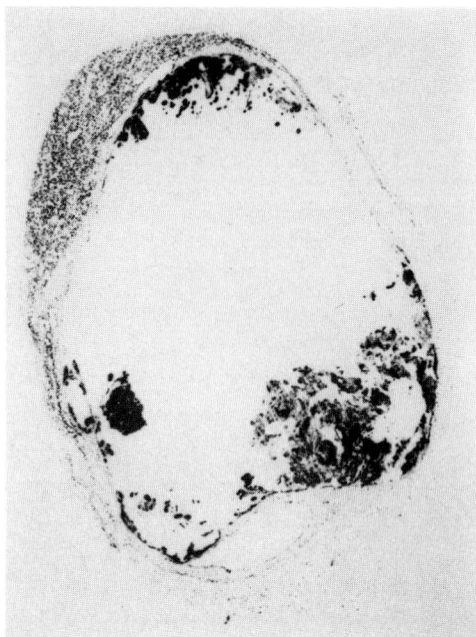

Fig. 7. Section of a choriocarcinoma of the testis after vascular perfusion with tritiated and ^{14}C-thymidine. Left, H & E stained section; right, unstained autoradiograph on X-ray film after contact exposure for 3 months. (×8).

Among the other nonseminomatous testicular tumours investigated by whole-tumour perfusion the Leydig cell tumour is characterized by a very slow rate of proliferation. The labelling index remains below 1%.

It is concluded that the proliferation pattern is highly different among seminomas and nonseminomatous germ cell tumours. Every tumour type shows its own peculiar growth characteristics which should be taken into account when evaluating the clinical tumour doubling time, estimating prognosis and planning therapeutic strategies.

Acknowledgements
Supported by grants from Wilhelm Sander-Stiftung and Dr Mildred Scheel-Stiftung für Krebsforschung.

References
Hilscher, W. & Maurer, W. (1962) Autoradiographische Bestimmung der Dauer der DNS-Verdopplung und ihres zeitlichen Verlaufs bei Spermatogonien der Ratte durch Doppelmarkierung mit C-14- und H-3-Thymidin. *Naturwissenschaften*, **49**, 352.

Hochstetter, A. R. von (1981) Mitotic count in seminomas — an unreliable criterion for distinguishing between classical and anaplastic types. *Virchows Archiv* [A], **390**, 63–69.

Malaise, E. P., Chavaudra, N. R. & Tubiana, M. (1973) The relationship between growth rate, labelling index and histological type of solid human tumors. *European Journal of Cancer*, **9**, 305–321.

Rabes, H. M., Rattenhuber, U., Carl, P., Staehler, G. & Löhrs, U. (1978) Wachstumskompartimente in menschlichen Hodentumoren. *Verhandlungen der Deutschen Gesellschaft für Urologie*, **30**, 296–298.

Rabes, H. M., Carl, P., Meister, P. & Rattenhuber, U. (1979) Analysis of proliferative compartments in human tumors. I. Renal adenocarcinoma. *Cancer*, **44**, 799–813.

Rabes, H. M. (1984) Die Zellkinetik in Metastasen. *Verhandlungen der Deutschen Gesellschaft für Pathologie*, **68**, 147–163.

Rabes, H. M., Schmeller, N., Hartmann, A., Rattenhuber, U., Carl, P. & Staehler, G. (1985) Analysis of proliferative compartments in human tumors. II. Seminoma. *Cancer*, **55**, 1758–1769.

Rattenhuber, U., Rabes, H. M., Carl, P. & Staehler, G. (1978) Methode der postoperativen Hodenperfusion zur Bestimmung zellkinetischer und metabolischer Parameter. *Verhandlungen der Deutschen Gesellschaft für Urologie*, **30**, 293–295.

Silvestrini, R., Pilotti, S. & Costa, A. (1981) Kinetic characterization of germ cell testicular tumors. (Abstract). UICC Conference on Clinical Oncology, Lausanne, Book of Abstracts, p. 115.

Silvestrini, R., Costa, A., Pilotti, S. & Pizzocaro, G. (1985) Cell kinetics in human germ cell tumors of the testis. *Testicular Cancer and Other Tumors of the Genitourinary Tract* (ed. by M. Pavone-Macaluso, P. H. Smith and M. A. Bagshow), pp. 55–62. Plenum Publishing Corporation, New York.

Steel, G. G. (1967) Cell loss as a factor in the growth rate of human tumours. *European Journal of Cancer*, **3**, 381–387.

Steel, G. G. (1977) *Growth Kinetics of Tumours*. Clarendon Press, Oxford.

Wimber, D. E. & Quastler, H. (1963) A ^{14}C- and ^{3}H-thymidine double labelling technique in the study of cell proliferation in tradescantia root tips. *Experimental Cell Research*, **30**, 8–22.

Discussion

Niemi In the normal testicular tissue around the tumour, do you see DNA replication in Sertoli cells or Leydig cells?

Rabes Very infrequently, in tumour-bearing testes, replication of Leydig cells has been seen. Obviously, we did not include perfectly normal testes in our perfusion programme.

Niemi Therefore the doctrine that Leydig cells do not divide is open to debate. Most histologists argue that mature Sertoli cells never undergo mitotic division.

Oliver In your patient with embryonal carcinoma did you study the residual seminiferous tubules and compare the labelling index of the *in-situ* carcinoma cells with that of the established tumour?

Rabes The labelling index was greatly increased in the foci of proliferating atypical intratubular spermatogonia, which we considered to be CIS, in comparison with the normal tubules.

This, however, was slightly lower than the labelling index of the primary seminoma, although there was very little difference between the seminoma-in-situ and the tumour cells at the periphery of the main tumour. Similar data for embryonal carcinoma are not yet available.

Skakkebæk A word of caution. I do not believe that your term 'seminoma-in-situ' is identical with our term 'carcinoma-in-situ'. It appeared to me that your slides showed the intratubular spread of seminoma. I think that in such cases the tumour cells have destroyed the tight junctions between the Sertoli cells which subsequently disappear from the tubules.

Rabes Intratubular spread of seminoma is certainly the most probable explanation of such foci of replicating intratubular atypical spermatogonia when they are found in close proximity to a seminoma. However, when a similar focus of intratubular cells is located at a considerable distance from the seminoma, as in our case, we tend to interpret this as a separate entity.

According to your definition, the foci which I showed in the autoradiograph should not be called CIS because there were no Sertoli cells present alongside the atypical spermatogonia.

Safirstein Did you quantify the degree of unscheduled DNA synthesis in your autoradiographs, and was this increased in comparison to normal?

Rabes Altering the exposure time of autoradiography can give quantitative results by differentiating the nuclei which have incorporated different amounts of tritiated thymidine thereby producing a different grain count in the autoradiographs. Therefore, unscheduled DNA synthesis (UDS) can, in principle, be determined apart from replicate DNA synthesis by counting the number of grains overlying the nuclei in the autoradiograph. Replicate DNA synthesis invariably shows a much higher silver grain number than unscheduled DNA synthesis because of the greater rate of precursor incorporation during DNA replication. However, we have not yet undertaken this time-consuming quantitative UDS determination in our autoradiographs.

A complication of the system if it is to be used for quantitation is that cells have low incorporation of thymidine and therefore a low grain count at the start and at the end of DNA synthesis, and this may be mistaken for UDS.

Ikinger Did you also perform angiography or microangiography in your tumours? I think it would be most interesting to compare your findings with the vascular pattern of the tumour.

Rabes We performed an angiographic evaluation of some of the testicular tumours which were used for perfusion experiments. This revealed that cell proliferation appears to be dependent on adequate vascularization. This can be demonstrated clearly in seminomas where proliferating cells have a homogeneous distribution provided there is sufficient vascularization. As the nodules increase in size, regular blood circulation in the central parts becomes deficient and the cells leave the proliferative compartment. Vascularization is preserved at the periphery, and there the cells actively proliferate. Apparently seminomas do not possess an angiogenic potential sufficient to induce vascularization of the inner parts of the nodules.

In advanced embryonal carcinomas, vascularization is also inadequate but cells do not enter G_O. Instead they become necrotic at a distance of greater than 200–250 µm from the supporting vessel. A quantitative determination of endothelial cell proliferation, using combined factor VIII immunohistochemistry and autoradiography, is in progress.

Comparative antitumour activity of cisplatin and two new cisplatin-analogues JM8 and JM9 in human testicular carcinoma xenografts

A. HARSTRICK, J. CASPER* and H.-J. SCHMOLL

Medizinische Hochschule Hannover, Abt. Hämatologie und Onkologie, Hannover, and *Southwest Foundation for Biomedical Research, San Antonio, Texas, U.S.A.

Summary

The comparative antitumour activity of cisplatin, JM8 and JM9 was tested using a panel of different heterotransplanted human testicular tumour cell lines. All drugs were applied at equitoxic doses in a 5 day schedule. In the two cisplatin sensitive cell lines 2102 EP and H 12.1 both analogues were inferior to cisplatin. No significant therapeutic effect was achieved with any of the three drugs in the cisplatin resistant line H 23.1. Thus JM8 and JM9 seem to be less active in cisplatin sensitive tumours and seem to be of no advantage in the case of cisplatin resistance.

Key words. Testicular tumour xenografts, platinum analogues.

Introduction

Most patients with nonseminomatous germ cell cancer can be cured by modern chemotherapy protocols. All combination chemotherapy protocols currently in use for the treatment of this tumour type are based on the very high antitumour activity of cisplatin (Einhorn & Donohue, 1977; Peckham et al., 1983; Seeber et al., 1979; Vugrin et al., 1981). Nevertheless, this excellent activity of cisplatin is accompanied by several severe toxic side effects especially nephrotoxicity (De Conti et al., 1973). Thus great efforts have been undertaken to develop platinum analogues which possess the high antineoplastic activity of cisplatin but are devoid of its severe nephrotoxicity. The two new cisplatin analogues JM8 and JM9 have recently been introduced into clinical phase I and II trials. Myelosuppression is the dose-limiting side effect while nephrotoxicity poses no problems in the use of both agents (Evans et al., 1983; Smith et al., 1985; Peckham, Harwich & Hendry, 1985; Creaven et al., 1983; Bramwell et al., 1985). Since most patients with testicular carcinomas respond to modern chemotherapy protocols, only few enter clinical phase II studies and thus it is difficult to assess the antitumour activity of new drugs in this tumour type.

Human tumours heterotransplanted in nude mice provide a good model for tumour orientated evaluation of antineoplastic drugs (Osieka et al., 1977; Steel, Courtenay & Peckham, 1983; Shorthouse et al., 1980). The aim of this study was to

Correspondence: Dr A. Harstrick, Medizinische Hochschule Hannover, Abt. Hämatologie und Onkologie, Postf. 610180, D-3000, Hannover 61, F.R.G.

investigate the cytotoxic activity of the new platinum analogues JM8 and JM9 in comparison to cisplatin using a panel of different human testicular carcinoma cell lines and thus to assess the possible role that both drugs may play in the treatment of nonseminomatous germ cell cancer.

Material and Methods

Mice

All experiments were performed using 6–8-week-old male congenitally athymic (nu/nu) nude mice of the NMRI strain obtained from the central breeding laboratory of the Medical School of Hannover. The mice were kept under pathogen free conditions and given free amounts of sterilized food and water.

Tumour cell lines

The three established human testicular carcinoma cell lines 2102 EP (kindly provided by Dr D. Bronson, San Antonio), H 12.1 and H 23.1 were used. The histological characteristics and pattern of tumour marker production after heterotransplantation on nude mice is shown in Table 1.

Table 1. Histology and tumour marker production

Cell line	Histology	AFP	β-hCG
2102 EP	EC	+	(+)
H 12.1	EC; STGC; IT	++	++
H 23.1	EC	−	−

EC: embryonal carcinoma; STGC: syncytiotrophoblastic giant cells; IT: immature teratoma

After transplantation on nude mice the tumour doubling times of the three lines are 15.5, 9.8 and 9.5 days, respectively.

Subcutaneously growing tumours were produced by subcutaneous injection of 1×10^7 cells per mouse into the right flank. The take rates are 55–75% for 2102 EP, 70–90% for H 12.1 and 95–100% for H 23.1.

Drugs

Cisplatin, JM8 and JM9 were obtained from Bristol Myers (Bristol-Arzneimittel, Rathenaustrasse 31, 6078 Neu-Isenburg and Bristol Myers Company, Pharmaceutical Research and Development Div., Brussels, Belgium). Cisplatin was dissolved in 0.9% NaCl, JM8 and JM9 were dissolved in sterile water. Equitoxic doses (approximate LD 20) determined in separate experiments in our laboratory were used. Doses and schedules are shown in Table 2.

Treatment and evaluation of therapeutic effect

Tumours were measured in 5-day intervals by a caliper and tumour volumes were calculated by the formula $a^2 \times b \times 0.5$ (a = width, b = length). Treatment was started when the majority of the tumours had reached a volume of 1–2 cm^3 (range

Table 2

Drug	Dose (mg/kg/day)	Schedule
Cisplatin	3	days 1–5 i.p.*
JM8	12.5	days 1–5 i.p.*
JM9	4.3	days 1–5 i.p.*

*Intraperitoneal.

of tumours included in the studies: 0.5–3.5 cm^3). Mice were stratified according to their tumour volume and divided into treatment groups of five or six animals. Five mice per line served as untreated controls. For each measurement point the relative tumour volumes were calculated by the formula V_t/V_0 (V_t = tumour volume at any given time; V_0 = tumour volume at initiation of treatment). The mean relative tumour volumes of each treatment group were used to construct growth curves. A

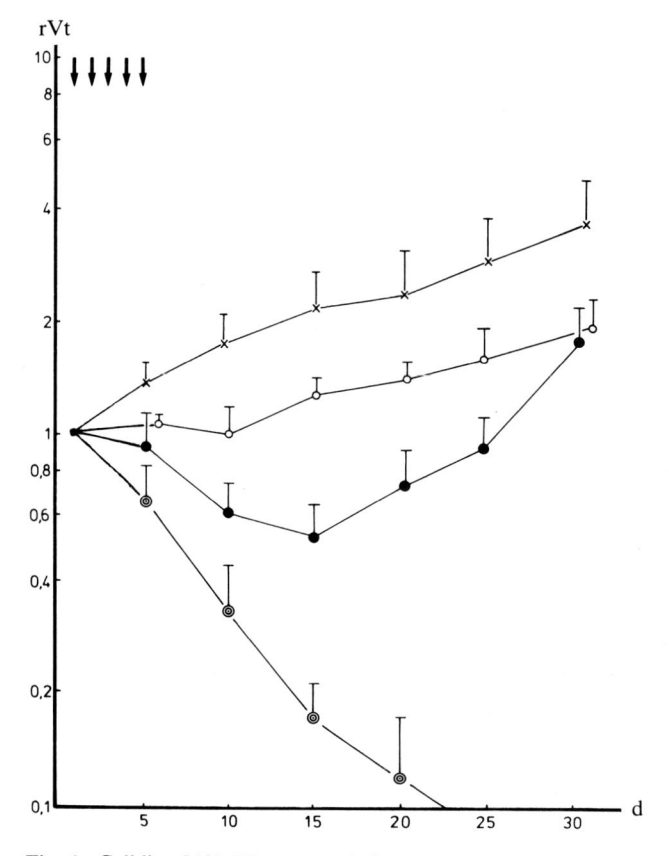

Fig. 1. Cell line 2102 EP; mean relative tumour volume (+ SD). The differences in antitumour activity between cisplatin and JM8 and between cisplatin and JM9 determined 30 days after initiation of treatment are statistically significant ($P < 0.01$).

In Figs. 1–3: abscissa: d = days after initiation of treatment; ordinate: rVt = relative tumour volume; ×—×, untreated control; ⊚—⊚, cisplatin; ●—●, JM8; ○—○, JM9; ↓, drug administration.

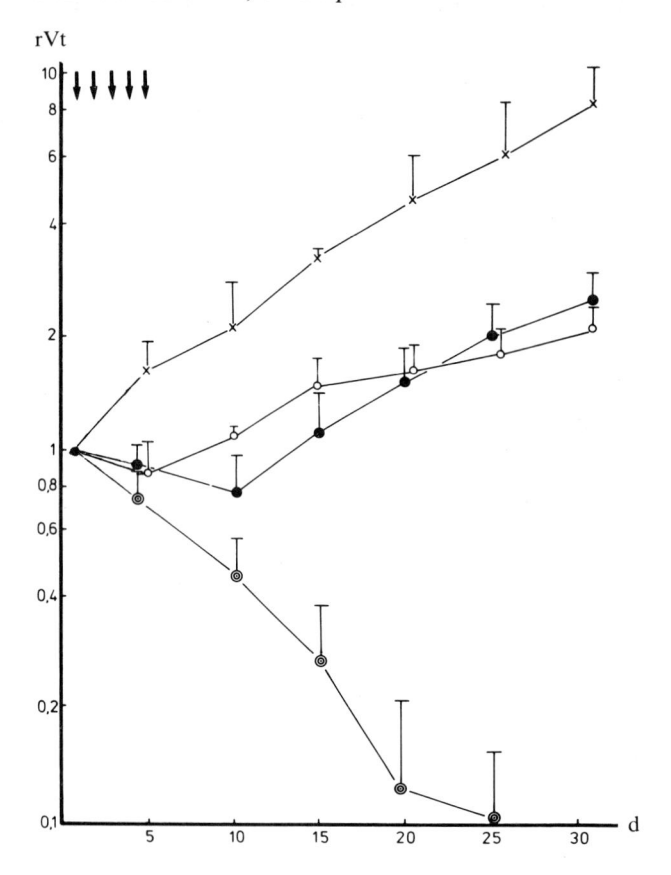

Fig. 2. Cell line H 12.1; mean relative tumour volume (+ SD). The differences in antitumour activity between cisplatin and JM8 and between cisplatin and JM9 determined 30 days after initiation of treatment are statistically significant ($P < 0.01$).

final assessment of antitumour activity was done 30 days after initiation of treatment. Differences in antitumour activity of cisplatin, JM8 and JM9 were analysed statistically by analysis of variance.

Results

The comparative activity of cisplatin, JM8 and JM9 against the two cisplatin-sensitive cell lines H 12.1 and 2102 EP is shown in Figs. 1 and 2. In both cell lines cisplatin produces a significant reduction of tumour volume and achieves complete disappearance of visible tumour in nearly half of the mice. The antitumour activities of JM8 and JM9 are much weaker in both lines. Treatment with JM8 results in an initial reduction of tumour volume which is followed by a rapid proliferation of all tumours while JM9 only achieves a moderate retardation of tumour growth.

The effects of the three agents against the cisplatin resistant line H 23.1 are shown in Fig. 3. None of the drugs are able to achieve a reduction of tumour volume. Only a slight retardation of tumour growth is produced by all three drugs in this cisplatin resistant cell line.

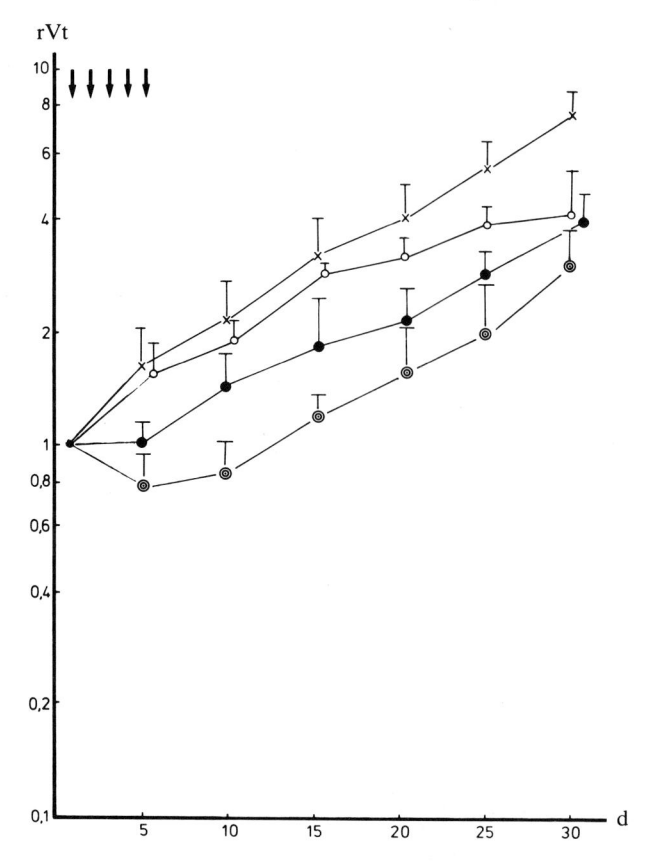

Fig. 3. Cell line H 23.1; mean relative tumour volume (+ SD). The differences in antitumour activity between cisplatin and JM8 and cisplatin and JM9 determined 30 days after initiation of treatment are statistically not significant ($P > 0.05$).

Discussion

Nonseminomatous germ cell cancers can be taken as a model for a curable malignant disease. All modern chemotherapy protocols are based on the outstanding activity of cisplatin in this tumour type (Einhorn & Donohue, 1977; Peckham *et al.*, 1983; Seeber *et al.*, 1979; Vugrin *et al.*, 1981). Nevertheless the high antineoplastic activity of cisplatin is biased by several severe toxic side effects including nephro- and ototoxicity (De Conti *et al.*, 1973) and peripheral neuropathy (Von Hoff, Reichert & Cuneo, 1979). Thus the development of new platinum components with the same antitumour activity but reduced toxicity would be of great advantage. JM8 and JM9 are two new platinum analogues which have recently been introduced into clinical studies. First experiences with these agents show some promising antitumour activity of both drugs which are devoid of the severe nephrotoxic effects observed after cisplatin treatment (Evans *et al.*, 1983; Smith *et al.*, 1985; Peckham *et al.*, 1985; Creaven *et al.*, 1983; Bramwell *et al.*, 1985). The aim of this study was to evaluate the antitumour activity of both drugs against a panel of heterotransplanted human germ cell cancer lines. Since most of the testicular carcinomas which have not previously been treated with cisplatin can be considered to be sensitive to this drug (Rozencweig et al., 1977), the two cisplatin sensitive lines 2102 EP and H 12.1 provide a good test system to assess the activity of JM8 and JM9 in nonpretreated testicular carcinomas. In both lines the antitumour activity of JM8 and JM9 is significantly lower than that of cisplatin when given at equitoxic doses. In contrast, xenografts originated from line H 23.1 are nearly resistant to cisplatin and thus can be taken as a model to evaluate antitumour activity of new drugs in the case of cisplatin resistance. As can be seen from Fig. 3, neither JM8 nor JM9 showed a significant therapeutic effect.

Thus both analogues seem to be inferior to cisplatin in the treatment of testicular carcinoma. Nevertheless much more work, involving additional cell lines and altered ways of drug administration, is necessary until a final assessment of the antitumour activity of JM8 and JM9 in testicular tumours can be made.

References

Bramwell, V. H. C., Crowther, D., O'Malley, S., Swindell, R., Johnson, R., Cooper, E. H., Thatcher, N. & Howell, A. (1985) Activity of JM9 in advanced ovarian cancer: A phase I–II trial. *Cancer Treatment Reports*, **69**, 409–416.

Creaven, P. J., Madajewicz, S., Pendyala, L., Mittelman, A., Pontes, E., Spaulding, M., Arbuck, S. & Solomon, J. (1983) Phase I clinical trial of cis-dichloro-transdihydroxy-isopropylamine platinum (IV) (CHIP). *Cancer Treatment Reports*, **67**, 795–800.

De Conti, R. C., Toftness, B. R., Lange, R. C. & Creasey, W. S. (1973) Clinical and pharmacological studies with cis-diamminedichloroplatinum (II). *Cancer Research*, **33**, 1310–1315.

Einhorn, L. H. & Donohue, J. P. (1977) Cisdiamminedichloroplatinum, vinblastin and bleomycin combination chemotherapy in disseminated testicular cancer. *Annals of Internal Medicine*, **87**, 293–298.

Evans, B. D., Raja, K. S., Calvert, A. H., Harland, S. J. & Wiltshaw, E. (1983) Phase II study of JM8, a new platinum analog in advanced ovarian carcinoma. *Cancer Treatment Reports*, **67**, 997–1000.

Osieka, R., Houchens, D. P., Goldin, A. & Johnson, R. K. (1977) Chemotherapy of human colon cancer xenografts in athymic nude mice. *Cancer*, **40**, 2640–2650.

Peckham, M. J., Barret, A., Liew, K. H., Horwich, A., Robinson, B., Dobbs, H. J., McElwain, T. J. & Hendry, W. F. (1983) The treatment of metastatic germ cell testicular tumours with bleomycin, etoposide and cisplatin (BEP). *British Journal of Cancer*, **47**, 613–619.

Peckham, M. J., Harwich, A. & Hendry, W. F. (1985) Advanced seminoma: Treatment with cisplatinum based combination chemotherapy or carboplatin (JM8). *British Journal of Cancer*, **52**, 7–15.

Rozencweig, M. D., von Hoff, D. D., Slavik, M. & Muggia, F. M. (1977) Cis-diamminedichloroplatinum (II) – A new anticancer drug. *Annals of Internal Medicine*, **86**, 803–812.

Seeber, S., Schilcher, R. B., Meier, C. R. & Schmidt, C. G. (1979) Sequential combination chemotherapy with velban-bleomycin and adriamycin-cisplatin in stage III testicular teratomas. *Proceedings of American Association for Cancer Research*, **20**, 282.

Shorthouse, A. J., Peckham, M. J., Smyth, J. F. & Steel, G. G. (1980) The therapeutic response of bronchial carcinoma xenografts: A direct patient–xenograft comparison. *British Journal of Cancer*, **41** (Suppl. IV), 142–145.

Smith, I. E., Harland, S. J., Robinson, B. A., Evans, B. D., Goodhart, C. C., Calvert, A. H., Yarnold, I., Glees, J. P., Baker, J. & Ford, H. J. (1985) Carboplatin: a very active new cisplatin analog in the treatment of small cell lung cancer. *Cancer Treatment Reports*, **69**, 43–46.

Steel, G. G., Courtenay, V. D. & Peckham, M. J. (1983) The response to chemotherapy of a variety of human tumour xenografts. *British Journal of Cancer*, **47**, 1–13.

Von Hoff, D. D., Reichert, C. M. & Cuneo, R. (1979) Demyelination of peripheral nerves associated with cisdiamminedichloroplatinum (II) therapy. *Proceedings of American Association for Cancer Research*, **20**, 91.

Vugrin, D., Whitmore, W. F., Sogani, P. C., Bains, M., Hen, H. & Golbey, R. (1981) Combined chemotherapy and surgery in treatment of advanced germ cell tumor. *Cancer*, **47**, 2228–2232.

Discussion

Niemi I was not quite clear what you meant by 'xenografts'. Did you graft tumour tissue or tumour cells grown *in vitro*?

Harstrick I think there is some confusion concerning the use of the term 'xenograft'.
 In all our experiments we used only a suspension of tumour cells grown *in vitro*. Injection of this into nude mice produces subcutaneously growing tumours. In our experience, this method gives rise to a more homogeneous population of tumours compared to transplantation of solid tumour pieces. Such solid pieces often consist of variable amounts of differentiated elements, undifferentiated elements and zones of necrosis.

Vogelzang What were the doses of JM8, JM9 and cisplatin which you used?

Harstrick We used

cisplatin	3 mg/kg/day
JM8	12.5 mg/kg/day
JM9	4.3 mg/kg/day

all for 5 days.

Safirstein Have you explored the reasons why the cell lines are resistant to JM8 and JM9 whereas they are sensitive to cisplatin?

Harstrick No. We have not investigated drug distribution, drug uptake, nor action of the drug at the subcellular level and thus we are not able to explain the observed differences as yet.

Andrews Do you have any comparable data on the cytotoxicity of these compounds on the same cells *in vitro*?

Harstrick No. We have not performed *in vitro* tests of the activity of the three drugs.

Schmoll Your results appear to be contradictory to the data from Professor Peckham's group. They report that JM8 is much better at treating xenografted tumours in mice compared to the data which you presented from the Hannover group.

Harstrick To my knowledge, Peckham has only investigated one testicular tumour xenograft regarding its sensitivity to JM8. It is perhaps possible that he has by chance used a tumour which is very sensitive to JM8. Nevertheless, I think that it is necessary to include more testicular xenografts in order to resolve our contradictory findings.

Oliver The Peckham data will be presented in a subsequent paper (Brada & Peckham, submitted).

The spermatocytic seminoma: views on pathogenesis

J. MÜLLER,[1] N. E. SKAKKEBÆK[1,2] and
M. CONSTANCE PARKINSON[3]   [1]*Laboratory of Reproductive Biology Y, Rigshospitalet, Copenhagen, Denmark,* [2]*University Department of Paediatrics, Hvidovre Hospital, Copenhagen, Denmark, and* [3]*Department of Histopathology, St Peter's Hospitals, London, U.K.*

Summary

The spermatocytic seminoma has clinical and histological characteristics which differ from those of other germ cell tumours of the testis. Classical seminomas and teratomas are believed to originate from intratubular carcinoma-in-situ (CIS), which is almost invariably found adjacent to these neoplasms. In addition, DNA analysis of these tumours and the surrounding CIS has shown both to have an aneuploid distribution. In order to throw light on the origin of the spermatocytic seminoma, we have examined the testicular tissue adjacent to fifteen spermatocytic seminomas for the presence of CIS and assessed the DNA content of the tumour cells densitometrically. In twelve specimens seminiferous tubules were present adjacent to the tumour, and in none of these cases was CIS seen. Nuclear DNA measurements were possible in eleven tumours and in five cases the distribution was diploid, in three cases tetraploid, and only in three cases aneuploid. Therefore, we suggest that the spermatocytic seminoma has a different cell of origin from that of other germ cell tumours of the testis.

Key words.   Spermatocytic seminoma, densitometry, DNA.

Introduction

The spermatocytic seminoma (Figs. 1a, 1b), a rare testicular germ cell tumour, was first described by Masson (1946). In contrast to classical seminoma, the spermatocytic neoplasm usually occurs in patients over 45 years of age, it is not seen in sites other than the testis, and has only been described in the normally descended organ. It rarely metastasizes and is not found in association with teratoma as a component of mixed germ cell tumours (Talerman, 1986). Masson (1946) suggested that the spermatocytic seminoma was composed of cells resembling spermatogonia and primary spermatocytes, constituting a distinct type of testicular germ cell tumour. Nevertheless, the spermatocytic seminoma is still regarded as a subgroup of the seminomas (Mostofi, 1980; Talerman, 1986), and Talerman, Fu & Okagaki (1984) concluded on the basis of ultrastructural and microspectrophotometric investigations that the spermatocytic seminoma is a better differentiated variant of the classical type.

Correspondence: Dr J. Müller, Laboratory of Reproductive Biology Y, Section 4052, Rigshospitalet, 9 Blegdamsvej, DK-2100 Copenhagen, Denmark.

Table 1. Densitometric data indicating the ploidy of the cells comprising eleven spermatocytic seminomas

Spermatocytic seminoma case no.	DNA ploidy distribution pattern*	Median DNA content†	Proportion of cells with greater DNA content than 2.5c
1	A	3.4c	0.78
2	T	4.2c	0.85
5	T	4.3c	0.98
6	D	1.9c	0.03
7	T	3.8c	0.91
8	D	1.7c	0.13
9	D	2.2c	0.39
10	D	2.4c	0.40
11	A	2.8c	0.58
14	A	2.6c	0.58
15	D	2.0c	0.25
CIS of the testis‡	A	3.0–5.0c	≥ 0.89

*D: diploid; T: tetraploid; A: aneuploid.
†2c denotes the diploid value.
‡Range of ploidy values in carcinoma-in-situ germ cells (from Müller & Skakkebæk, 1981).

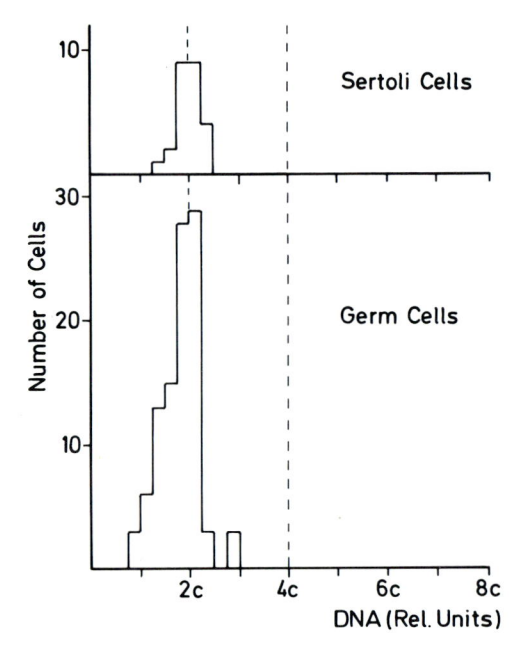

Fig. 2. Nuclear DNA distribution histogram of spermatocytic seminoma cells. Diploid pattern.

It has been suggested that the so-called 'intratubular change' adjacent to spermatocytic seminomas could represent spermatocytic carcinoma-in-situ rather than intratubular tumour spread. If the former is the correct interpretation, the morphological appearances clearly differ from that of CIS associated with semi-

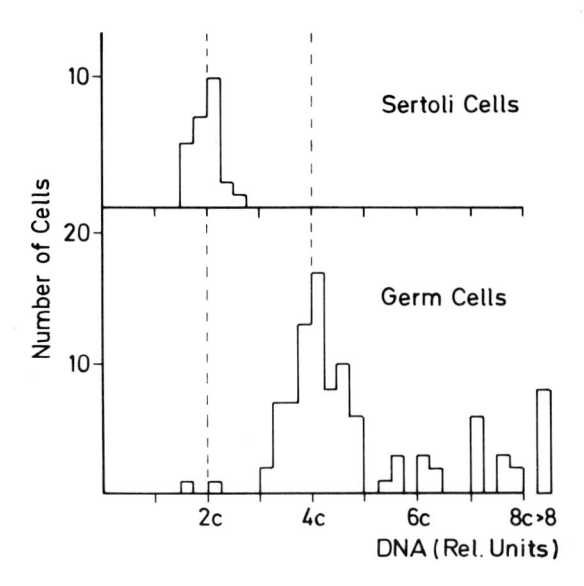

Fig. 3. Nuclear DNA distribution histogram of spermatocytic seminoma cells. Tetraploid pattern.

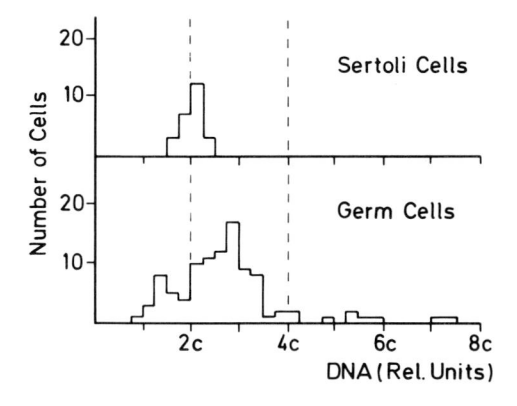

Fig. 4. Nuclear DNA distribution histogram of spermatocytic seminoma cells. Aneuploid pattern. Note the high proportion of cells with diploid DNA content.

noma and teratoma and would support our suggestion that the cell of origin of spermatocytic seminoma differs from that of seminoma and teratoma. The possible premalignant nature of these intratubular changes could only be proved by biopsy evidence of their existence prior to the development of a tumour.

Additional support for the suggestion that the pathogenesis of the spermatocytic seminoma differs from that of other germ cell tumours was given by the densitometric measurements. Only three of the eleven spermatocytic seminomas had an aneuploid DNA distribution resembling that of CIS of teratoma and seminoma. In a previous study (Talerman et al., 1984) the DNA distribution of spermatocytic seminomas has also been found to differ from that of classical seminomas. Although the spermatocytic seminoma most likely originates from a cell of the spermatogenic line, the specific cell type (spermatogonium, spermatocyte, spermatid) from which the tumour develops, remains to be identified. The results of the DNA measurements suggest that the tumours arise from several different levels. Normal spermatogonia and secondary spermatocytes are diploid, whereas primary spermatocytes are tetraploid. We found several different DNA patterns including diploid and tetraploid distributions.

In conclusion, our study supports the theory that the spermatocytic seminoma has a different origin from that of other germ cell tumours of the testis which may explain its different clinical characteristics.

Acknowledgements

This study was made possible by the work originally carried out by the British Testicular Tumour Panel and Registry and the preservation of their records. The work was supported by grants from the Danish Cancer Society (26/82 and 86-044).

References

Atkin, N. B. (1973) High chromosome numbers of seminomata and malignant teratomata of the testis: a review of data on 103 tumours. *British Journal of Cancer*, **28**, 275–279.

Jacobsen, G. K., Henriksen, O. B. & von der Maase, H. (1981) Carcinoma-in-situ of testicular tissue adjacent to malignant germ cell tumors. *Cancer*, **47**, 2660–2662

Masson, P. (1946) Études sur le séminome. *Revue Canadienne de Biologie*, **5**, 361–387.

Mostofi, F. K. (1980) Pathology of germ cell tumors of the testis. *Cancer*, **45**, 1735–1754.

Müller, J. & Skakkebæk, N. E. (1981) Microspectrophotometric DNA measurements of carcinoma-in-situ germ cells in the testis. *International Journal of Andrology*, Suppl. 4, 211–221.

Müller, J. & Skakkebæk, N. E. (1984) Abnormal germ cells in maldescended testes: A study of cell density, nuclear size and deoxyribonucleic acid content in testicular biopsies from 50 boys. *Journal of Urology*, **131**, 730–733.

Pugh, R. B. C. (1976) Testicular tumours: Introduction. *Pathology of the Testis* (ed. by R. B. C. Pugh), pp. 139–159. Blackwell Scientific Publications, Oxford.

Sigg, C. & Hedinger, C. (1981) Atypical germ cells in testicular biopsy in male sterility. *International Journal of Andrology*, Suppl. 4, 163–171.

Skakkebæk, N. E. (1975) Atypical germ cells in the adjacent 'normal' tissue of testicular tumours. *Acta Pathologica et Microbiologica Scandinavica*, A, **83**, 127–130.

Skakkebæk, N. E. & Berthelsen, J. G. (1981) Carcinoma-in-situ of the testis and invasive growth of different types of germ cell tumours. A revised germ cell theory. *International Journal of Andrology*, Suppl. 4, 26–33.

Talerman, A. (1986) Germ cell tumors. *Pathology of the Testis and its Adnexa* (ed. by A. Talerman and L. Roth), pp. 29–65. Churchill Livingstone, New York.

Talerman, A., Fu, Y. S. & Okagaki, T. (1984) Spermatocytic seminoma. Ultrastructural and microspectrophotometric observation. *Laboratory Investigation*, **51**, 343–349.

Thackray, A. C. T. (1976) Seminoma. In: *Pathology of the Testis* (ed. by R. C. B. Pugh), pp. 164–198. Blackwell Scientific Publications, Oxford.

Weibel, E. R. (1979) *Stereological Methods*, Vol. 1, *Practical methods for biological morphometry*, pp. 101–161. Academic Press, London.

Discussion

Holstein I would like to obtain some material from spermatocytic seminoma fixed in glutaraldehyde and embedded in Epon. This is the only way to determine the morphological features of such tumours. My problem is that I have never found spermatocytic seminoma in my material. Therefore, I address my question to you and to the audience. Do the cells of spermatocytic seminoma have nuclei which exhibit chromosomes in meiotic prophase, i.e. zygotene? This is a necessary finding in order to make the diagnosis. However, I think that tumour cells performing meiosis is a contradiction in terms.

Müller We have not performed electron microscopical studies ourselves. Some studies in the literature report that it is possible to demonstrate characteristics of spermatocytes in the tumour cells of spermatocytic seminoma. However, this is not the case in other investigations. Talerman *et al.* (1984, *Laboratory Investigation*, **51**, 343–349) could not demonstrate typical mature spermatocytes capable of meiotic division, but stated that the features of spermatocytic seminoma were certainly not similar to these of classical seminoma. This report also emphasizes the different macroscopic appearances and different clinical features of spermatocytic seminoma as opposed to classical seminoma.

Niemi If spermatocytic seminoma is not similar to classical seminoma, should it be called 'atypical seminoma'? In order to use the term 'spermatocytic', we should really be able to identify some signs that the cells have entered meiosis.

Müller The present nomenclature is difficult and we do not yet have a proper term. The so-called 'classical seminoma' is not really a seminoma and if this tumour could be renamed, the term 'seminoma' could be reserved to the tumour we now call 'spermatocytic seminoma', and we could forget about 'spermatocytic'.

Friedman Spermatocytic seminoma does exist and is completely different from ordinary germinoma (Talerman, 1980, *Cancer*, **45**, 2169; Walter, 1980, *Virchows Archiv (Pathological Anatomy)*, **386**, 175; Schoborg *et al.*, *Journal of Urology*, **124**, 1980, 739). Specific ultrastructural studies have been performed and well described by Rosai *et al.* (1969, *Cancer*, **24**, 103–116).

Niemi But do the tumour cells have the characteristics of spermatocytes?

Friedman Yes. All the changes in the chromatin which are seen in spermatocytic elements are present.

G. K. Jacobsen Do you know if spermatocytic seminomas stain for placental alkaline phosphatase (PlAP)?

Grigor I have found that spermatocytic seminoma does not stain for PlAP by immunoperoxidase.

Skakkebæk I believe that you have seen intratubular changes in association with spermatocytic seminoma.

Grigor Yes. The tumour was characteristic of the spermatocytic type of seminoma. Tumour cells were identified in many of the surrounding seminiferous tubules. These tubules were completely filled with cells similar in appearance to the cells of the main tumour mass. The CIS pattern as described by Professor Skakkebæk and as seen in association with other types of germ cell tumour except spermatocytic seminoma, was not seen.

G. K. Jacobsen I have studied two cases of spermatocytic seminoma for PlAP, both with negative reactions. I may add that I have looked for the 'CIS pattern' in seminiferous tubules adjacent to 10 spermatocytic seminomas and have never seen it, but I have seen intratubular spermatocytic seminoma.

Niemi I urge pathologists to prepare semithin sections from all future examples of spermatocytic seminoma which you will receive.

Lectin binding sites in human seminiferous epithelium, in CIS cells and in seminomas

RAIJA MALMI *and* K.-O. SÖDERSTRÖM *Department of Pathology, University of Turku, SF-20520 Turku, Finland*

Summary

The distribution of glycoconjugates in germ cells during spermatogenic differentiation, in carcinoma-in-situ (CIS) cells and in seminoma were studied by lectin histochemistry. The results show that human germ cells are rich in carbohydrate-containing compounds with specific alterations in the expression of glucosyl moieties during germ cell development. CIS cells reveal different lectin binding sites from spermatogenic cells, but the distribution of glycosubstances in CIS cells is similar to that of seminoma cells which supports the suggestion of the malignant nature of CIS germ cells.

Key words. Lectins, human testis, CIS cells, seminoma, glycoconjugates.

Introduction

Lectins have been introduced as histochemical markers to study the distribution of glycosubstances in various normal and malignant cells and tissues. Many reports on the interaction of lectins with sperm from various animal species have been published (Koehler, 1981). The changes in the glycoconjugates occurring during germ cell differentiation are less studied although the periodic acid–Schiff staining has widely been used to follow the development of acrosomes (Clermont & Leblond, 1955). Only a few studies have been conducted using modern histochemical methods to examine the glycoconjugate distribution of seminiferous epithelium (Söderström, Malmi & Karjalainen, 1984; Lee & Damjanov, 1985).

According to the present conception, both seminomatous and nonseminomatous germ cell tumours develop from intratubular carcinoma-in-situ (CIS) cells (Skakkebæk & Berthelsen, 1981). The glycocompounds found in normal germ cells may also be expressed in the malignant cells of germ cell origin. To define more precisely the alterations in the glycosubstances that occur during germ cell differentiation and malignant transformation, we have stained tissue sections containing normal testicular tissue, CIS cells and invasive seminoma with various fluorochrome-coupled lectins.

Materials and Methods

Tissues

Frozen sections of human testis were obtained from three men, aged 20–40 years, within 20 h after accidental death and from an adult brain death patient during

Correspondence: Dr Raija Malmi, Department of Pathology, University of Turku, Kiinanmyllynkatu 10, SF-20520 Turku 52, Finland.

kidney transplantation. The samples were snap-frozen in liquid nitrogen, stored at −80°C, cut in 8 μm thick sections and fixed in acetone at −20°C for 10 min. Histologically normal spermatogenesis was found in all cases.

Several testicular biopsy specimens, which were taken for investigation of infertility and showed normal spermatogenesis, were studied, as well as testicular specimens from different patients with carcinoma-in-situ of the testis. For routine histology, testicular tissue was fixed either in Bouin's or Cleland's fluid, embedded in paraffin and sections of 4–5 μm were stained with iron haematoxylin and eosin. In seven cases CIS cells were found inside the seminiferous tubules in the biopsies. In addition to CIS, in three cases tubules with normal spermatogenesis were also present and in two cases there was invasive seminoma.

Lectins
FITC-labelled lectins of different sugar binding specificities (Table 1) were obtained from Vector Laboratories (Burlingame, Calif.). The specificity of the observed binding patterns was tested with the appropriate inhibitory saccharides, as described earlier (Söderström *et al.*, 1984). The frozen and deparaffinized sections were covered with a drop of lectin solution (lectin concentration 150 μg/ml) and incubated in a moist chamber at room temperature for 30 min, washed in phosphate buffered saline (PBS) and twice in distilled water and mounted with Aquamount.

Table 1. Labelled lectins used in the study

Lectin	Carbohydrate specificity	Inhibiting sugar
Concanavalin A (Con A)	α-D-Mannosyl-, α-D-glucosyl-	α-Methyl mannoside
Lens culinaris (LCA)	α-D-Mannosyl-, α-D-glucosyl-	α-Methyl mannoside
Triticum vulgaris (wheat germ) (WGA)	(β-N-Acetylglucosaminyl-)$_n$, sialic acid	N-Acetylglucosamine
Ricinus communis I (RCA I)	D-Galactosyl-	α-Lactose
Arachis hypogaea (peanut) (PNA)	β-D-Galactose-(1→3)-N-acetyl galactosamine; β-D-galactosyl-	D-Galactose
Glycine maximum (soybean) (SBA)	N-Acetylgalactosaminyl- β-D-galactosyl-	N-Acetylgalactosamine
Helix pomatia (HPA)	N-Acetylgalactosaminyl-	N-Acetylgalactosamine
Ulex europaeus I (UEA I)	L-Fucosyl-	Fucose

For references, see Goldstein & Hayes (1978).

Results
In frozen sections of human testis each lectin presented a typical binding pattern, though minor variations in the intensity of fluorescence was observed in different testes. The Bouin- and Cleland-fixed paraffin embedded testicular tissue biopsies presented similar lectin staining patterns as observed in acetone-fixed frozen sections, but a slight decrease in the labelling intensity, evidently due to the tissue processing, was noticed with some lectins. Lectin binding sites in CIS cells were

Table 2. Staining of normal spermatogonia, normal spermatids, CIS cells and seminoma cells with lectins

	Spermatogonia	Spermatids (acrosomes)	CIS cells	Seminoma cells
Con A	+	++	++	++
LCA	+	++	++	++
WGA	+	++	+	+
RCA I	−	++	+	+
PNA	+	++	+/−	−
SBA	−	+	+/−	+/−
HPA	−	+*	−	−
UEA I	+/−	+/−	+	+/−

*Late spermatids

differently distributed from germ cells during normal spermatogenic development but were similar to those in seminoma cells. The staining of the seminiferous epithelium with normal spermatogenesis, the CIS cells and the seminoma cells are summarized in Table 2. Other testicular structures also presented a typical binding pattern but they will not be reported in this study.

Lectin binding during germ cell differentiation
In the seminiferous epithelium all types of germ cells expressed a large number of receptors for Con A (Fig. 1) and LCA in their cytoplasm, but the reaction was most pronounced in spermatid acrosomes. WGA was also positive for all the germ cells, and especially the acrosomes were brightly fluorescent (Fig. 4). RCA I was bound to germ cell surfaces from spermatocytes onwards and particularly to developing acrosomes. The intensity of the reaction increased adluminally. PNA stained faintly the cytoplasm of spermatogonia and spermatocytes, but the main binding sites were expressed in the acrosomal region of spermatids. SBA was not bound to spermatogonia and primary spermatocytes were rarely labelled, but the postmeiotic cells were fluorescent, as well as developing acrosomes. HPA binding sites were expressed selectively only in the acrosomes of late spermatids. UEA I was brightly fluorescent in all germinal cells in frozen sections, but showed a variable staining reaction in paraffin embedded tissue.

Lectin binding to carcinoma-in-situ cells and seminoma cells
In all the seven cases of CIS a bright, granular staining in the cytoplasm and along the cell borders of CIS cells was observed by Con A (Fig. 2). Invading malignant cells presented an identical granular staining (Fig. 3). LCA gave a strong, often also granularly distributed reaction in the cytoplasm of CIS cells and seminoma cells, but in most cases the fluorescence was less intense than with Con A. WGA was bound to the cytoplasm of CIS and seminoma cells, particularly to the perinuclear region, but the fluorescence was less intense than with Con A and LCA (Figs. 5 and 6). With RCA I a faint or moderate perinuclear fluorescence of CIS and seminoma cells was also observed. In four cases PNA failed to stain testicular tissue with carcinoma-in-situ, although the adjacent tubules with normal germ cell differentiation presented acrosomal binding characteristic for PNA. In the other three cases

and seminoma cells supports the suggestion that CIS cells are precursors of invasive seminoma. However, the staining of CIS cells differs from that of germ cells because they contain binding sites for RCA 1 and SBA, not found in spermatogonia. On the other hand, both lectins were positive in spermatid acrosomes during germ cell maturation. During malignant transformation of CIS cells, glucosyl moieties not observed in spermatogonia are expressed. Although it is probable that changes in the composition of cytoplasmic glycoconjugates would follow the malignant transformation of spermatogonia to CIS cells, the difference in lectin binding between the two cell types also suggests that the adult spermatogonia are not necessarily the direct precursors of CIS cells, but a more primitive cell type, possibly an embryonal or prepubertal spermatogonium, may be involved.

Acknowledgments

Professor M. Niemi and Professor N. E. Skakkebæk are kindly acknowledged for providing testicular biopsy specimens. This study was supported by the Finnish Cancer Organization.

References

Clermont, Y. & Leblond, C. P. (1955) Spermatogenesis of man, monkey, ram and other mammals as shown by the periodic acid–Schiff technique. *American Journal of Anatomy*, **96**, 229–250.

DeBray, H., Decout, D., Strecker, G., Spik, G. & Montreuil, J. (1981) Specificity of twelve lectins towards oligosaccharides and glycopeptides related to N-glycosyl proteins. *European Journal of Biochemistry*, **117**, 41–55.

Goldstein, I. J. & Hayes, C. E. (1978) The lectins: carbohydrate binding proteins of plants and animals. *Advances in Carbohydrate Chemistry and Biochemistry*, **35**, 127–340.

Gondos, B., Berthelsen, J. G. & Skakkebæk, N. E. (1983) Intratubular germ cell neoplasia (carcinoma-in-situ): a preinvasive lesion of the testis. *Annals of Clinical and Laboratory Science*, **13**, 185–192.

Koehler, J. K. (1981) Lectins as probes of the spermatozoon surface. *Archives of Andrology*, **6**, 197–217.

Lee, M. C. & Damjanov, I. (1985) Lectin binding sites on human sperm and spermatogenic cells. *Anatomical Record*, **212**, 282–287.

Skakkebæk, N. E. & Berthelsen, J. G. (1981) Carcinoma-in-situ of the testis and invasive growth of different types of germ cell tumours. *International Journal of Andrology*, Suppl. 4, 26–34.

Söderström, K. O., Malmi, R. & Karjalainen, K. (1984) Binding of fluorescein isothiocyanate conjugated lectins to rat spermatogenic cells in tissue sections. *Histochemistry*, **80**, 475–479.

Discussion

Niemi Have you used your lectins to stain normal embryonic gonads, and if not yourself, do you know anyone who has?

Malmi I have no information as yet on this particular aspect but I hope to have results in the future.

Analysis of the autoimmune response in an '*in situ*' carcinoma of the testis

D. LEHMANN *and* Hj. MÜLLER   *Laboratory of Human Genetics, Department of Research of the University Clinics, Kantonsspital, CH-4031 Basel, Switzerland*

Summary

Immune response in a patient with an *in-situ* seminoma of the testis was studied. Immunohistochemical examination of the testicular biopsy demonstrated remarkable intracellular and membraneous accumulation of IgG antibodies in the atypical spermatogonia. Using FITC-conjugated Concanavalin A, an abnormally high binding of Concanavalin A was detected in the transformed cells. Circulating antibodies directed against an antigenic determinant (60 kD) which is expressed on normal human spermatozoa and lymphocytes were found only in the patient's serum and not in 500 control sera. The role and possible diagnostic value of this autoimmune reactivity in testicular malignancies are discussed.

Key words.   Carcinoma-in-situ, seminoma, immune surveillance.

Introduction

Most of the research work which has been done on human testicular cancer has examined the role of endocrine and metabolic factors. Immunological aspects, however, may also be relevant for the development or the restriction of tumours as proposed by the immune surveillance theory (Burnet, 1971). Immunological factors should thus also be taken into account when considering malignancy of the testis. Transformed cells, according to the immune surveillance theory, are generally eliminated. In a few cases, where the immune system functions inefficiently, they may develop into a proliferative malignancy. This theory is based on two propositions: (1) transformed cells have, in general, different antigenic properties from normal cells; (2) the immune response to transformed cells is the same as that to infected cells or invasive micro-organisms.

In this study *in-situ* carcinoma of the testis was used to study immune reactions which might play an important role in the restriction of malignancies. A few characteristics of seminoma-in-situ make it an interesting model: (1) it involves constantly proliferating stem cells; (2) germ cells express antigenic determinants which are common to the embryo and also to a few carcinogenic cells (Goldberg & Tokuda, 1977; Gabel, Eddy & Shapiro, 1979); (3) the seminiferous tubule is known to be an immuno-privileged site (Head, Neaves & Billingham, 1983).

An immunochemical and immunohistochemical approach to the examination of a seminoma-in-situ is described in this paper.

Correspondence: Dr Dan Lehmann, Laboratory of Human Genetics, Department of Research of the University Clinics, Kantonsspital, CH-4031 Basel, Switzerland.

Materials and Methods

Patient

A 29-year-old infertile man suffered from a large varicocele in the left testicle and had an oligo-astheno-teratospermia. Tissue specimens were removed. Seminoma-in-situ was diagnosed on the right site. The left testicle showed reduced spermatogenesis. Multiple numerical and structural chromosome aberrations were evident from chromosome preparations of the mitotically dividing cells of the right gonad. The tumour markers α-fetoprotein and β-hCG were within the normal range in the serum. The right testis was removed and post-operative follow-up revealed no recurring conditions. One year after operation the patient fathered a healthy child (see Lehmann et al., 1986a).

Immunohistochemistry

Biopsy specimens were fixed in 3.5% paraformaldehyde, embedded in glycolmethacrylate, and stained immunologically (see Lehmann et al., submitted).

Blot-immunobinding assay

Spermatozoa extracts were separated by polyacrylamide gel electrophoresis and transferred to nitrocellulose filter paper. The binding test for antisperm antibodies was performed according to a procedure previously described (Lehmann et al., 1985).

Trypsin digestion

Washed spermatozoa (10^9) were incubated in trypsin (10 µg/ml PBS) for 30 min at 37°C. The digestion was terminated by the addition of PMSF/DMSO (1 mM final concentration). The preparation was immediately frozen in liquid nitrogen or used for further investigations.

Results

Immunohistochemistry

Histological and cytogenetical evaluation of the patient's testicular biopsy specimens indicated the existence of atypical spermatogonia in the right testis. Analysis of the tissue by immunohistochemistry revealed immune deposits which were located only in the atypical germ cells. IgG but not IgA or IgM were detected predominantly in cytoplasmic vesicles within the abnormal germ cells (see Fig. 1) and in some of the tubules attached to the membrane of the abnormal cells. These antibodies could fix complement as indicated by the accumulation of C3 complement component in the atypical cells. PAS-staining of the patient's testicular sections showed that the atypical cells possessed intracytoplasmic vesicles which contained considerable amounts of stained material, probably glycogen. Since defects in glycosylation and glycoprotein transport are known to occur in transformed cells, the binding capacity of different fluorescein labelled lectins having various glycoprotein-binding specificities (Vector Kit 2100) was examined. Concanavalin A, which is known to bind to mannose residues, showed an abnormal higher binding capacity to the atypical cells as compared to its binding to testicular tissue from healthy fertile persons (Fig. 2). All the other tested lectins did not show abnormal changes in their binding pattern. Upon incubation of the patient's testicular section with anti-albumin antibodies,

Autoimmunity in seminoma-in-situ 165

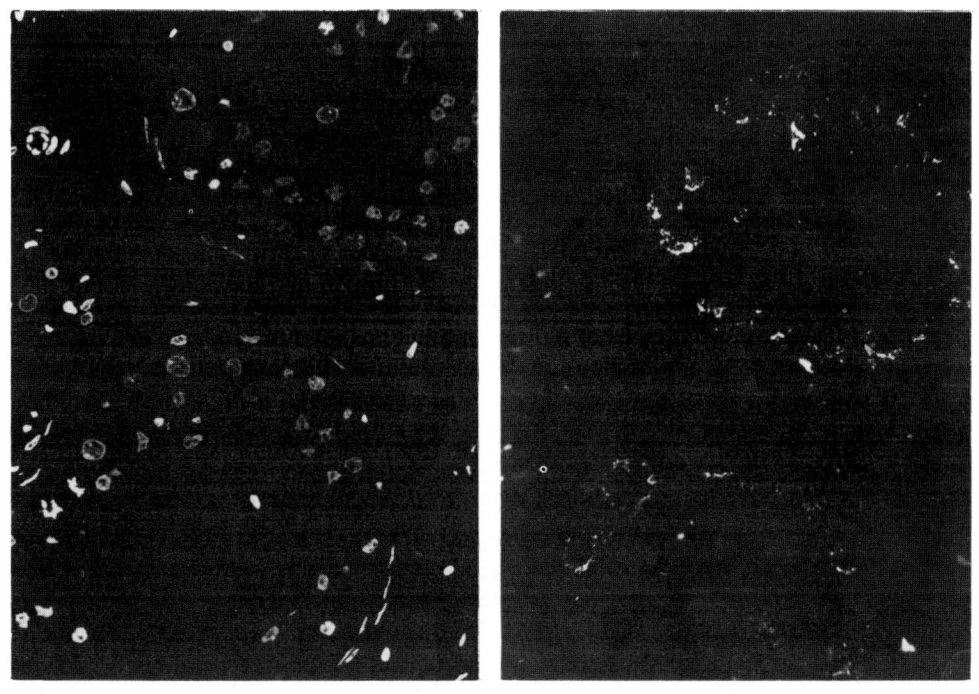

Fig. 1. Immunofluorescence micrographs of the right testicular biopsy of a patient with seminoma-in-situ showing (a) a section through the seminiferous tubules with atypical spermatogonial nuclei stained with the DNA-specific dye Hoechst 33258, and (b) the same section stained with FITC conjugate, demonstrating remarkable IgG deposits restricted to the atypical cells.

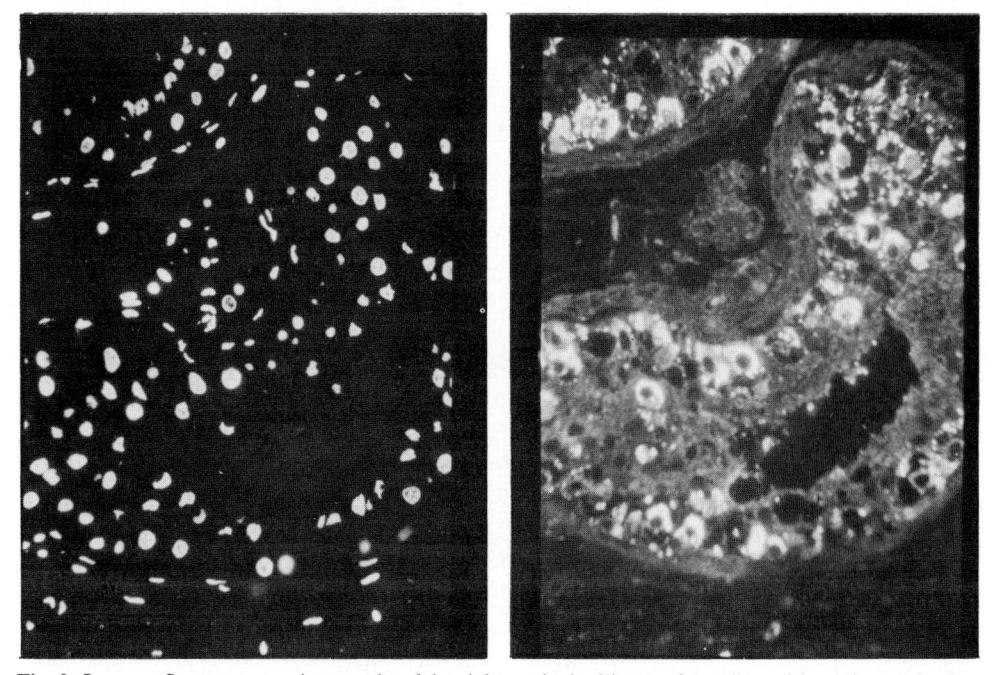

Fig. 2. Immunofluorescence micrographs of the right testicular biopsy of a patient with seminoma-in-situ, showing (a) a section through the seminiferous tubules with the abnormal nuclei of the atypical spermatogonia stained with the DNA-specific dye Hoechst 33258, and (b) the same section stained with FITC conjugated Concanavalin A.

massive intracellular uptake of albumin by the atypical spermatogonia was demonstrated.

Immunochemistry

To examine further the humoral autoimmune response the patient's serum was tested by the blot immunobinding test for the detection of antisperm antibodies. Antibodies were found to a single antigenic determinant with the approximate M.W. of 60,000 kD using iodinated protein A probe (Fig. 3). Interestingly, antibody to this particular antigen was not detected in the sera of more than 500 infertile patients and healthy controls. The antigen, however, seems not to have been peculiar for the patient's spermatozoa, as it could also be extracted by SDS/urea treatment from spermatozoa and lymphocytes of normal human donors. This antibody binding reactivity could not be absorbed by AB positive erythrocytes. Treatment of spermatozoa from pooled healthy donors with trypsin released a soluble molecule possessing a similar mobility in SDS-PAGE to that of the antigen which has been extracted from spermatozoa with SDS/urea. This molecule preserved the antigenic determinant for the specific antibody as was shown using the blot immunobinding test. This indicates that the molecule is probably located on the outer sides of the cell membrane of normal spermatozoa and lymphocytes.

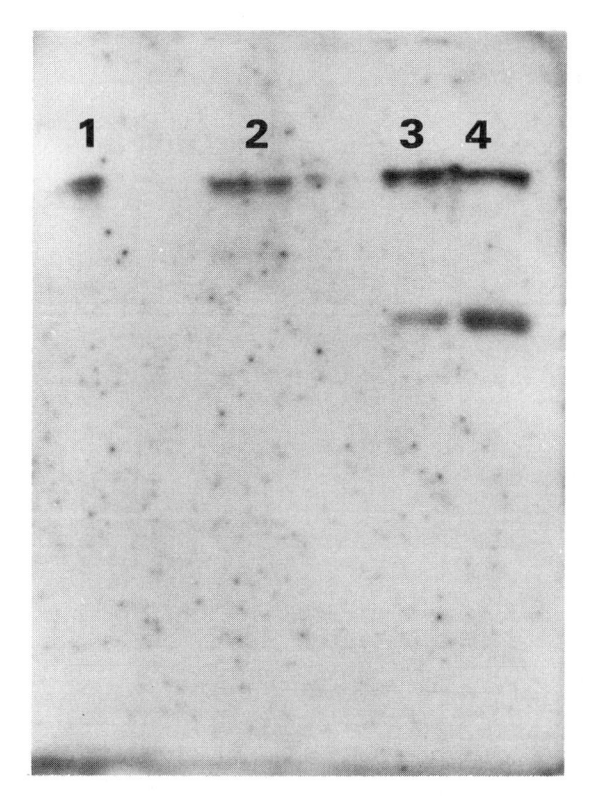

Fig. 3. Autoradiogram of an immunobinding blot test with the patient's serum. Lane 1: normal pooled spermatozoa extracted with trypsin; lane 2: normal pooled spermatozoa extracted with SDS/urea; lane 3; normal pooled lymphocytes, blood group O, extracted with SDS/urea; lane 4: normal pooled lymphocytes, blood group A, extracted with SDS/urea.

Discussion

Immunochemistry and immunohistochemistry used in the investigation of the immune reactivity to seminoma-in-situ both resulted in new findings which may well lead to a better understanding of the involvement of humoral immunity in testicular malignancy. Mononuclear infiltrations were not observed in the vicinity of the deteriorated cells, nor elsewhere in the patient's testicular tissue.

The immune deposits detected in the patient's seminiferous tubules seem to be specific to an antigen which is expressed only on the transformed atypical germ cells. Although the cell membrane was shown to be permeable to albumin which indicates that some degree of degeneration had already occurred, the fact that only IgG molecules and not IgA or IgM antibody were detected in the cells shows that the antibodies are indeed directed specifically to an antigen. It is, however, not yet possible to answer the question of whether the antibody detected by the blot immunobinding test in the serum of the patient and those found intracellularly in the abnormal spermatogonia are directed to the same antigenic determinant. In our study on the expression of glycoproteins on germ cells during spermatogenesis using binding of lectins with different sugar specificity to testis sections from healthy men, it was shown that Concanavalin A could bind with a high affinity to germ cells in various stages of differentiation. It may thus be that the abnormal accumulation of material with a high affinity to Concanavalin A in the atypical spermatogonia represents a germ cell specific molecule with a function in the differentiation of germ cells. This would imply a defective processing and/or transport of high mannose type oligosaccharide chain, a phenomenon which has been observed in tumorigenic cells (Bramwell & Harris, 1978). The 60,000 kD M.W. antigen to which antibodies were found only in the patient's serum could not be localized in normal human testicular tissue nor could it be detected using immunofluorescence on ethanol fixed or alive spermatozoa. Two theories for the involvement of surface molecules in malignancy development could explain why the antigen is undetectable in normal tissue or cell:

1. Cancer may be caused by a differential rate of expression and thus in normal cells where the antigen is expressed in minute amounts it is undetectable.
2. Proteins which are normally masked are in cases of transformation unmasked and can be regarded as non-self antigens (Springer, 1984). The reductive condition used in the SDS-PAGE may result in unmasking of proteins which are otherwise masked and thus permit their detection by the blot immunobinding test.

Preliminary results from the immunofluorescence test using spermatozoa treated with neuraminidase and the patient's serum, indicate that the patient has a circulating antibody to a molecule on the surface of spermatozoa which is unmasked upon treatment with neuraminidase. Such a humoral autoimmune response may provide an explanation to the local restriction of seminoma-in-situ into the inner side of the seminiferous tubule. This is in agreement with the present report of C3 accumulation in the deteriorated cells. If the antibodies are really directed to a differentiation molecule, it is possible that such antibodies are common to patients with *in-situ* malignancy of the testis. This fact will thus be useful diagnostically and perhaps even therapeutically. Early detection of carcinoma-in-situ is of special clinical importance, since it has been shown to develop into invasive tumours in a high percentage of patients (Nüesch-Bachman & Hedinger, 1977; Sigg & Hedinger, 1980).

Acknowledgements

The authors wish to thank: Drs B. Leibundgut for supplying the biopsy specimens and F. Hadziselimovic and J. Wegman for the histological evaluation and Mr N. Koeth and Mrs A. Krauss for their help with the manuscript. This study was supported by the Stanley Thomas Johnson Foundation, the Freiwillige Akademische Gesellschaff Basel and by the Swiss National Foundation (Grant No. 3.818.0.84).

References

Bramwell, M. E. & Harris, H. (1978) An abnormal membrane glycoprotein associated with malignancy in a wide range of different tumours. *Proceedings of the Royal Society of London*, B, **201**, 87.

Burnet, F. M. (1971) Immunological surveillance in neoplasia. *Transplantation Reviews*, **7**, 3.

Gabel, C. A., Eddy, E. M. & Shapiro, B. M. (1979) Persistance of sperm surface components in the early embryo. *The Spermatozoon*, pp. 219–229. Urban and Schwarzenberg Inc., Baltimore.

Goldberg, E. H. & Tokuda, S. (1977) Evidence for related antigens on sperm, tumor and fetal cells in the mouse. *Transplant Proceedings*, **9**, 1363–1365.

Head, J. R., Neaves, W. B. & Billingham, R. E. (1983) Immune privilege in the testis. *Transplantation*, **36**, 423–431.

Lehmann, D., Temminck, B., Leibundgut, B., Da Rugna, D. & Mueller, Hj. (1986) Immunological infertility in men: immunohistological and serological evidence (Manuscript submitted.)

Lehmann, D., Temminck, B., Lilmanen, K., Leibuidput, B., Hadziselinovic, T. & Miller, Hj.: (1986) Autoimmune phenomena and cytopenetic findings in a patient with carcinoma (seminoma) in situ. *Cancer*, **58** (in press).

Lehmann, D., Temminck, B., Leibundgut, B., Da Rugna, D. & Mueller, Hj. (1985) Blot immunobinding test for detection of antisperm antibodies. *Journal of Reproductive Immunology*, **8**, 329–336.

Nüesch-Bachmann, H. & Hedinger, C. (1977) Atypische Spermatogonien als Präkanzerose. *Schweizensche Medizinische Wochenschrift*, **107**, 795–801.

Sigg, C. & Hedinger, C. (1981) Atypical germ cells in testicular biopsy in male sterility. *International Journal of Andrology*, suppl. 4, 163–171.

Springer, G. F. (1984) T and Tn, general carcinoma autoantigens. *Science*, **224**, 1198–1206.

Discussion

Oliver There is a known association between mumps and testicular atrophy and also with testicular tumour. Did you study your sera for activity against cells infected by the mumps virus?

Lehmann We have not tried that.

Niemi Did you screen all the 500 men with the blots made of spermatozoa?

Lehmann Yes, and only one case was positive — that of intratubular seminoma.

Walt In the adult patient with CIS what was the reaction of the antisperm antibody to the main tumour mass away from the area of CIS, and have you any other information about the reaction with tumour tissue?

Lehmann The patient you refer to had his biopsy for infertility and no solid tumour was identified in our material. We have no information as yet on the staining of tumour tissue, but this is part of our future plans.

Niemi Did you see any lymphocytic reaction around the seminiferous tubules?

Lehmann No. We did not see any.

General discussion on the biology of malignant germ cells

Chairman M. NIEMI

Hargreave We have heard today of many elegant techniques for examining tumours and testicular biopsy samples including semithin sections, electron microscopy, HLA, lectins and many others. What is the concensus about the best routine method for handling and fixing a freshly excised testicular tumour? What should the surgeon and pathologist do routinely?

Holstein I am involved with morphological methods. In the first instance, it is necessary to obtain the testicular tissue or the orchidectomised testis immediately after surgery. Fixation should be performed by immersion in, or perfusion with, glutaraldehyde/phosphate buffer/OsO_4. The whole testis or tumour is cut into 7–10 transverse slices and several specimens are taken for embedding in Epon. This will give high quality information about the nuclear and cytoplasmic details of the cells, and will permit an excellent evaluation of the testicular tumours. Following this procedure there is then the possiblity of electron microscopical investigation if required.

Niemi Part of the tumour tissue should be kept frozen for immunological staining. Frozen sectioning is the safest starting procedure when investigating an antibody because often it is not known how well an antigen will resist fixation and embedding in paraffin wax or plastics.

G. K. Jacobsen A correct morphological diagnosis is of paramount importance when considering the optimal method of handling the orchidectomy specimen. In the first instance, the entire specimen must be carefully examined macroscopically. Serial slices should be cut through the whole tumour to look for different types of tissue. Blocks of tumour tissue should be taken from all parts with different appearances, and haemorrhagic, jelly-like (myxomatous) or oedematous areas should not be avoided.

For routine microscopical examination, formalin-fixed paraffin-embedded material will suffice and such material can also be used for immunohistochemical examination of AFP and hCG. If certain antigens are to be studied, various other fixatives may be used. Other investigations can be performed by (a) making imprint specimens, (b) taking blocks for electron microscopy, (c) taking fresh tissue for frozen sections (to be kept in case this will be required for specific examinations) and (d) taking portions of tissue for snap-freezing, xenografting in nude mice, preparing cell cultures, or other special studies to be performed.

All the tissue which is not taken initially for diagnosis and special studies should be retained at least until the diagnosis has been made and the results of marker studies are known.

Grigor First I shall answer Professor Holstein's comments. I agree that Epon-embedding and semithin sections give ideal cytological detail, but the average clinical pathologist is more familiar with formalin-fixed paraffin-embedded sections and such material is more meaningful for giving a histopathological diagnosis. It would not be wise to use only semithin Epon-embedded sections unless we all had the experience and expertise of Professor Holstein.

Secondly, it is important to realize that formalin is the best general fixative for handling routine surgical biopsies in a general pathology department, although other fixatives offer many advantages under special circumstances. Unfortunately, formalin is a poor fixative for many studies which we perform on testicular tumours.

My advice to surgeons who perform orchidectomies is to give prior notification to the pathologist that a testis is about to be removed. My advice to the pathologist is to collect personally the specimen completely fresh and unfixed from the operating theatre as soon as it is removed. The pathologist should then immediately cut the specimen taking representative samples for electron microscopy, special fixation (e.g. Bouin's, Carnoy's or other fixatives suitable for immunohistochemical localization of relevant antigens and tumour markers) and special studies requiring frozen or fresh tissue. The remainder should be fixed in formalin for routine histology and for long-term storage. Many representative blocks of the tumour must be taken and samples taken from surrounding testis, rete, epididymis and cord, including the upper resection margin.

A testicular tumour submitted to the pathologist after a day's fixation in formalin – either intact, which reduces penetration of fixative through the tunicas and allows autolytic changes in the important part of the specimen, or irregularly sectioned which precludes an accurate examination of the gross appearances – has very little investigative potential and may even be unsatisfactory for histological assessment and diagnosis.

Walt I agree that it is important to receive fresh, unfixed tissue. For many purposes it is also important to receive the specimen under sterile conditions. The pathologist can then decide if there is suitable tumour tissue available for purposes other than diagnosis – for example, tissue and cell culture, transplantation into nude mice, chromosomal studies, etc. There will also be the possibility of appropriate fixation for light and electron microscopical analyses.

Skakkebæk I agree that Epon-embedded material gives good preservation of cellular structures. However, what is really important is the amount of information which can be obtained from the investigations. Malignant characteristics of various structures in Epon may be more difficult for many pathologists to interpret and diagnose.

Hargreave How useful is formalin fixation in the diagnosis of CIS?

Skakkebæk Formalin is a poor fixative for the preservation of the diagnostic features of CIS. We recommend Stieve's fixative* which allows excellent morphological demonstration of cell structures and preserves the antigenicity of P1AP in the CIS cells which can then be demonstrated by immunocytochemistry. Bouin's fixative is adequate for morphological details.

G. K. Jacobsen In many laboratories, fixatives containing mercurial compounds are not allowed to be used.

Engström In-situ hybridization as a method of examining gene expression in histological sections from human tumours will provide a unique diagnostic tool for pathologists in the future. One serious drawback with formaldehyde fixation is the rapid destruction of mRNA which makes it virtually impossible to apply this powerful technique to conventionally processed specimens. Therefore, I hope it will be possible to use a mild fixation procedure (for example 4% paraformaldehyde overnight, which is used for preparing tissue for *in-situ* hybridization) without the risk of threatening a firm histopathological diagnosis in parallel slides.

Skakkebæk I have no information about the use of paraformaldehyde as a fixative.

Niemi There may be growing a new generation of pathologists who will use semithin sections routinely in diagnostic pathology. In germ cell tumours in particular this will be an important step forward, because then cytological criteria can be used for classification.

---

*Stieve's fixative: 40 g mercuric chloride in 1430 ml distilled water added to 80 ml glacial acetic acid in 400 ml of 40% formaldehyde just prior to use (38 ml of the former added to 12 ml of the latter).

Screening for carcinoma-in-situ of the testis

A. GIWERCMAN,[1] J. G. BERTHELSEN,[1] J. MÜLLER,[1] H. von der MAASE[2] and N. E. SKAKKEBÆK[1,3]

[1]Laboratory of Reproductive Biology, University Department of Obstetrics and Gynaecology, Rigshospitalet, [2]Department of Oncology ONB, Finsen Institute, Rigshospitalet, and [3]University Department of Paediatrics, Hvidovre Hospital, Copenhagen, Denmark

Summary

Germ cell neoplasia detected at the preinvasive stage of carcinoma-in-situ (CIS) can be cured by orchidectomy or by localized irradiation of the testis. Therefore, screening for carcinoma-in-situ of the testis has been applied to groups of individuals known to have an increased risk of testicular cancer. A high (5.5%) incidence of CIS was found in the contralateral testis of men with a unilateral cancer of the testis. An increased incidence of CIS was also found among men with a history of cryptorchidism. We recommend routine screening for CIS of the testis in both groups of men. The role of screening for CIS among subfertile men remains to be elucidated.

Key words. CIS testis, screening, risk groups, testicular cancer.

Introduction

Since the association between carcinoma-in-situ (CIS) of the testis and invasive testicular neoplasia was described in 1972 (Skakkebæk, 1972) screening for CIS of the testis has been applied to groups of individuals with an increased risk of testicular cancer (Krabbe *et al.*, 1979; Berthelsen *et al.*, 1982; von der Maase *et al.*, 1986).

Germ cell neoplasia detected at the stage of CIS can be cured by orchidectomy alone. In addition, recent investigations indicate that localized irradiation can eradicate CIS of the testis without significantly affecting Leydig cell function (von der Maase, Giwercman & Skakkebæk, 1986). These results emphasize the importance of screening for CIS.

The aim of the present paper is to review the results of screening for carcinoma-in-situ of the testis and to discuss future perspectives.

Maldescended testis

It has been known for several years that men with a history of maldescent of the testis have an increased risk of developing testicular malignancy (Gilbert & Hamilton, 1940).

Correspondence: Dr Aleksander Giwercman, Laboratory of Reproductive Biology, Rigshospitalet 4052, Blegdamsvej 9, DK-2100 Copenhagen Ø, Denmark.

Krabbe et al. (1979) asked 180 patients to participate in a study of men with a history of testicular maldescent. CIS was found in four men among fifty who agreed to have a testicular biopsy.

This observation prompted us to investigate testicular biopsies from a larger group of 20–30-year-old men previously treated for testicular maldescent. Preliminary results based on histological examination of testicular specimens from more than 200 men indicate that the incidence of CIS among 20–30-year-old men with a history of maldescent is lower than that found by Krabbe and co-workers. We now estimate the risk to be approximately 2%. A similar figure of invasive testicular tumours was estimated in a cohort study of young men with prior maldescent (Giwercman et al., 1987), where a risk of 4–5 times the normal life-time risk (Prener & Østerlind, 1985) of 0.5% was found.

Contralateral testis in men with unilateral testicular cancer

During the past 8 years Danish men previously treated for unilateral testicular cancer have been offered the opportunity of having a biopsy from the contralateral testis analysed for CIS (Berthelsen et al., 1982). Six hundred men have been investigated and CIS was found in thirty-four of these patients (von der Maase et al., 1987). Thus, the incidence of CIS in the contralateral testis of Danish men with unilateral testicular cancer was approximately 5.5%.

Twenty per cent of patients with unilateral testicular cancer have a history of cryptorchidism and/or atrophic contralateral testis. Biopsies from these patients reveal a 23% incidence of CIS in the remaining testicle, and this constitutes 85% of all the cases of CIS found in the remaining testis of unilateral testicular tumour patients (Berthelsen et al., 1982).

Somatosexual ambiguity

The frequency of gonadal tumours in intersex patients with a karyotype which includes a Y chromosome is very high (Scully, 1981). Two subgroups of patients with somatosexual ambiguity have been the subject of a search for CIS of the testis.

Among twelve consecutive patients with the androgen insensitivity (testicular feminization) syndrome, Müller & Skakkebæk (1984) found three cases of CIS. All three were found among eight patients with the incomplete form of the androgen insensitivity syndrome.

CIS was also found in all testicular specimens from four children and adolescents with gonadal dysgenesis and a 45,XO/46,XY mosaic karyotype (Müller et al., 1985).

Subfertile men

No systematic screening for CIS of the testis has been performed in subfertile men. However, retrospective studies of testicular tissue from men submitted for testicular biopsy because of subfertility indicate that even this group of men have an increased risk of having CIS of the testis. The frequency of CIS was found to be 0.55%, 1.1% and 0.4% in a Swiss, Danish and English study, respectively (Nüesch-Bachmann & Hedinger, 1977; Skakkebæk, 1978; Pryor et al., 1983).

The groups of men in these studies were very inhomogeneous and included some men known to have a very low risk of testicular cancer (i.e. men with Klinefelter's syndrome or Sertoli-cell-only syndrome). Thus, it seems reasonable to assume that it is possible to define a group of subfertile men who have a higher risk of having CIS of the testis than suggested by the three studies mentioned above. Based on the experience from biopsies of other risk groups (Berthelsen et al., 1982), we expect that the highest frequency of CIS will be found among men with very poor semen quality, atrophic testes and/or a history of cryptorchidism.

Methods of screening
Surgical testicular biopsy is the only established method of screening for CIS of the testis. Although the standard biopsy specimen is only 3–4 mm in diameter, the efficiency in diagnosing CIS is very high because the changes are usually dispersed throughout the testis and will appear in a random biopsy (Berthelsen & Skakkebæk, 1981). The CIS pattern is easily recognized by light microscopical examination if the specimen is fixed in a suitable fluid (Bouin's, Cleland's or Stieve's fixative). CIS may be difficult, or impossible, to diagnose in routine formalin-fixed material. However, a positive staining reaction for glycogen or for placental-like alkaline phosphatase (PlAP) supports the diagnosis of CIS (Beckstead, 1983; Jacobsen & Nørgard-Petersen, 1984).

A surgical testicular biopsy, which may be performed under local anaesthesia (Rowley & Heller, 1966), is well accepted as an outpatient procedure and is associated with complications in only very few cases (Bruun et al., 1987). Local spread of CIS cells has never been observed after this procedure. However, it must be emphasized that a trans-scrotal biopsy should be avoided if the patient is suspected of having a testicular tumour.

The surgical testicular biopsy is somewhat discomforting for the patient and too resource-consuming for screening of large populations. Consequently, efforts should be made to find non-invasive methods of identifying groups with a high risk of having CIS and thereby to reduce the number of individuals submitted for testicular biopsy. Recent results of ultrasound scanning for the diagnosis of early testicular neoplasia are promising and may aid in selecting patients for testicular biopsy (Lenz et al., 1987). Preliminary studies indicate that magnetic resonance imaging may also have a role in the diagnosis of CIS of the testis (Thomsen et al., 1987).

Conclusion
Men with unilateral cancer of the testis should be offered screening for CIS of the contralateral testis, particularly in the light of the recent encouraging results of localized irradiation treatment which eradicates CIS cells (von der Maase et al., 1987). Our preliminary data indicate that androgen production is not significantly affected by the application of a radiation dose of 20 Gy (von der Maase et al., 1987).

The screening biopsy of the contralateral testis should preferably be carried out during anaesthesia for removal of the primary tumour.

It remains to be established whether men with a history of cryptorchidism should routinely be offered testicular biopsy as screening for CIS of the testis. Our preliminary results indicate that the risk of having CIS in this group is about 2%. We propose that screening for CIS of the testis should be carried out routinely in these patients if this figure is confirmed. As the risk of having testicular cancer in men with a history of cryptorchidism is not significantly increased before the age of 20 years (Giwercman *et al.*, 1987), we suggest that screening should be performed at the age of 18–20 years. Testicular biopsy in prepubertal boys cannot be recommended as a screening procedure for CIS because the usefulness of this method at that time of life has not yet been verified.

No firm conclusion concerning indications for screening can be made with regard to subfertile men, as this group has not been thoroughly investigated.

In individuals with somatosexual ambiguity and a Y chromosome in their karyotype, screening for CIS may be recommended because radiation treatment of CIS may turn out to be an alternative therapy to orchidectomy in these patients. However, individual assessment should be made for each patient in this group.

The testicular biopsy, when performed postpubertally, is a very sensitive method of diagnosing CIS of the testis (Berthelsen & Skakkebæk, 1981). In addition, out of more than 1500 men who did not have CIS changes in their testicular biopsy, which was examined in our laboratory, only one single patient developed cancer of the testis during an observation period up to 8 years (Skakkebæk, Berthelsen & Müller, 1982; von der Maase *et al.*, 1986). Therefore a postpubertal testicular biopsy which does not show CIS changes does not, in general, need to be repeated later in life, as the risk of a subsequent germ cell tumour of the testis is extremely low.

Only a small proportion of testicular cancers develop in men who belong to a risk group. Therefore, effective prevention of testicular cancer can only be obtained if men outside the risk groups are also offered screening for CIS of the testis. This will only be possible if the methods of screening for CIS of the testis can be improved.

Acknowledgements

This work was supported by grants from The Danish Cancer Society (87-007, 86-017, 86-044, 86-065) and from P. Carl Petersens Fund (B1322).

References

Beckstead, J. H. (1983) Alkaline phosphatase histochemistry in human germ cell neoplasms. *American Journal of Surgical Pathology*, **7**, 341–349.

Berthelsen, J. G. & Skakkebæk, N. E. (1981) Distribution of carcinoma-in-situ in testes from infertile men. *International Journal of Andrology*, Suppl. 4, 172–184.

Berthelsen, J. G., Skakkebæk, N. E., von der Maase, H., Sørensen, B. L. & Mogensen, P. (1982) Screening for carcinoma in situ of the contralateral testis in patients with germinal testicular cancer. *British Medical Journal*, **285**, 1683–1686.

Bruun, E., Frimodt-Møller, C., Giwercman, A., Lenz, S. & Skakkebæk, N. E. (1987) Testicular biopsy as an out-patient procedure, complications and the patient's acceptance. *International Journal of Andrology*, **10**, 199–202.

Gilbert, J. B. & Hamilton, J. B. (1940) Studies in malignant testis tumors III. Incidence and nature of tumors in ectopic testes. *Surgery, Gynecology and Obstetrics*, **71**, 731–743.

Giwercman, A., Grindsted, J., Hansen, Jensen, O. M. & Skakkebæk, N. E. (1987) Testicular cancer risk in boys with maldescended testis. A cohort study. (Submitted.)

Jacobsen, G. K. & Nørgaard-Pedersen, B. (1984) Placental alkaline phosphatase in testicular germ cell tumours and in carcinoma-in-situ of the testis. An immunohistochemical study. *Acta Pathologica et Microbiologica Scandinavica*, Sect. A, **92**, 323–329.

Krabbe, S., Berthelsen, J. G., Volsted, P., Eldrup, J., Skakkebæk, N. E., Eyben, F. V., Mauritzen, K. & Nielsen, A. H. (1979) High incidene of undetected neoplasia in maldescended testes. *Lancet*, **i**, 999–1000.

Lenz, S., Giwercman, A., Skakkebæk, N. E., Bruun, E. & Frimodt-Møller, C. (1987) Ultrasound in detection of early neoplasia of the testis. *International Journal of Andrology*, **10**, 187–190.

Müller, J. & Skakkebæk, N. E. (1984) Testicular carcinoma in situ in children with the androgen insensitivity (testicular feminization) syndrome. *British Medical Journal*, **288**, 1419–1420.

Müller, J., Skakkebæk, N. E., Ritzen, M. & Ploen, L. (1985) Carcinoma in situ of the testis in children with 45,X/46,XY gonadal dysgenesis. *Journal of Pediatrics*, **106**, 431–436.

Nüesch-Bachmann, I. H. & Hedinger, C. (1977) Atypische Spermatogonien als Präkanzerose. *Schweizerische Medizinische Wochenschrift*, **107**, 795–801.

Prener, A. & Østerlind, A. (1985) *Cancer in Denmark*. Danish Cancer Registry, Copenhagen

Pryor, J. P., Cameron, K. M., Chilton, C. P., Ford, T. F., Parkinson, M. C., Sinokrot, J. & Westwood, C. A. (1983) Carcinoma in situ in testicular biopsies from men presenting with infertility. *British Journal of Urology*, **55**, 780–784.

Rowley, M. J. & Heller, C. G. (1966) The testicular biopsy: surgical procedure, fixation, and staining technics. *Fertility and Sterility*, **17**, 177–186

Scully, R. E. (1981) Neoplasia associated with anomalous sexual development and abnormal sex chromosomes. *Pediatric and Adolescent Endocrinology*, **8**, 203–217.

Skakkebæk, N. E. (1972) Possible carcinoma-in-situ of the testis. *Lancer*, **i**, 516–517.

Skakkebæk, N. E. (1978) Carcinoma in situ of the testis: Frequency and relationship to invasive germ cell tumours in infertile men. *Histopathology*, **2**, 157–170.

Skakkebæk, N. E., Berthelsen, J. G. & Müller, J. (1982) Carcinoma-in-situ of the undescended testis. *Urologic Clinics of North America*, **9**, 377–385.

Thomsen, C., Jensen, K. E., Giwercman, A., KJær, L., Henriksen, O. & Skakkebæk, N. E. (1987) Magnetic resonance: *In vivo* tissue characterization of the testis in patients with carcinoma-in-situ testis by magnetic resonance imaging. *International Journal of Andrology*, **10**, 191–198.

von der Maase, H., Giwercman, A. & Skakkebæk, N. E. (1986) Radiation treatment of carcinoma-in-situ of testis. *Lancet*, **i**, 624–625.

von der Maase, H., Rørth, M., Walbom-Jørgensen, S., Sørensen, B. L., Christophersen, I. S., Hald, T., Jacobsen, G. K., Berthelsen, J. G. & Skakkebæk, N. E. (1986) Carcinoma in situ of the contralateral testis in patients with testicular germ cell cancer. A study of 27 cases in 500 patients. *British Medical Journal*, **293**, 1398–1401.

von der Maase, H., Giwercman, A., Müller, J. & Skakkebæk, N. E. (1987) Management of carcinoma-in-situ. *International Journal of Andrology*, **10**, 209–220.

Discussion

Hargreave How many of your infertile patients had testicular maldescent? In my experience, it is difficult to get accurate figures for this because the operation is often done in childhood and the patient may not even be aware that he has a scar, and also the operation notes may not describe exactly where the testis was located. Do the incidence figures of 0.4% (English), 0.55% (Swiss) and 1.1% (Danish) of infertile patients with CIS include or exclude infertile patients who had previous testicular maldescent?

It is important to realize that testicular maldescent is not a single entity and we should differentiate between those who have true undescended testes, located in the abdomen or within the inguinal canal, and those who have ectopic testes such as in the superficial inguinal pouch. Perhaps it is only the patients with true undescended testes who are at risk of having CIS. Unfortunately, these two different conditions are not always categorized and the site of the testis is not always accurately documented. They probably have a different pathogenesis, undescent being related to fetal hormonal defects whereas ectopia is due more to mechanical problems.

Giwercman I agree with the necessity of distinguishing between ectopic and undescended testes, and indeed retractile testes. It is often difficult to do so because of inaccurate case documentation. We had access to the case records of all the patients participating in our study, but the findings of the physical examinations and the details of the surgical procedures were not always made clear. The determination of the relative significance of ectopia and undescent as factors associated with CIS will, I believe, require prospective studies.

We are looking at the difference between maldescent and retractile testes and we are hoping to determine if the size of the testis should be taken into account before recommending a biopsy.

Patients with a history of maldescent have been included in the three studies from different countries of infertile patients with CIS.

Skakkebæk In our studies we were not performing a biopsy as a screening test for CIS in infertile males. All our patients were infertile males referred for testicular biopsy for various different reasons from several different urologists and andrologists. Therefore, these biopsies were taken from a mixture of highly selected patients including those with Sertoli-cell-only syndrome (who should not be expected to have CIS), undescended testis, Klinefelter's syndrome and various other conditions. The reports from the other countries also refer to a heterogeneous group of infertile patients.

Hargreave Therefore, you do not recommend testicular biopsy programmes to screen for CIS in patients with infertility in general, but you try to identify which patients are more likely to have CIS?

Skakkebæk That is absolutely correct. We have no data to suggest that routine testicular biopsy is indicated for infertility.

Bannwart Does the age of operation for maldescent of the testis influence the occurrence of CIS?

Giwercman In our series of men with a history of cryptorchidism only five patients had CIS out of a total of 255 who were biopsied. It was therefore not possible to assess if the time of orchidopexy had any relevance to the occurrence of CIS. However, a recent report (Pike *et al.*, 1986, *Lancet*, **i**, 1246–1248) suggests that the age of surgical correction of undescended testes has no bearing on the subsequent incidence of testicular cancer.

Rankin You say that a single biopsy at the age of 18 years is all that is required for the screening of cryptorchids. In patients with unilateral testicular cancer, is a single biopsy of the contralateral testis at the time of operation sufficient, or may these patients develop CIS in that remaining testis at a later date?

Giwercman In patients who have CIS detected in one testis, we recommend a biopsy of the contralateral testis prior to treatment of the first testis, and this treatment depends on whether the disease is unilateral or bilateral. If CIS is not found in the contralateral testis, the biopsy does not need to be repeated as the risk of developing CIS and subsequent invasive testicular cancer is extremely low. This advice is also relevant for the patients you are referring to. A single biopsy is sufficient. We have only seen one patient in a series of 1500 who developed testicular cancer following a negative biopsy.

Dieckmann Patients with unilateral cryptorchidism have an increased risk of developing testicular cancer in the contralateral normally descended testis. If your patients have one undescended testis do you only biopsy the affected side or do you also recommend a contralateral biopsy?

Giwercman Bilateral testicular biopsy is recommended but if your resources are limited, perhaps only the affected side requires biopsy. Testicular tumours developing in patients with unilateral cryptorchidism usually appear in the affected side, and in only 5–10% of cases does the tumour develop in the contralateral testis which is only a small increase over the background incidence.

Vogelzang Do patients with congenital inguinal hernia and other congenital anomalies such as spina bifida, supernumerary nipples, require screening testicular biopsies?

Giwercman We have not studied patients with congential inguinal hernia. However, all men with a history of cryptorchidism were asked about previous inguinal hernia but our data has not yet been analysed.

Some subtypes of intersex patients with a Y chromosome have a very high incidence of gonadal CIS and these patients represent a special problem. Each patient should be individually assessed before recommending investigation for CIS.

Hargreave It must be remembered that children with inguinal hernia may have associated undescended testis, and the operation note concerning the repair of the hernia does not always describe the location of the testis.

Oliver Dr Berthelsen's first report on biopsy of the contralateral testis in patients with testicular tumour suggested that the incidence of CIS was highest in those patients with small volume testis, poor semen quality, and a history of previous cryptorchidism. Does your extended series corroborate this finding?

Giwercman Our latest results are not yet available but atrophy of the contralateral testis and a history of cryptorchidism are factors which are of particular interest to us. Berthelsen found that 85% of patients with CIS in the contralateral testis had a small testis less than 12 ml or a history of cryptorchidism although such patients constituted only 20% of the total number of patients who had unilateral testicular cancer.

Skakkebæk Perhaps testicular biopsy from the contralateral testis should only be performed if that testis is small, but we have found that it is extremely difficult to assess relative testicular size except in specialized centres. Even with the help of an orchidometer, different urologists can produce quite varied estimates of testicular size. Therefore, we recommend that routine biopsy of the contralateral testis should always be performed in local hospitals where expertise in measuring testicular volume is not available.

Jackson Did your measure serum PlAP in patients who had CIS?

Giwercman Serum PlAP was only measured in two or three patients and none had elevated levels.

Ikinger I have a comment on ultrasound screening. We have performed ultrasound in an attempt to detect small intratesticular lesions.

Walker carcinoma was induced within the testes of a series of Wistar rats in a randomized manner. Using an 8 MHz ultrasound scanner we found an echo-rich area 2 mm in size and this corresponded to the tumour. In our study, 85% of tumours of this size could be detected.

In a man with a history of seminoma removed 3 years previously, routine screening of the remaining testis revealed a 2.5 mm echo-poor area. This testis was removed and a second tumour was found confirming the presence of bilateral seminoma.

In our experience, I think it is not possible to detect tumours smaller than 2 mm in diameter, and in particular I do not think that CIS can be detected with ultrasound.

Hargreave Your results are impressive. In my experience ultrasound is very much an operator-dependent technique, and I believe this will limit the use of ultrasound as an effective screening method for CIS except in centres with special expertise where small lesions and subtle changes can be defined.

Experience of screening for carcinoma-in-situ of the testis among young men with surgically corrected maldescended testes

K. V. PEDERSEN, P. BOIESEN *and* C. G. ZETTER-LUND *Departments of Urology and Pathology, County Hospital of Jönköping, Sweden*

Summary

One hundred and twelve young men with maldescended testes which had been surgically corrected were examined for premalignant/malignant changes in the testes. Bilateral testicular biopsies were made in ninety-four patients. Three had carcinoma-in-situ of the testis in the biopsy. Invasive tumour of seminomatous type was found in two of these testes after orchidectomy had been performed. No correlation was found with testicular localization pre- or postoperatively, with testicular volume or with tumour markers.

Key words. Testicular cancer, carcinoma-in-situ testis, testicular maldescent.

Introduction

During the last two decades the prognosis of testicular cancer has changed for the better due to improved treatment. Furthermore, the description of premalignant changes in the testicles by Skakkebæk (1978) has stimulated the interest of searching for early testicular cancer in so-called risk groups.

It is well known that patients with maldescended testes have an increased incidence of testicular cancer (Martin, 1982). In our area ten of eighty patients with testicular cancer had maldescended testes.

In 1979 Krabbe *et al.* reported four cases of carcinoma-in-situ in the testis among fifty men earlier operated upon for maldescended testes.

The first symposium on 'Early Detection of Testicular Cancer' (1981) stressed the need for further investigations of this group of patients to make a better understanding of frequency, risk and treatment.

In the following paper we present the results of a screening programme for the detection of premalignant changes in the testes of young men operated upon for maldescended testes in our urological department between 1965 and 1970.

Materials and Methods

During the period 1965–70, 189 patients were operated upon for maldescended testes. Forty patients had moved from the area and were questioned by mail about any testicular disease. None answered confirmatory. The remaining 149 patients were offered an examination for detection of testicular malignancy and 112 patients accepted. Eighty-five patients had unilaterally, and twenty-seven patients had

Correspondence: Dr Knud V. Pedersen, Department of Urology, Regionsjukhuset, 581 85 Linköping, Sweden.

bilaterally, maldescended testes. The mean age for the unilaterally operated group was 10.1 years and for the bilaterally operated group 8.8 years.

We performed a clinical examination, and determined testicular localization and testicular volume using Prader's orchidometer. Serum concentrations of alpha-fetoprotein (AFP) and human chorionic gonadotrophin (hCG) were determined. Ninety-four patients accepted an open surgical testicular biopsy on both sides. The biopsy material was fixed in Bouin's fixative and embedded in EFL-67 embedding medium (SERVA, Feinbiochemica, Heidelberg, New York). 2 μm sections were cut at twelve levels and stained with a modified Weigert's haematoxylin and eosin. The biopsies were examined by one pathologist (P.B.) and classified according to the recommendations of Skakkebæk (1978). Special attention was paid to premalignant changes in the seminiferous tubules, the so-called carcinoma-in-situ.

Results

Surgical corrections were planned for 139 testes. Thirteen testes were removed either initially or at a later stage. At the screening examination, 122 testes were located in the scrotum, two in the subcutaneous inguinal ring, and two were not found. These two testes were thought to be aplastic after exploration in childhood, but both were found in the abdomen and removed.

We defined testicular volume of more than 12 ml as normal and testes measuring 12 ml or less were classified as atrophic. Thirty-two testes (26%) were smaller than normal. All patients had normal serum concentration of AFP and hCG.

Ninety right-sided and ninety left-sided testicular biopsies were examined by light microscopy. Three patients had carcinoma-in-situ in the testis and fifty-four patients had varying degrees of intratubular atrophy. The correlation between testicular localization and histology is shown in Table 1 (preoperatively) and Table 2 (postoperatively). Testicular volume and histology are correlated in Table 3.

Unilaterally operated patients with normal testicular biopsy histology were operated upon at a mean age of 8.6 years, while those with intratubular atrophy were on average 10 years old at operation. The two patients with carcinoma-in-situ were

Table 1. The histological picture of testicular biopsies in relation to the preoperative localization of the testes

	Localization	Intratubular atrophy	Carcinoma-in-situ	Normal histology
Unilaterally operated testes ($n = 66$)	Abdominal	2	—	1
	Inguinal canal	7	—	15
	Superficial inguinal ring	13	2	23
	Scrotal base	2	—	1
Bilaterally operated testes ($n = 43$)	Abdominal	2	—	—
	Inguinal canal	7	—	13
	Superficial inguinal ring	8	1	10
	Scrotal base	2	—	—

Table 2. The histological picture of testicular biopsies in relation to the postoperative localization of the testes

	Localization	Intratubular atrophy	Carcinoma-in-situ	Normal histology
Unilaterally operated testes ($n = 66$)	Abdominal	2	—	—
	Inguinal canal	—	—	—
	Superficial inguinal ring	1	—	—
	Scrotal base	22	2	39
Bilaterally operated testes ($n = 44$)	Abdominal	1	—	—
	Inguinal canal	—	—	—
	Superficial inguinal ring	1	—	—
	Scrotal base	17	1	24

Table 3. The histological picture of testicular biopsies in relation to testicular volume

	Volume	Intratubular atrophy	Carcinoma-in-situ	Normal histology
Unilaterally operated testes ($n = 67$)	12 ml or less	11	1	6
	More than 12 ml	14	1	34
Bilaterally operated testes ($n = 44$)	12 ml or less	11	—	4
	More than 12 ml	8	1	20

operated upon in the 8th and 13th year of life. Bilaterally operated patients with normal testicular biopsy histology were operated upon at a mean age of 9.6 years, while those with intratubular atrophy were 8.9 years old on average. One patient with carcinoma-in-situ was operated on at the age of 10 years.

All three testes with carcinoma-in-situ were removed. Two of them had additional invasive malignant tumours of seminomatous type.

Seventy-one testes had descended normally to the scrotum and were biopsied. Eleven (16%) had varying degrees of intratubular atrophy. None had premalignant or malignant changes.

Discussion

In a population where 12.5% of patients with testicular cancer had a history of maldescended testes, we screened young men 'the other way around' by examining those operated on for testicular maldescent about 15 years earlier. The purpose was to detect possible premalignant changes in the presumably 'high risk' testes. 60% of the operated patients underwent a clinical examination and ninety-four patients (50%) accepted a bilateral testicular biopsy. The histological findings were related to age of operation, testicular localization before and after surgical correction and testicular volume.

Recommendation for orchidectomy was given to the patients with carcinoma-in-situ of the testis. Two of the three patients with premalignant changes also had invasive malignant tumour. In all the biopsies with carcinoma-in-situ there was intratubular atrophy, which also appeared in the majority of the rest of the biopsies. The three patients with carcinoma-in-situ had their testes in the scrotum and two of them were of normal size.

Since no signs of testicular malignancy were found either by clinical examination or by determination of tumour markers, the only way of detecting premalignant changes is by open surgical biopsy. Berthelsen & Skakkebæk (1981) have shown that a surgical testicular biopsy is well representative of the histological pattern in the testicle.

Our findings confirm the finding that patients with maldescended testes have a high risk of developing testicular cancer. We assert the necessity of offering this group of patients at least one follow-up examination to exclude testicular malignancy. At present the only reliable diagnostic procedure is open surgical biopsy. At what time in life and how often this has to be done is still an open question. More experience in this field will hopefully create recommendations for handling patients with a history of testicular maldescent.

This study was accepted by the Committee of Ethics, University of Linköping, Sweden.

References

Berthelsen, J. G. & Skakkebæk, N. E. (1981) The distribution of carcinoma-*in-situ* in testes from infertile men. *International Journal of Andrology*, Suppl. 4, 172.
Krabbe, S., Berthelsen, J. G., Volsted, P., Eldrup, J. Skakkebæk, N. E., Eyben, F., Mauritzen, K. & Nielsen, A. H. (1979) High incidence of undetected neoplasia in maldescended testes. *Lancet*, i, 999–1000.
Martin, D. (1982) Malignancy in the cryptorchid testis. *Urologic Clinics of North America*, 9(3), 371–376.
Skakkebæk, N. E. (1978) Carcinoma-*in-situ* of the testis: frequency and relationship to invasive germ cell tumour sin infertile men. *Histology*, 2, 157–170.

Discussion

Hargreave Do you recommend biopsy for patients with normal sperm analysis and a past history of undescended testis, or can you use sperm analysis as a method for selecting cryptorchid patients for biopsy?

Pedersen Our patients had seminal fluid analysis prior to biopsy, but we cannot be sure that all our patients who were labelled as having previous undescended testis did, in fact, have true undescent. Precisely 50% of our patients who had been previously operated on for bilateral testicular maldescent had a normal seminal analysis and none of these had CIS. Perhaps patients with a history of bilateral testicular maldescent and a normal sperm analysis need not have a biopsy.

Giwercman Seminal analysis may be of value in selecting patients for biopsy. Most (60–70%) of our CIS patients had very poor semen quality but many of these were selected for biopsy because of infertility and/or testicular cancer, so that our series is biased. In some recent studies of men with unilateral undescended testis and CIS, a relatively good semen quality (>30 million spermatozoa per ml) was found in some of the patients.

Hargreave Your results indicate that CIS may be associated with good semen analysis so that this cannot be used as a universal screening method for excluding the possibility of CIS.

Pedersen Most of our patients with a history of unilateral cryptorchidism had normal semen analysis.

Wahlqvist In some of our patients who had a previous operation for unilateral cryptorchidism, a tumour developed in the nonoperated testis. If a screening programme is to be of value should a bilateral biopsy be performed to exclude CIS?

Skakkebæk You are correct. The normally descended testis in unilateral cryptorchidism also carries an increased risk of developing testicular cancer, although much lower than in the undescended testis. I do not think that we have enough evidence yet to decide whether unilateral or bilateral biopsy is indicated. However, if the results presented by Dr Giwercman and Dr Pedersen are confirmed in larger series, then in my opinion bilateral biopsies should be considered.

It is important to realize that we do not know the true incidence of CIS in patients with cryptorchidism, although we think it is in the region of 2–3%, and 20% of those who develop testicular cancer will do so in the normally descended testis. The only way to detect this 20% of tumours at a preinvasive stage is to perform bilateral biopsies.

Hargreave We still have to decide on the exact criteria for testicular biopsy but it appears that biopsy of all cryptorchids will show CIS in 2% of cases. However, if we concentrate on cryptorchids with poor sperm analysis then possibly 4% of biopsies may reveal CIS and this figure would seem to make biopsy mandatory in such cases.

Ultrasound in detection of early neoplasia of the testis

SUZAN LENZ,[1] A. GIWERCMAN,[2] N. E. SKAKKEBÆK,[2,3] E. BRUUN and C. FRIMODT-MØLLER[4] [1]*Department of Diagnostic Ultrasound, Rigshospitalet, Copenhagen,* [2]*Laboratory of Reproductive Biology, University Department of Gynaecology and Obstetrics, Rigshospitalet, Copenhagen,* [3]*University Department of Paediatrics, Hvidovre Hospital, Copenhagen, and* [4]*University Department of Urology, Gentofte Hospital, Copenhagen*

Summary

Testicular ultrasound scanning was performed in 192 men with a history of cryptorchidism. The ultrasonic tissue pattern was evaluated and each testis was accordingly given a score on a scale from 1 to 4, 1 representing the normal uniform pattern and 4 being a very irregular pattern. Testicular biopsy of the previously maldescended testicle(s) was carried out in 143 of the scanned men and from two contralateral testicles where the score 4 was given at the ultrasound examination. Two biopsies showed carcinoma-in-situ pattern. Both were found among testes with a very irregular echo pattern. This pattern was found in only 3.2% of all scanned testes.

Key words. Ultrasound, testis, early neoplasia.

Introduction

Ultrasound scanning has successfully been used to visualize nonpalpable tumours (Rifkin *et al.*, 1984). The detection limit for neoplasia in the testis is, according to our experience, a tumour of 4 mm in diameter. The diagnosis of earlier stages of malignancy still requires testicular biopsy. In the present study we have evaluated the use of ultrasound in the detection of early malignancy in the testis by consecutive ultrasound scanning and biopsy of the testes of men with a history of cryptorchidism.

Material and Methods

Patients

Two hundred and eighty men, aged 18–30 years, admitted consecutively to two hospitals in Copenhagen (Gentofte and St. Joseph) during the years 1966–77 for treatment of uni- or bilateral testicular maldescent were offered testicular ultrasound scanning and biopsy. Eighty-eight of them turned down the offer.

Correspondence: Dr Suzan Lenz, Department of Diagnostic Ultrasound, Rigshospitalet 4023, 9 Blegdamsvej, DK-2100 Copenhagen, Denmark.

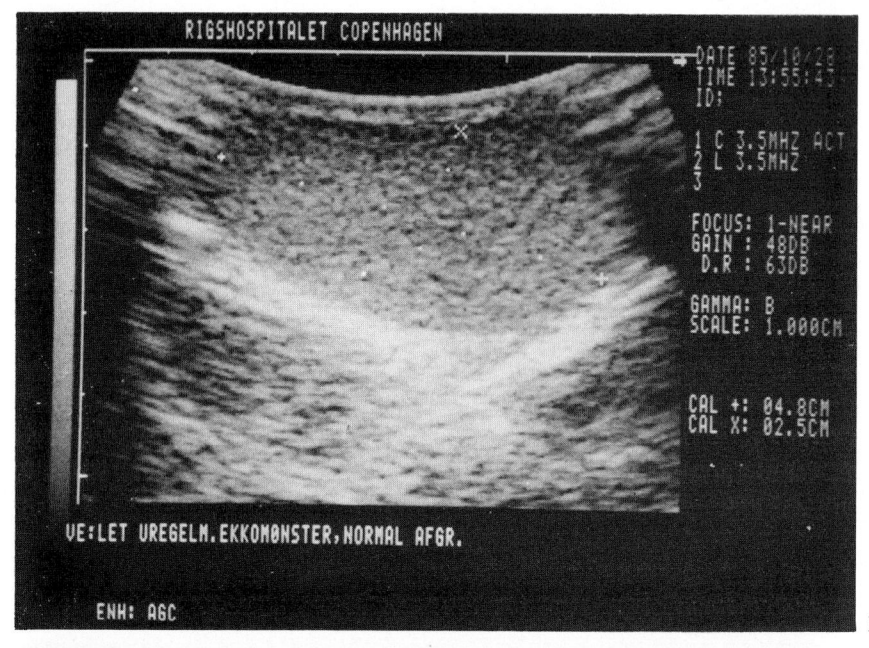

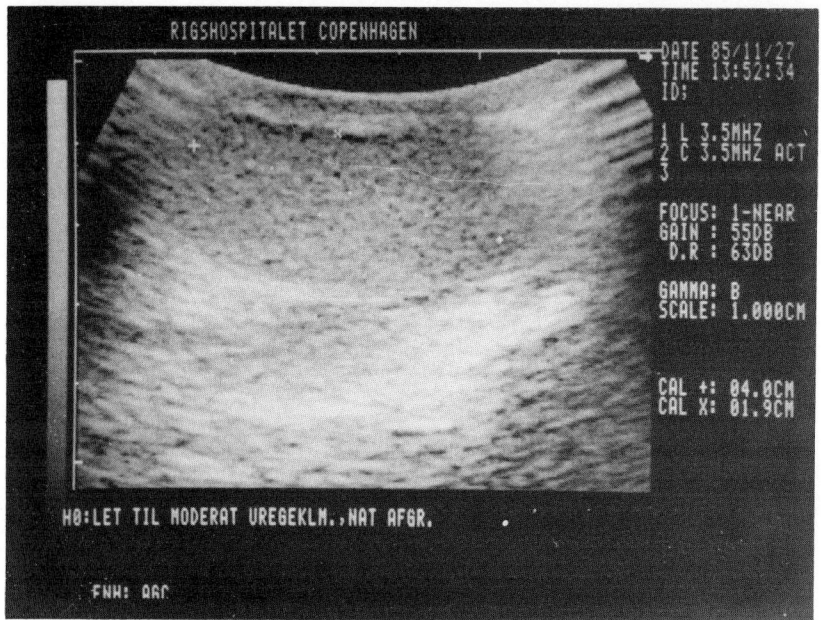

Figs. 1–4. Ultrasound scans of testicles showing echopattern 1–4. Electronic calipers are inserted for measurements given at the lower right of each picture. Fig. 1 demonstrates score 1, Fig. 2 score 2, Fig. 3 score 3 and Fig. 4 score 4.

Additionally forty-nine refused to have the biopsy performed after being ultrasound scanned. The preliminary nature of the investigation was explained to all men and they were given the free choice to participate.

Ultrasound in detection of early neoplasia 189

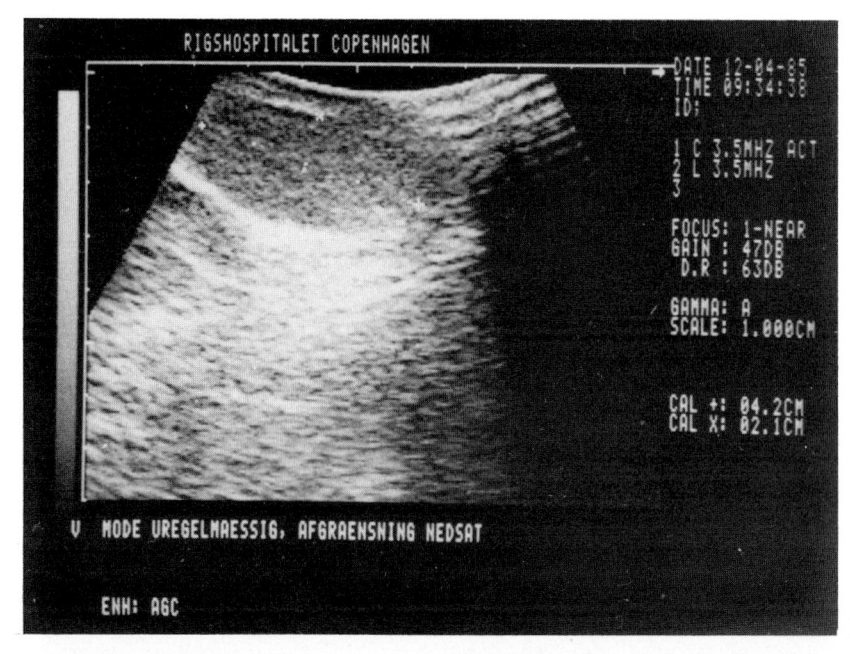

Fig. 3.

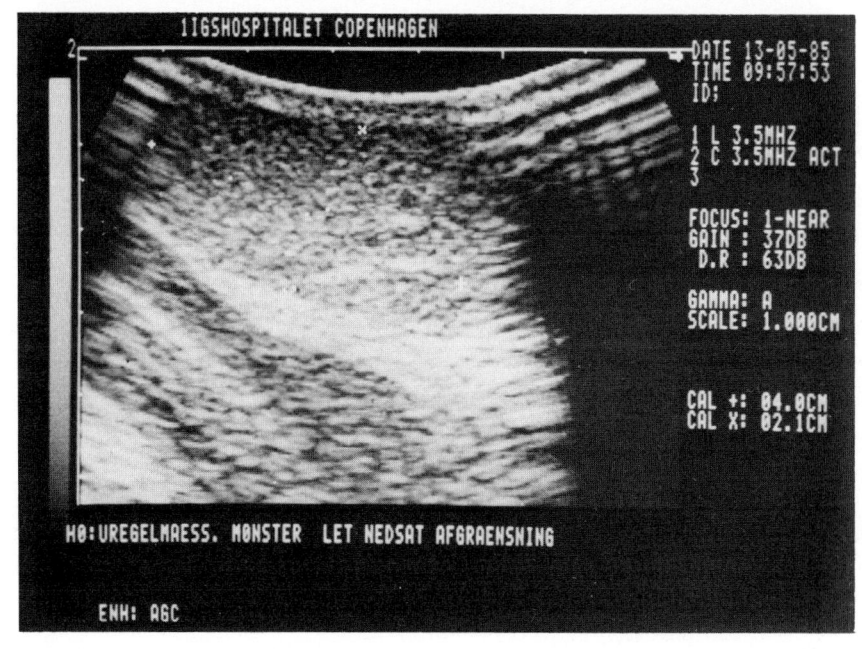

Fig. 4.

Scanning
Ultrasound scanning of both testicles was performed using a curved array 3.5 MHz transducer and an Aloka 270 dynamic scanner. The nearfield focus was chosen and the transducer placed directly on the skin of the scrotum. The ultrasonic tissue pattern was evaluated and each testis was accordingly given a score on a scale from 1 to 4, 1 representing the normal uniform pattern and 4 being a very irregular

pattern (Figs. 1–4). All ultrasound investigations were carried out by the same sonologist and preceded testicular biopsy in all but two patients.

Biopsy

In men with bilateral maldescent, biopsy of both testes was performed. Men with unilateral maldescent had only the testis in question examined except two patients in whom biopsy of the contralateral testis was also done as a very irregular echopattern was observed. The tissue was fixed in Stieve's fixative and stained with iron-haematoxylin and eosin. Light microscopic examination was performed by one person (NES) to whom the scanning results were unknown. A detailed report on testicular biopsy findings will be published elsewhere.

Results

Scanning of 379 testicles from 192 men was performed. Echopattern 1 was found in 241 testes, pattern 2 in ninety-two testes, pattern 3 in thirty-three testes and pattern 4 in twelve testes.

In one patient, physical examination as well as ultrasound revealed testicular tumour. Therefore, the planned testicular biopsy was not performed. An embryonal carcinoma was found by histological examination of the orchidectomy specimen.

A total of 197 biopsies were performed in 143 (74.5%) of the scanned men. Carcinoma-in-situ (CIS) was found in two testes, one from each of two men. Both testes had echopattern 4 by ultrasound. Among the biopsied men echopattern 4 was found in eleven testes from nine men. One of the testes with CIS pattern was normally descended. Testicular biopsy was performed because a very irregular echopattern was observed.

All but one testis with score 4 had severely impaired spermatogenesis. The histological picture was dominated by a Sertoli cell only pattern.

Discussion

Both cases of CIS were found among the testes with a very irregular echopattern. This pattern was found in only 3.2% (12/379) of all scanned testes.

Access to a simple, non-invasive method of identifying men with a high risk of having early testicular malignancy would make it possible to perform large-scale screening for testicular CIS. As only two cases of CIS were found we cannot make any firm conclusion. However, ultrasound may be a new lead in the search for a method of selecting patients who should be offered testicular biopsy. Additional groups of men must be investigated. Furthermore the relationship between echopatterns and testicular histology remains to be explained.

Acknowledgement

This study was supported by The Danish Cancer Society, grants 84-007, 87-017, 86-044 and 86-065 and by P. Carl Petersen's fund, grant B1322.

Reference

Rifkin, M. D., Kurtz, A. B., Pasto, M. E. *et al.* (1984) The sonographic diagnosis of focal and diffuse infiltrating intrascrotal lesions. *Urological Radiology*, **6**, 20–26.

Magnetic resonance: *in vivo* tissue characterization of the testes in patients with carcinoma-in-situ of the testis and healthy subjects

C. THOMSEN, K. E. JENSEN, A. GIWERCMAN,†
L. KJÆR, O. HENRIKSEN and N. E. SKAKKEBÆK,*†
*Department of Magnetic Resonance and *Department of Pediatrics,
Hvidovre Hospital, and †Laboratory of Reproductive Biology,
Department of Gynecology and Obstetrics, Rigshospitalet,
University of Copenhagen, Denmark*

Summary

Six patients with carcinoma-in-situ (CIS) of the testis and five healthy volunteers were examined with magnetic resonance imaging (MRI), relaxation time measurements (T_1 and T_2) and magnetic resonance spectroscopy. The study was carried out on a Siemens Magnetom (1.5 Tesla) whole body MR scanner. All patients with CIS had a biopsy taken before MR examination and histology was compared with the MR results. Significant difference between T_1 relaxation processes for normals and patients with CIS was shown. It remains to be seen whether these findings are related to the neoplasia or the reduced spermatogenesis.

Introduction

Carcinoma-in-situ (CIS) of the testis is a lesion in the germinative epithelium of the testis (Nüesch-Bachmann & Hedinger, 1977; Skakkebæk, 1972). Follow-up of patients with CIS have shown that 50% developed testicular cancer over a 5-year period (Skakkebæk, Berthelsen & Müller, 1982).

Several groups are at risk of harbouring CIS and subsequent development of invasive testicular cancer: (1) In patients who have been operated on for testicular cancer on one side, approximately 5% harbour CIS in the contralateral testis (Berthelsen *et al.*, 1982). (2) Patients with a history of a maldescended testis (Krabbe *et al.*, 1979). (3) Infertile male patients with oligozoospermia (Skakkebæk, 1978). At present, a surgical biopsy is the only reliable method for the detection of CIS, and only a limited number of patients can be examined with this invasive method.

Magnetic resonance imaging (MRI) is a non-invasive diagnostic method with which high resolution images of the testes can be obtained. By measuring the

Correspondence: Dr Carsten Thomsen, Department of Magnetic Resonance, Hvidovre Hospital, DK 2650 Copenhagen, Denmark.

proton relaxation processes it may be possible to differentiate between normal and pathological tissue even if no lesion is seen in the images.

Magnetic resonance spectroscopy is another aspect of this technique where it is possible to obtain phosphorus spectra from the testes. To our knowledge *in vivo* spectroscopy of the human testis has not been reported previously.

The aims of the present study were: (1) to determine the T_1 and T_2 relaxation processes in patients with CIS and to compare them with those obtained from healthy subjects, and (2) to obtain phosphorus spectra from patients with CIS and controls in order to evaluate the possible role of MR in detecting CIS.

A number of studies (Araki *et al.*, 1984; Moore *et al.*, 1986) have shown that the T_1 relaxation time is prolonged in malignancy.

Material and Methods

Patients

Six patients with CIS, aged 24–37 years (median 26 years), and five healthy volunteers matched for age were included in the study. Of the six patients, three had been operated on previously for testicular cancer on the other side and the other three had a history of an undescended testis. The diagnosis of CIS was based on surgical biopsies in all cases (Skakkebæk *et al.*, 1982). The volunteers had no history of maldescended testes and were found to be normal on physical examination. All had fathered children. The study has been approved by the local ethical committee.

MR investigations

The study was carried out on a Siemens Magnetom whole body MR scanner, operating at 1.5 Tesla. The testes were imaged using a spin echo sequence with a repetition time (TR) of 1.8 s and echo times (TE) of 30 and 90 ms. The slice thickness was 7 mm and the matrix size 256 × 256 giving a voxel size of 1.2 × 1.2 × 7 mm^3.

T_1 relaxation processes. Twelve inversion recovery pulse sequences were applied with the repetition time varying from 0.24 to 8 s. Inversion time was kept constant at 150 ms. The echo time of the 180° rephasing pulse was 30 ms.

T_2 relaxation processes. A combined Carr-Purcell and Carr-Purcell-Meibom-Gill multiple spin echo pulse sequence with thirty-two echoes was applied. The echoes were read out at 30 ms intervals from 30 to 960 ms. The repetition time was 6 s.

Phosphorus spectroscopy was performed with a surface-coil placed over the testis, a 90° pulse was applied and the free induction decay signal was read out after a delay of 1 ms. In the volunteers both testes were examined using an 8 cm surface coil. In the patients, the testes with CIS were examined using a 4 cm surface coil. To increase the signal-to-noise ratio, 512 samples were obtained with a repetition time of 8 s giving a total acquisition time of 70 min.

Calculations and statistics

Assuming a simple mono-exponential model, T_1 was calculated from the following formula (Hendrick, Nelson & Hendee, 1984):

$$S\alpha\varrho(H) \times e^{-TE/T_2}[1 - 2e^{-TI/T_1} + 2e^{-(TR-TE/2)/T_1} - e^{-TR/T_1}]$$

where S = MR signal, $\varrho(H)$ = proton density, TI = inversion time, TR = repetition time, and TE = echo time of the rephasing 180° pulse.

For the bi-exponential analyses, the signal was the sum of the two expressions as above. T_2 was calculated from

$$S\alpha\varrho(H) \times e^{-TE/T_2}[1 - 2e^{-(TR-TE/2)/T_1} + e^{-(TR+TE)/T_2}]$$

The MR signal used for evaluation of the relaxation processes was read out from a central region of interest (2×2 cm^2) in the testis.

A bi-exponential model for T_1 or T_2 was accepted if the ratio between the unexplained variance for the mono- and bi-exponential fit was significant in an F-test at the 1% level.

Comparison between the results obtained from the two different testes in the normals was done using a linear correlation analysis. Mann-Whitney rank sum test for unpaired samples was used for comparison between groups, the normals contributing with the mean value for both sides.

Results

The testis and epididymis were, in all cases, well demonstrated using the spin echo sequence described above (Figs. 1 and 2). Focal lesions were not seen in any of the patients with CIS. However, in one patient (no. 0272) with unilateral CIS and fibrosis the testis was small and had an inhomogeneous signal intensity. A similar

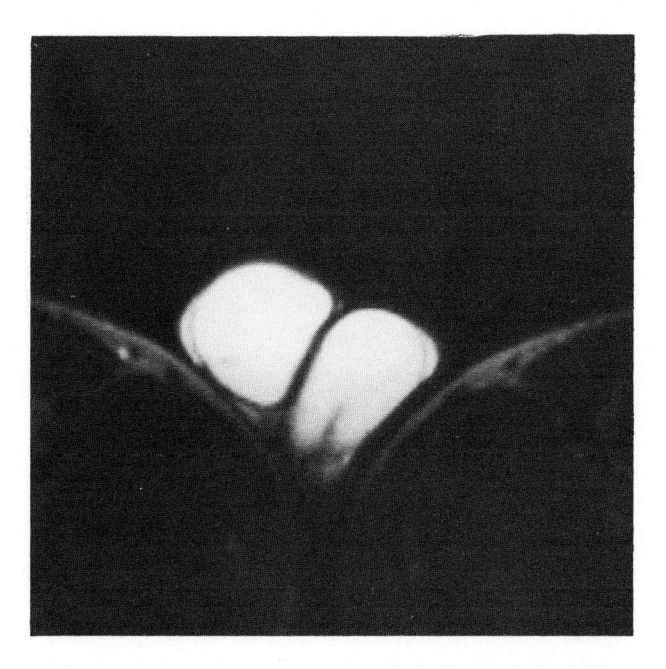

Fig. 1. MR image of the testes in the axial plane from a normal volunteer. On the left side (image left) the epididymis is clearly seen below the testis. On the right side the rete testis is seen as an area with decreased signal intensity. Below this the epididymis is seen.

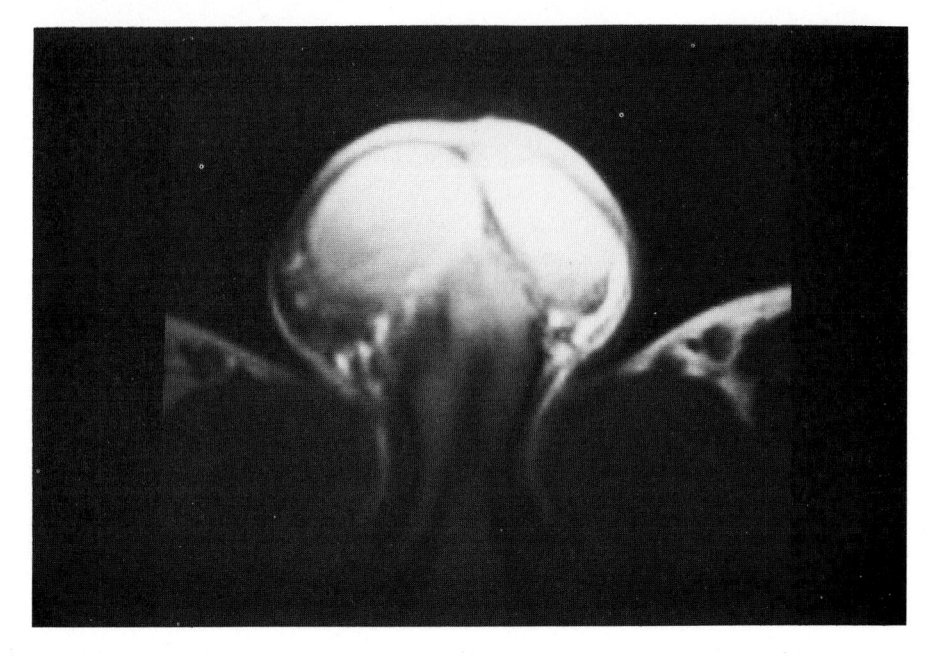

Fig. 2. MR image of the testes from patient 0272 with carcinoma-in-situ, fibrosis and atrophy of the right testis (image right). The right testis is small with inhomogeneous signal intensity. The left testis is normal.

signal pattern was obtained from one testis of patient no. 0222; this testis was contralateral to the one with CIS and had pronounced fibrosis (Fig. 2 and Table 1).

The longitudinal T_1 relaxation process differed from a mono-exponential function in all but one case (no. 0222): a bi-exponential model was therefore applied. The results of these analyses are seen in Table 1. The correlation between the fast component, $T_{1,fast}$, obtained from the right and the left testis in the normals was 0.997 ($P < 0.01$): the corresponding figure for the slow component, $T_{1,slow}$, was 0.860 ($P < 0.10$). Fig. 3 shows the slow component, $T_{1,slow}$, from the normals and patients: the results obtained in the contralateral testis are also shown. It is seen that the $T_{1,slow}$ is significantly prolonged in the testes with CIS ($P < 0.01$). The $T_{1,slow}$ values from the contralateral testes of the patients were within the range of the normals except in one case where histological examination showed oedema of the testis.

The transverse relaxation process did, in all cases, fit to a mono-exponential function, the time constants T_2 being seen in Fig. 4 and Table 1. It is seen that the T_2 times for the patients were lower than the values obtained in the normals ($P < 0.05$). The correlation between the values for T_2 obtained on the right and the left side in the normals was statistically significant ($r = 0.940$, $P < 0.05$). The T_2 time from the contralateral testis of the three patients in whom this was measured was below the range of the normals. In all three cases other pathologies were seen histologically in these contralateral testes.

Spectroscopy was carried out in four volunteers. All spectra showed the same pattern (Fig. 5) with a large sugar phosphate/2,3-diphosphoglycerate peak. These

Table 1. MRI findings compared to pathological findings in human testes.

No.	Right testis Biopsy	MRI	$T_{1,fast}$	%	$T_{1,slow}$	%	T_2	Left testis Biopsy	MRI	$T_{1,fast}$	%	$T_{1,slow}$	%	T_2	Comments
0222	Carcinoma-in-situ	No focal lesions, normal size	—	0	1802	100	189	Atrophy and fibrosis	Inhomogeneous, small	—	0	1289	100	105	Left side cryptorchism
0272	Atrophy, fibrosis, carcinoma-in-situ	Inhomogeneous, small	181	39	2667	61	109	Normal spermatogenesis, oedema	No focal lesions, normal size	147	41	2956	59	181	Right side cryptorchism
0321								Carcinoma-in-situ	No focal lesions, normal size	249	26	2404	74	222	Right side testicular cancer, operated
0353								Fibrosis, carcinoma-in-situ	No focal lesions, normal size	99	24	1594	65	232	Right side testicular seminoma, operated
0508	Atrophy, carcinoma-in-situ	No focal lesions, small	137	25	1673	75	222	Atrophy	No focal lesions, small	144	20	1559	80	160	Right side cryptorchism
0510								Carcinoma-in-situ	No focal lesions, normal size	150	20	1627	80	183	Right side testicular cancer
0652			135	16	1438	84	264		No focal lesions, normal size	130	14	1382	86	254	Normal volunteer
0653		No focal lesions, normal size	115	22	1501	78	199		No focal lesions, normal size	112	29	1574	71	216	Normal volunteer
0682		No focal lesions, normal size	103	52	1295	48	234		No focal lesions, normal size	104	48	1298	62	234	Normal volunteer
0683		No focal lesions, normal size	75	13	1157	87	264		No focal lesions, normal size	75	17	1238	73	263	Normal volunteer
0684		No focal lesions, normal size	129	25	1586	75	251		No focal lesions, normal size	125	25	1459	75	262	Normal volunteer

$T_{1,fast}$, $T_{1,slow}$: The fast and slow component in the T_1 relaxation process in ms. % gives the fraction of the two components. T_2: The T_2 relaxation time in ms.

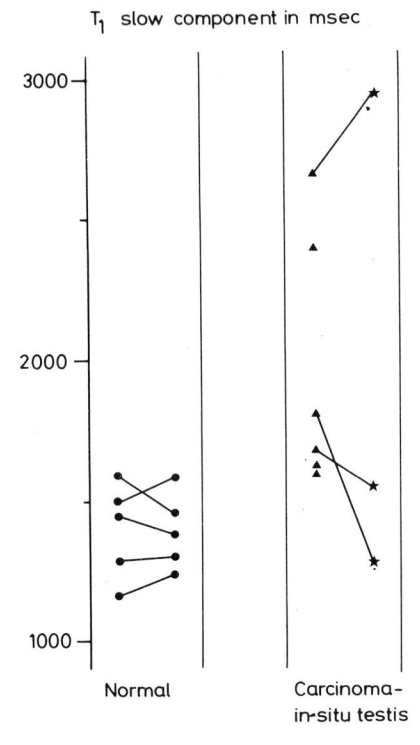

Fig. 3. The slow component of the T_1 relaxation process of the testes. In the normals the T_1 relaxation time is given for both testes, whereas in the patients the T_1 time is given for the testis with carcinoma-in-situ and the contralateral testis. ●—●, $T_{1,\text{slow}}$ relaxation time for the two testes in the normal volunteers. ▲—★, $T_{1,\text{slow}}$ relaxation time for testis with carcinoma-in-situ and the contralateral testis, respectively.

metabolites are known to be present in high concentrations in tissues with much metabolic activity and rapid growth.

By looking at the chemical shift of inorganic phosphate, the pH was calculated varying from 7.0 to 7.1 in the normal testes. In the three patients studied no phosphorous signal was obtained.

Discussion

The main results of the present study were a significantly longer $T_{1,\text{slow}}$ and a shorter T_2 relaxation time in testes with CIS as compared to normal testes.

The T_1 relaxation process showed a clearly multi-exponential pattern both in the patients and in the normals. By a bi-exponential analysis it was possible to get two components which in the normals showed a good correlation when the two tests were compared. The fast and slow components differed by a factor of about 10, and our experiences from phantom studies are that with a difference in this order it is possible to get an accurate estimation of the components and their relative weights.

The biological event underlying the multi-exponential T_1 relaxation process cannot be deduced from the present study. The T_2 relaxation process could be

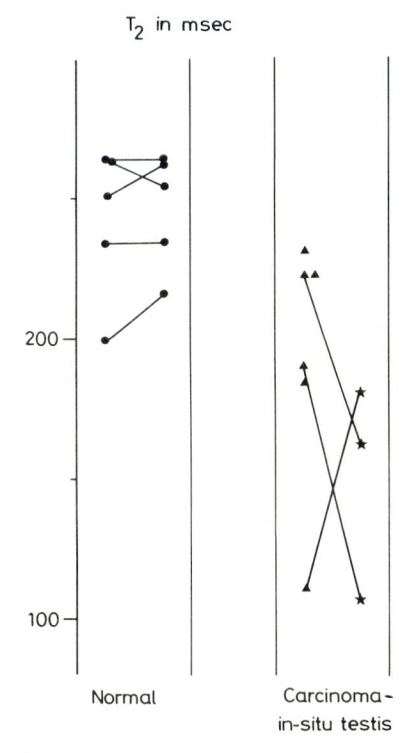

Fig. 4. The T_2 time of the testes. In the normals the T_2 relaxation time is given for both testes, and in the patients the T_2 time is given for the testis with carcinoma-in-situ and for the contralateral testis. ●—●, T_2 time for the two testes in the normal volunteers. ▲—★, T_2 time for the testis with carcinoma-in-situ and the contralateral testis, respectively.

described as a mono-exponential function. To get reliable estimation of the T_2 time in the multi-echo experiment, the repetition time, TR, has to be at least twice the T_1 time of the slow component.

We found no difference in the images between the patients with CIS and the normals. This is not surprising, as CIS is a diffuse non-invasive disorder of the germinative epithelium.

The spectra from the normal testes showed all the same pattern with a large sugar-phosphate/2,3-diphosphoglycerate peak which is characteristically seen in tissues with rapid cell growth and marked metabolic activity. It was not possible to get useful spectra from the patients with CIS, possibly due to a low concentration of phosphorus in these testes. Further studies have to be done in order to increase the sensitivity, for example by designing special coils for testicular spectroscopy.

Thus, these preliminary results indicate that measurements of the proton relaxation processes may give useful information about the patients at risk. It remains to be seen whether the findings are related to the neoplasia or the reduced spermatogenesis. To date no health hazards have been reported due to MR examination, and this technique might be suitable for screening investigations. In such studies it is necessary to take the multi-exponential T_1 behaviour into account.

Surgical procedure

Premedication was not regularly used as the patients themselves had to manage their transport home.

Local anaesthesia was established by means of a nerve block using 5 ml of 1% lidocaine around the spermatic vessels, and by means of infiltration anaesthesia with 1% lidocaine in the scrotal skin and Dartos layer.

All biopsies were done single-handedly by one of two urologists (E.B. or C.F.M.). The testis was held firmly by the other hand until the visceral layer of tunica vaginalis had been closed with a running baseball stitch after the biopsy. The Dartos layer and the skin were closed by continuous locked sutures. The first 38 patients were closed with absorbable sutures in the skin (catgut or Dexon), but thereafter we changed to nonabsorbable sutures.

All statistical analyses were performed using the chi-square test.

Results

Three patients were lost to follow-up, and replies were received from 150 (73%) of the 206 patients contacted.

According to the questionnaire, 72% of the patients expressed no desire for admittance to hospital nor for general anaesthesia, whereas the other 28% would have preferred hospital admittance for general anaesthesia (Table 1). A significant number of the patients wanting hospitalization complained of discomfort during the procedure. Analysis of the data suggests that the unpleasant sensation in the flanks caused by traction of the spermatic cord during the procedure was significantly related to the feeling of insufficient local anaesthesia ($P < 0.01$).

Table 1. The effects of testicular biopsy as an outpatient procedure reported by 150 patients responding to the questionnaire

Adverse side effects	Outpatient procedure acceptable (108 patients; 72%)	Outpatient procedure not acceptable (42 patients; 28%)	Significance between the two groups*
Sense of insufficient local anaesthesia	22 (20%)	22 (52%)	$P < 0.001$
Unpleasant flank sensation during cord traction	42 (39%)	33 (79%)	$P < 0.001$
Minor postoperative complications	35 (32%)	20 (48%)	$P > 0.05$

*Chi-square test

Postoperative pain in the wound lasted from a few hours up to 30 days with a median duration of 3.5 days. However, the median absence from work did not exceed 1 day.

Three patients were admitted postoperatively to hospital to ensure adequate drainage of pus from the scrotal sac.

Superficial serous exudation, or localized induration around the stitch puncture sites, was encountered in 23% of the patients, but an established wound infection was only seen in a few patients, and this could be handled on an outpatient basis. These cases and those with local swelling or bleeding from cicatrix are listed under 'minor complications' in Table 1.

When we adopted nonresorbable skin sutures, the wound afflictions were significantly reduced from 41% to 17% ($P < 0.01$). Two patients received penicillin as prophylaxis after a troublesome biopsy. In addition, fifteen patients received penicillin postoperatively; two patients because of suspected epididymal infection. Persistent sequela caused by the biopsy were not encountered.

Discussion

Apart from a single case with a temporary haematoma in the spermatic cord, we are not aware of any complications due to the local anaesthesia.

Concerning the biopsy technique, no serious complications were encountered and no complications could be ascribed to the outpatient procedure as such.

Seventy-two per cent of the patients found the method acceptable, and the absenteeism from work was minimal compared to the procedure being carried out with hospitalization.

Transseptal orchidopexy (Ombrédanne, 1910) has been the surgical method used most frequently in our patients for the previous correction of their maldescended testis. In cases where the biopsy incision was performed over the epididymis and where it was impossible to rotate the testis within the scrotum because of adhesions, we found the best solution was to widen the scrotal incision and exteriorize the testis. The biopsy was then easily performed, although a little more infiltration anaesthesia was sometimes needed, but the procedures have been without complications.

An unpleasant sensation in the flanks seems to be an inherent feature of our biopsy method. It is possible that nursing assistance during the biopsy or use of premedication could minimize this inconvenience, but not without a certain consumption of resources, especially if costs of transportation become a part of the procedure.

In conclusion, we find the results and complications from testicular biopsy as an outpatient procedure comparable with similar operations upon hospitalized patients. However, both for society and for the patients, the outpatient procedure implies considerable cost savings.

Acknowledgement

This study was supported by The Danish Cancer Society, grants 84-007, 87-017, 86-044 and 86-065 and by P. Carl Petersen's fund, grant B1322.

References

Blandy, J. (1976) Technique of testicular biopsy. *Urology*, pp. 1262–1263. Blackwell Scientific Publications, Oxford.

Ombrédanne, L. (1910) Indications et technique de l'orchiopexie transscrotale chez l'enfant. *Presse Medicale*, **18**, 745–750.

Rowley, M. J. & Heller, C. G. (1966) The testicular biopsy: surgical procedure, fixation, and staining techniques. *Fertility and Sterility*, **17**, 177–186.

Discussion

Hargreave One reason given in the UK for not doing a testicular biopsy in cryptorchids or in the contralateral testis of tumour patients is that the procedure may leave a palpable lump in the testis and this may make follow-up clinical or ultrasound examination very difficult. Would you care to comment?

Bruun We have not performed clinical follow-up after the biopsy. We are aware of only one patient complaining of a little fibrosis at the site of the biopsy.

Schraffordt Koops Is it not possible to do a needle biopsy rather than an open biopsy?

Bruun We have performed a Trucut core biopsy and aspiration of testicular tissue concomittant with the surgical biopsy, but the material has not yet been evaluated.

Skakkebæk We have had a look at Dr Bruun's material comparing the Trucut biopsy with the routine surgical biopsy and we have seen the CIS lesion. But we have only looked at five cases so far so we cannot yet assess how reliable is this method.

Incidence of bilateral testicular germ cell cancer in Denmark, 1960–84: preliminary findings

ANNE ØSTERLIND,[1] J. G. BERTHELSEN,[2] N. ABILDGAARD,[3] S. O. HANSEN,[4] H. JENSEN,[5] B. JOHANSEN,[6] J. MUNCK-HANSEN[7] and L. H. RASMUSSEN[5]   [1]*The Danish Cancer Registry, Institute of Cancer Epidemiology under the Danish Cancer Society, Copenhagen,* [2]*Laboratory of Reproductive Biology, Rigshospitalet and Department of Gynaecology and Obstetrics, Herlev Hospital, Copenhagen,* [3]*Department of Oncology, The Municipal Hospital, Aarhus,* [4]*Department of Oncology, Odense Hospital, Odense,* [5]*Department of Oncology, Finsen Institute, Copenhagen,* [6]*Department of Oncology, Aalborg Hospital, Aalborg, and* [7]*Department of Oncology, Herlev Hospital, Copenhagen, Denmark*

Summary

The incidence of a second primary testicular germ cell cancer in the contralateral testicle among 2338 men with a first primary testicular germ cell cancer diagnosed in the years 1960–79 in Denmark was established in this preliminary report. The material represents 83% of the total cohort followed until 31 December 1984. The relative risk for a patient with testicular cancer to get yet another testicular cancer was studied, taking into account the histology of the first primary testicular germ cell cancer. Based on fifty-eight nonsimultaneous contralateral testicular cancer cases and 19,995 'person-years at risk', the overall relative risk of invasive germ cell cancer in the contralateral testicle following a first germ cell testicular cancer was found to be 23.3 (95% confidence interval: 18–30). Among men with nonseminoma the risk was higher (relative risk = 27.5) than among men with seminomas (relative risk = 20.1). Overall, sixty-two (2.7%) patients developed a second cancer. In four of these patients bilateral tumours occurred simultaneously.

Key words. Cancer incidence, germ cell cancer, bilateral testicular cancer.

Introduction

Patients with testicular germ cell cancer have an increased risk of developing a new primary cancer in the contralateral testis as well (Kleinerman, Liebermann & Li, 1985; Østerlind, Rørth & Prener, 1985). The incidence of bilateral cancer has been reported, mostly in hospital-based series, to be 1–5% (Pugh, 1976; Sokal, Peckham & Hendry, 1980; Dieckmann *et al.*, 1986), and only a few population based studies have been reported (Kleinerman *et al.*, 1985; Østerlind *et al.*, 1985). Reporting to cancer registries of multiple cancer in the same individual is, however, often

Correspondence: Dr A. Østerlind, The Danish Cancer Registry, Institute of Cancer Epidemiology under the Danish Cancer Society, Landskronagade 66, 4th floor, DK-2100 Copenhagen, Denmark.

deficient (Storm *et al.*, 1986) and may be suspected to be so in particular for paired organs. A second explanation for the low incidence reported from the registry material is the coding practice. In the registry material, bilateral nonsimultaneous testicular tumours with identical histology are recorded as one tumour with the date of the first cancer taken as the date of diagnosis. Therefore only cases in whom the morphology of the first and of the second primary tumours are different were included in the analysis reported (Østerlind *et al.*, 1985). The true incidence of bilateral cancer is unknown since no long-term large cohort studies with validation of nationwide and unselected material has been reported. Furthermore, the figures available in the population based studies do not take into account the histology of the first tumour and only a few studies take into account the length of observation after the first tumour.

We therefore found it relevant to evaluate the incidence of bilateral testicular cancer in Denmark. A population based cohort study is feasible in Denmark where the national Cancer Registry has recorded practically all primary testicular cancers since 1943 and where the treatment of testicular cancer is centralized at five oncological centres.

The present report gives preliminary results from a study of the incidence of contralateral testicular germ cell cancer in men who had their first primary testicular cancer diagnosed in the years 1960–79 in Denmark.

Material and Methods

All notified testicular germ cell cancer cases diagnosed between 1 January 1960 and 31 December 1979 were included in the study. The records of these cases were identified in the registry card file from where the personal data were drawn. A few additional patients were found in the files of the oncological centres during the investigation.

For each case information on treatment and stage was abstracted from the hospital records and to verify the testicular germ cell cancer diagnoses, pathology reports were examined (Table 1). Through these hospital records and by the use of

Table 1. Some clinical data of the 2338 testicular cancer patients where follow-up has been completed

Histology	Stage	No. of patients	Age (years), mean	No. of person-years
Seminoma	I	890		
	II	226		
	III	62		
	Unknown	44		
All seminoma		1,222	41.3	12,293
Nonseminoma	I	631		
	II	216		
	III	235		
	Unknown	34		
All nonseminoma		1,116	31.8	7,702

the Danish Central Population Register, death certificates and autopsy reports each patient was followed until: (1) time of the diagnosis of a germ cell cancer in the contralateral testicle, (2) 31 December 1984 if there was no evidence of a contralateral tumour, (3) date of death or emigration, (4) date of removal of the contralateral testis for a reason other than germ cell cancer.

Person-years at risk were calculated from time of diagnosis of the first testicular cancer until one of the four above-mentioned events, whichever occurred first. Expected numbers of testicular cancer were computed by multiplying the person-years at risk in 5-year age and calendar periods with the corresponding incidence rates for testicular cancer in all of Denmark, thereby adjusting indirectly for age and calendar time effects when summed over the cells (Monson, 1974). Relative risks were obtained by dividing the observed by the expected number of cases and 95% confidence limits of relative risks calculated, assuming a Poisson distribution (Rothman & Boice, 1982).

Results

Among the 2338 men for whom the records are completed (83%), sixty-two developed a contralateral cancer within the follow-up time of 5–25 years (Fig. 1, Table 2). The median time interval between first and second tumour was 3.7 years for patients with a seminoma as first tumour and 4.7 years for patients with a nonseminoma as the first tumour. This difference is not statistically significant (Mann-Whitney test). Three seminoma patients and one nonseminoma patient had the second tumour diagnosed simultaneously with the first, while the longest observed interval between the two tumours was 20 years in a patient with a nonseminoma as first and second tumour.

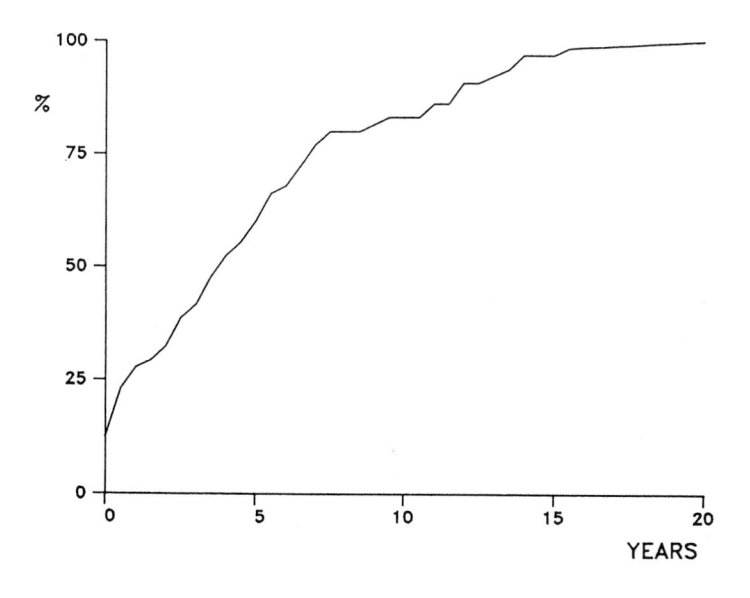

Fig. 1. Time interval between first and second testicular germ cell cancer (cumulative percentage).

Table 2. Number of contralateral testicular cancer cases by histology and time since a first testicular germ cell cancer

Histology	Simultaneous	Years since first testicular cancer				Total
		< 1	1–4	5–9	10+	
Seminoma	3	4	11	7	6	31
Nonseminoma	1	3	10	12	5	31

Based on the presently available data from the 2338 men with a total of 19,995 person-years at risk, the preliminary overall relative risk has been calculated to be 23.3 (95% confidence interval: 18–30) (Fig. 2). For patients with a seminoma as the first tumour, the relative risk was found to be 20.1 (95% confidence interval: 13–29), while for patients with a nonseminoma as the first tumour, a relative risk of 27.5 (95% confidence interval: 18–39) was found. The relative risk of developing a second cancer is increased in all time periods and did not vary by time after initial diagnosis (Fig. 2). The lifetime risk of developing a germ cell tumour is approximately 0.6% in Danish men (Prener & Østerlind, 1985). The lifetime risk of developing a second tumour in these men has not yet been calculated.

Of the thirty-one patients with a seminoma as the first tumour, twenty-three also had a seminoma as the second tumour, while nineteen of thirty-one patients had a nonseminoma both as first and second tumour.

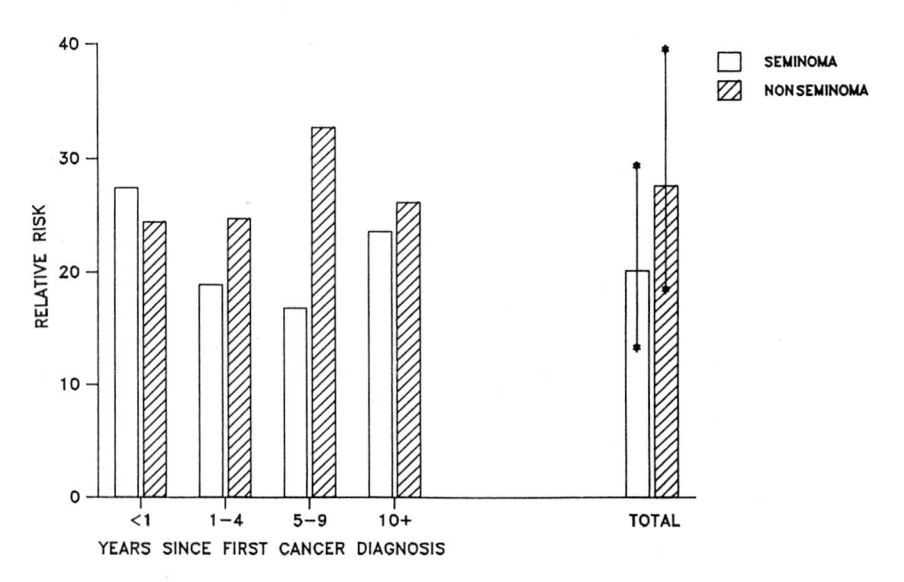

Fig. 2. Relative risk of contralateral cancer, by histology of the first tumour and time since the first testicular cancer.

Discussion

The present cohort study shows that at least sixty-two of 2338 Danish men (2.7%) with a testicular germ cell cancer develop a contralateral cancer within an observation period up to 25 years. This incidence is in accordance with those previously found in the often smaller hospital-based studies. However, in the large population based studies less than 1% of the testicular cancer patients were recorded with a contralateral testicular cancer. This lower estimate is expected and explainable by the deficient reporting of multiple tumours (Storm *et al.*, 1986) and limitations in the coding practice in the registry (Østerlind *et al.*, 1985). For the above-mentioned reasons the relative risk of 23.3 found in our study is also higher than those previously reported.

Although the follow-up of the patients has been very thorough, the sixty-two bilateral cases may represent a minimum estimate figure for development of neoplasia for the following reasons: (1) potent chemotherapeutic treatment for the first tumour may have eradicated some early stages of contralateral tumours (von der Maase, Giwercman & Skakkebæk, 1986), (2) some patients may have died with an unrecognized tumour in the contralateral testis, (3) we may have missed some contralateral tumours in the follow-up. The presently available results do not allow any conclusion as to whether radiotherapy for the first cancer increases the risk of a tumour in the contralateral testis. Neither is it possible to show whether potent chemotherapy for the first cancer decreases the risk for a contralateral tumour.

The incidence of testicular germ cell cancer in Denmark is higher than in most other countries (Waterhouse *et al.*, 1982). Whatever is the cause of this may also increase the incidence of a tumour in the contralateral testis and thereby cause a higher risk of bilateral testicular tumours in Denmark than in most other countries.

The present study confirms that men with testicular germ cell cancer are at an increased risk of developing a new clinically manifest primary cancer of the contralateral testis. The preliminary estimate of the risk of developing a tumour in the contralateral testis is 23 times the normal risk of developing testicular cancer.

Acknowledgments

We wish to thank the large number of clinical departments who have willingly placed their case records at our disposal. We wish to thank Andrea Meehrsohn for data processing assistance, Aase Larsen for preparing the graphs and Pia Kristiansen for preparing the manuscript.

References

Dieckmann, K.-P., Boeckmann, W., Brosig, W., Jonas, D. & Bauer, H.-W. (1986) Bilateral testicular germ cell tumors. Report of nine cases and review of the literature. *Cancer*, **57**, 1254–1258.

Kleinerman, R. A., Liebermann, J. V. & Li, F. P. (1985) Second cancer following cancer of male genital system in Connecticut, 1935–82. *National Cancer Institute Monograph*, **68**, 139–148.

Monson, R. R. (1974) Analysis of relative survival and proportional mortality. *Computer and Biomedical Research*, **7**, 325–332

Prener, A. & Østerlind, A. (1985) Cancer in Denmark. A summary description of selected cancers. The Danish Cancer Registry under the Danish Cancer Society, Copenhagen.

Pugh, R. C. B. (1976) *Pathology of the Testis*. Blackwell Scientific Publications, Oxford.

Rothman, K. J. & Boice, J. D., Jr (1982) Epidemiologic analysis with a programmable calculator. Epidemiology Resources Inc., Boston.

Sokal, M., Peckham, M. J. & Hendry, W. F. (1980) Bilateral germ cell tumours of the testis. *British Journal of Urology*, **52**, 158–162.

Storm, H. H., Lynge, E., Østerlind, A. & Jensen, O. M. (1986) Multiple primary cancers in Denmark 1943–80, influence of possbile underreporting and suggested risk factors. *Yale Journal of Biology and Medicine* (in press).

von der Maase, H., Giwercman, A. & Skakkebæk, N. E. (1986) Radiation treatment of carcinoma-in-situ of testis. *Lancet*, **i**, 624–625.

Waterhouse, J. A. H., Muir, C. S., Shangumaratnam, K. & Powell, J. (ed.) (1982) Cancer incidence in five continents. IV. *IARC Scientific Publications*, No. 42, IARC, Lyon.

Østerlind, A., Rørth, M. & Prener, A. (1985) Second cancer following cancer of the male genital system in Denmark, 1943–80. *National Cancer Institute Monograph*, **68**, 341–347.

Management of carcinoma-in-situ of the testis

H. VON DER MAASE,[1,2] A. GIWERCMAN,[3] J. MÜLLER[3] and N. E. SKAKKEBÆK[3,4] [1]*Department of Oncology ONB, Finsen Institute, Rigshospitalet,* [2]*Department of Oncology, Herlev University Hospital,* [3]*Laboratory of Reproductive Biology, Rigshospitalet, and* [4]*University Department of Paediatrics, Hvidovre Hospital, Copenhagen, Denmark*

Summary

Carcinoma-in-situ (CIS) of the testis progresses to invasive cancer within 5 years in 50% of cases, and therefore requires therapeutic intervention. CIS is probably eradicated by intensive cancer chemotherapy but this is too toxic for the management of non-invasive disease. Eight patients with unilateral testicular cancer and contralateral CIS received localized irradiation (20 Gy in ten fractions of 2 Gy) to the remaining testis: after 3 months the CIS cells had disappeared and 'Sertoli-cell-only' tubules were found. LH and FSH levels were elevated but testosterone levels remained fairly constant. Localized irradiation should be considered as the treatment of CIS in the contralateral testis of testicular tumour patients unless chemotherapy is indicated for the primary tumour.

Unilateral orchidectomy is recommended for unilateral CIS associated with infertility or testicular maldescent. Localized testicular irradiation should now be considered for bilateral disease. Patients with the androgen insensitivity syndrome should normally be treated with bilateral orchidectomy, but irradiation may be useful in selected cases.

Key words. Carcinoma-in-situ, germ cell cancer, testicular neoplasm.

Introduction

Carcinoma-in-situ (CIS) of the testis represents a characteristic pattern of intratubular atypical germ cells (Skakkebæk, 1972a, b, 1978; Nüesch-Bachmann & Hedinger, 1977a). The risk for CIS to progress to invasive growth has been estimated to be about 50% within 5 years (Skakkebæk, Berthelsen & Müller, 1982; von der Maase *et al.*, 1986a). Spontaneous disappearance of CIS has never been documented, but it is still not known whether all cases of CIS will progress into invasive growth or if some cases may persist as intratubular disease. However, the risk of progression to invasive tumour has justified the change from the early 'wait-and-see' policy to therapeutic intervention either by immediate orchidectomy or by some other form of treatment. The aim of the following review is to elucidate the present guidelines for the management of CIS of the testis depending on the patient category in question.

Correspondence: Dr Hans von der Maase, Department of Oncology ONB, Finsen Institute, Rigshospitalet, DK-2100 Copenhagen, Denmark.

Carcinoma-in-situ of the testis in infertile men

The incidence of CIS in testicular biopsies from infertile men has been reported to be from 0.55% (Nüesch-Bachmann & Hedinger, 1977) to 1.1% (Skakkebæk, 1978) The CIS changes may progress into either seminomatous or nonseminomatous invasive tumour (Nüesch-Bachmann & Hedinger, 1977; Skakkebæk, 1978) or local invasion into the interstitial tissue may occur at a stage in which they cannot be identified as either seminomatous or nonseminomatous tumour cells—a phenomenon denoted as early invasive growth (Skakkebæk et al., 1982).

Before knowing the natural history of CIS in these patients, the general management of infertile men with CIS was by careful follow-up at 3-monthly physical examination. Orchidectomy was then performed at the first sign of invasive growth. However, in 1978 Skakkebæk & Berthelsen recommended removal of the testis as soon as a diagnosis of CIS was made. This recommendation was based on the data reported by Nüesch-Bachmann & Hedinger (1977) and Skakkebæk (1978) showing development of nine germ cell tumours in eighteen testes after a period of 1 month to 6 years following the diagnosis of CIS. Thereafter immediate orchidectomy has been the management of CIS in our institutions for this group of patients.

Immediate or subsequent orchidectomy is, however, inappropriate in patients with bilateral CIS, as has been observed in three of seventeen infertile men in whom bilateral biopsies were performed (Sigg & Hedinger, 1981; Skakkebæk et al., 1982). The high frequency of bilateral CIS indicates that all patients with CIS of one testis should always have a testicular biopsy performed on the other side. If the contralateral testicular biopsy is free of CIS, the condition may be considered as truly unilateral as none of approximately 1000 infertile men without CIS have developed a testicular cancer within an observation period of up to 8 years (Skakkebæk et al., 1982). In such unilateral cases of CIS where sufficient androgen production can be expected from the other testis, the recommended treatment is still immediate orchidectomy. However, an alternative approach should be considered for cases of bilateral CIS in order to avoid subsequent androgen insufficiency. This matter will be discussed in detail below in relation to the management of CIS of the contralateral testis in patients with unilateral testicular germ cell cancer where attempts should also be made to preserve testicular tissue.

Carcinoma-in-situ of the maldescended testis

CIS of the testis has been demonstrated in patients with a maldescended testis (Waxman, 1976; Williams & Brendler, 1977; Dorman et al., 1979) or with a history of previously corrected cryptorchidism (Skakkebæk, 1972b; Krabbe et al., 1979). In the study by Krabbe et al. (1979) testicular biopsies revealed CIS in four of fifty men previously treated for undescended testes. In patients with unilateral testicular cancer and CIS in the remaining contralateral testis, cryptorchidism had been present unilaterally or bilaterally in about half of the cases (Berthelsen et al., 1982). Thus, cryptorchid patients represent a group at risk of having CIS of the testis, although the exact magnitude of that risk is as yet unknown. Nor is the natural progression of CIS in this group of patients known. However, there is no reason to believe that the risk of developing a testicular cancer in this patient category is different from that of 50% within 5 years observed for other patient categories with CIS of the testis (Skakkebæk et al., 1982; von der Maase et al., 1986a).

Ipsilateral orchidectomy should be performed for the presence of unilateral CIS of the testis of postpubertal boys or men soon after the diagnosis has been made. If, as occasionally occurs, CIS is diagnosed in a prepubertal boy it may be sufficient to institute close follow-up and confirm the diagnosis in a repeat biopsy after puberty before performing an orchidectomy. The treatment policy for bilateral CIS of cryptorchid patients has been bilateral orchidectomy. However, we now recommend localized bilateral irradiation of the testes as an alternative therapy in such cases (see below).

Carcinoma-in-situ of the contralateral testis in patients with unilateral testicular germ cell cancer

From July 1972 to June 1986, CIS of the contralateral testis was diagnosed in thirty-four of 600 patients with unilateral testicular germ cell cancer (5.7%), an incidence which has been consistent throughout the study (Berthelsen et al., 1979, 1982; von der Maase et al., 1986a). This group of patients with CIS is characterized by a high frequency of cases with a small testicular volume of 12 ml or less, and/or a history of cryptorchidism (Berthelsen et al., 1982). Otherwise, patient characteristics do not differ from those of the population of patients with testicular cancer in general (von der Maase et al., 1986a).

The risk of developing a contralateral testicular cancer when CIS is present in the remaining testis has been estimated at being 40% within 3 years, and 50% within 5 years (von der Maase et al., 1986a). These calculations were based on the development of contralateral testicular cancer in seven of nineteen untreated patients. One further patient has now developed a contralateral tumour 30 months after the initial orchidectomy at which time a simultaneous diagnosis of CIS of the contralateral testis was made. This patient neglected the recommended close follow-up and reappeared with a grossly enlarged testis and markedly elevated pre-operative serum alphafetoprotein concentration. Orchidectomy was performed revealing a mixed germ cell tumour containing seminoma and elements of endodermal sinus tumour. Alphafetoprotein levels returned to normal post-operative levels and routine staging procedures did not reveal any signs of metastases.

Thus, a total of eight out of nineteen patients have developed a contralateral cancer, either as early invasive growth, or as seminomatous or nonseminomatous tumour. The second tumour in all patients has been classified as stage I and has probably been cured by orchidectomy alone (von der Maase et al., 1986a). Development of a contralateral testicular cancer has only occurred in untreated patients, whereas invasive growth has not been observed in ten patients receiving chemotherapy for their initial testicular cancer (median observation time 25 months, range 4–96 months). None of the 566 patients without CIS in the screening biopsy of the remaining testis has developed a contralateral testicular tumour (median observation time 45 months, range 1–101 months).

Patients with CIS of the contralateral testis receiving chemotherapy for the initial testicular cancer should be offered continuous clinical surveillance including follow-up biopsies, but without further specific treatment for the CIS itself. The strategy for management of patients with CIS not receiving chemotherapy is, however, more controversial. One could choose either to continue the 'wait-and-see' policy and perform an orchidectomy at the first sign of invasive growth or perform an orchidectomy immediately after the diagnosis of CIS. It is, however, important, if at all possible, to avoid a second orchidectomy which results in subsequent androgen insufficiency. Presently, two treatment strategies seem to be of potential interest in this respect: systemic cancer chemotherapy and localized irradiation of the testis.

Systemic cancer chemotherapy
Intensive chemotherapy given for the initial testicular cancer eradicates CIS from the contralateral testis (von der Maase et al., 1985, 1986a). Ten patients have received combination chemotherapy based on the drugs cisplatin (cis-diamminedichloroplatinum II), vinblastine and bleomycin (PVB). Eight of these patients have had one or more follow-up biopsies performed after cessation of the chemotherapy and in all these cases the CIS changes had disappeared. However, these biopsy specimens have contained small areas of germ cells which may indicate that a few CIS cells have also survived the treatment. In fact, the possibility of relapse in these patients should be expected, as development of contralateral germ cell tumours has been observed despite prior or on-going intensive chemotherapy for the initial cancer (Fowler et al., 1979). This would also be in accordance with the report by Greist et al. (1984) which provided evidence that the testis, as for childhood acute leukaemia, may act as a sanctuary during intensive chemotherapy with PVB for disseminated testicular germ cell cancer. Even intensive chemotherapy may thus not be sufficient to avoid eventual progression of CIS and, moreover, such treatment is too toxic for the management of pre-invasive disease. Chemotherapy should consequently only be given if indicated because of dissemination of the initial testicular cancer and not because of CIS of the contralateral testis.

Localized irradiation of the testis
In May 1985 we started to investigate the efficacy of localized irradiation for CIS of the testis (von der Maase, Giwercman & Skakkebæk, 1986b). Radiotherapy was given as 14–18 MeV electrons to the scrotum placed in a cup of lead. The total dose was 20 Gy delivered as ten fractions of 2 Gy, five fractions per week. Eight patients with unilateral testicular cancer have received localized irradiation for CIS of the contralateral testis. All patients have had a minimum observation time of 3 months and selected data from these patients are given in Table 1. A follow-up biopsy at about 3 months after irradiation has revealed that the CIS changes had disappeared in all eight cases. The seminiferous tubules were well preserved, but only Sertoli cells and no germ cells nor CIS cells were present within the tubules. The Leydig cells were morphologically normal (Fig. 1). Compared with the pretreatment values, the serum LH and FSH values were elevated 3–4 months after irradiation in most cases, whereas the serum testosterone values were not significantly changed in any of the patients (Table 1). Three of the patients have reached an observation time of 12 months with a continuous unchanged serum testosterone value. None of

Table 1. Data from eight patients receiving localized irradiation for carcinoma-in-situ of the testis

Patient identification	Age (years)	Histological diagnosis of follow-up biopsy 3 months after irradiation	Serum testosterone (nmol/l) Before irradiation	Serum testosterone (nmol/l) 3–4 months after irradiation	Serum LH (IU/l) Before irradiation	Serum LH (IU/l) 3–4 months after irradiation	Serum FSH (IU/l) Before irradiation	Serum FSH (IU/l) 3–4 months after irradiation
4	45	Sertoli cell only	7.0	9.2	8.7	15.3	29	46
20	46	Sertoli cell only	15.6	15.5	6.7	12.4	22	29
21	29	Sertoli cell only	14.0	17.5	14.7	25.0	40	52
25	26	Sertoli cell only	24.8	28.6	10.2	15.3	26	36
26	27	Sertoli cell only	17.9	17.1	6.6	13.1	18	43
29	38	Sertoli cell only	7.7	15.4	7.5	12.4	16	26
30	31	Sertoli cell only	17.6	15.6	17.7	27.0	42	56
32	25	Sertoli cell only	13.5	11.9	27.0	27.0	37	34

95% reference for: serum testoterone: 10.3–27.4 nmol/l; serum LH: 1.5–10.5 IU/l; serum FSH: 1.1–7.9 IU/l.
Wilcoxon test for paired data: for serum testosterone: $P > 0.10$; serum LH: $P \leq 0.05$; serum FSH: $P \leq 0.05$.

the eight patients have complained of disturbance of libido or of other sexual dysfunctions, nor has the irradiation been associated with any discomfort.

Thus, the present radiation schedule seems to eradicate CIS of the testis without significantly affecting testosterone production. Recurrence of the CIS changes is not expected as no germ cells were present in the follow-up biopsies after irradiation. It is, of course, not possible to state categorically that germ cells are not present in small areas elsewhere in the testis, but the biopsy specimens are usually representative for the whole testis (Berthelsen & Skakkebæk, 1981). Nor do we expect a significant decrease in the Leydig cell function as the maximum effect on the testosterone production seems to occur within 3 months after irradiation (Tomic et al., 1983). The raised LH values may, however, represent subtle Leydig cell dysfunction. Alteration of Leydig cell function after a lower dose of radiation to the testis, in the range 2–10 Gy, has been reported (Rowley et al., 1974; Tomic et al., 1983; Shapiro et al., 1985). Whether this has long-term influence on the endocrine function has not yet been clarified and requires a longer observation time. We are at present making a more detailed ongoing evaluation of the endocrine function of the irradiated testis.

We recommend that all patients with unilateral testicular germ cell cancer should be offered a testicular biopsy. If the biopsy specimen is without CIS the risk of developing a contralateral cancer is negligible. Patients with CIS receiving chemotherapy because of dissemination of the initial testicular cancer should be offered continuous clinical control without further treatment. For patients with CIS not receiving chemotherapy it seems that we have devised an effective and non-toxic treatment, and these patients are now offered localized irradiation of the testis.

Carcinoma-in-situ of the testis in patients with androgen insensitivity (testicular feminization) syndrome
CIS of the testis in a patient with the androgen insensitivity syndrome was first described by Skakkebæk (1979) and Nogales et al. (1981). Subsequently, Müller & Skakkebæk (1984) have reported CIS in three of twelve patients with androgen insensitivity. These findings are in accordance with the fact that patients with the androgen insensitivity syndrome have an increased risk of developing germ cell tumours (Scully, 1981). Thus, we recommend gonadectomy when the diagnosis of androgen insensitivity syndrome has been established (Müller & Skakkebæk, 1984). However, the management of this group of individuals is difficult and further investigations are clearly needed to clarify whether localized irradiation of the testis has a place in the treatment of girls with the complete androgen insensitivity syndrome. This procedure would allow pubertal development and maintenance of sufficient levels of sex steroids throughout adulthood without oestrogen replacement therapy.

In summary, management of CIS of the testis depends on the patient category and whether CIS is found in one or both testes. Orchidectomy is the treatment of choice in unilateral cases of CIS whereas localized irradiation of the testes is an alternative treatment in bilateral cases. Similarly, localized irradiation of the testis should also be applied for CIS of the contralateral testis in patients with unilateral testicular cancer, with the exception that patients receiving chemotherapy because of dissemination of the initial testicular cancer should be offered continuous clinical monitoring without further treatment.

The ultimate goal in the management of CIS of the testis is to diagnose the disease early and to cure it by orchidectomy alone, or perhaps even to avoid orchidectomy by eradicating the CIS germ cells without causing unacceptable systemic side effects.

Acknowledgement
This study was supported by The Danish Cancer Society, grants 84-007, 87-017, 86-044 and 86-065 and by P. Carl Petersen's fund, grant B1322.

References
Berthelsen, J. G. & Skakkebæk, N. E. (1981) Distribution of carcinoma-in-situ in testes from infertile men. *International Journal of Andrology*, Suppl. 4, 172–184.
Berthelsen, J. G., Skakkebæk, N. E., Mogensen, P. & Sørensen, B. L. (1979) Incidence of carcinoma in situ of germ cells in contralateral testis of men with testicular tumours. *British Medical Journal*, ii, 363–364.
Berthelsen, J. G., Skakkebæk, N. E., von der Maase, H., Sørensen, B. L. & Mogensen, P. (1982) Screening for carcinoma in situ of the contralateral testis in patients with germinal testicular cancer. *British Medical Journal*, 285, 1683–1686.
Dorman, S., Trainer, T. D., Lefke, D. & Leadbetter, G. (1979) Incipient germ cell tumor in a cryptorchid testis. *Cancer*, 44, 1357–1362.
Fowler, J. E., Jr, Vugrin, D., Cvitkovic, E. & Whitmore, W. F., Jr (1979) Sequential bilateral germ cell tumors of the testis despite interval chemotherapy. *Journal of Urology*, 122, 421–425.
Greist, A., Einhorn, L. H., Williams, S. D., Donohue, J. P. & Rowland, R. G. (1984) Pathologic findings at orchiectomy following chemotherapy for disseminated testicular cancer. *Journal of Clinical Oncology*, 9, 1025–1027.
Krabbe, S., Skakkebæk, N. E., Berthelsen, J. G., Eyben, F. V., Volsted, P., Mauritzen, K., Eldrup, J. & Nielsen, A. H. (1979) High incidence of undetected neoplasia in maldescended testes. *Lancet*, i, 999–1000.
Müller, J. & Skakkebæk, N. E. (1984) Testicular carcinoma in situ in children with the androgen insensitivity (testicular feminization) syndrome. *British Medical Journal*, 288, 1419–1420.
Nogales, F. F., Jr, Toro, M., Ortega, I. & Fulwood, H. R. (1981) Bilateral incipient germ cell tumours of the testis in the incomplete testicular feminization syndrome. *Histopathology*, 5, 511–515.
Nüesch-Bachmann, I. H. & Hedinger, C. (1977) Atypische Spermatogonien als Präkanzerose. *Schweizerische Medizinische Wochenschrift*, 107, 795–801.
Rowley, M. J., Leach, D. R., Warner, G. A. & Heller, C. G. (1974) Effect of graded doses of ionizing radiation on the human testis. *Radiation Research*, 59, 665–678.
Scully, R. E. (1981) Neoplasia associated with anomalous sexual development and abnormal sex chromosomes. *Pediatric and Adolescent Endocrinology*, 8, 203–217.
Shapiro, E., Kinsella, T. J., Makuch, R. W., Fraas, B. A., Glatstein, E., Rosenberg, S. A. & Sherins, R. J. (1985) Effects of fractionated irradiation on endocrine aspects of testicular function. *Journal of Clinical Oncology*, 3, 1232–1239.
Sigg, C. & Hedinger, C. (1981) Atypical germ cells in testicular biopsy in male sterility. *International Journal of Andrology*, Suppl. 4, 163–171.
Skakkebæk, N. E. (1972a) Abnormal morphology of germ cells in two infertile men. *Acta Pathologica et Microbiologica Scandinavica*, A, 80, 374–378.
Skakkebæk, N. E. (1972b) Possible carcinoma-in-situ of the testis. *Lancet*, i, 516–517.
Skakkebæk, N. E. (1978) Carcinoma in situ of the testis: Frequency and relationship to invasive germ cell tumours in infertile men. *Histopathology*, 2, 157–170.
Skakkebæk, N. E. (1979) Carcinoma-in-situ of testis in testicular feminization syndrome. *Acta Pathologica et Microbiologica Scandinavica*, A, 87, 87–89.

Skakkebæk, N. E. & Berthelsen, J. G. (1978) Carcinoma-in-situ of the testis and orchidectomy. *Lancet*, **ii**, 204–205.

Skakkebæk, N. E., Berthelsen, J. G. & Müller, J. (1982) Carcinoma-in-situ of the undescended testis. *Urologic Clinics of North America*, **9**, 377–385.

Tomic, R., Bergman, B., Damber, J.-E., Littbrand, B. & Löfroth, P. O. (1983) Effects of external radiation therapy for cancer of the prostate on the serum concentrations of testosterone, follicle-stimulating hormone, luteinizing hormone and prolactin. *Journal of Urology*, **130**, 287–289.

von der Maase, H., Berthelsen, J. G., Jacobsen, G. K., Hald, T., Rørth, M., Christophersen, I. S., Sørensen, B. L., Walbom-Jørgensen, S. & Skakkebæk, N. E. (1985) Carcinoma-in-situ of testis eradicated by chemotherapy. *Lancet*, **i**, 98.

von der Maase, H., Rørth, M., Walbom-Jørgensen, S., Sørensen, B. L., Christophersen, I. S., Hald, T., Jacobsen, G. K., Berthelsen, J. G. & Skakkebæk, N. E. (1986a) Carcinoma in situ of the contralateral testis in patients with testicular germ cell cancer. A study of 27 cases in 500 patients. *British Medical Journal*, **293**, 1398–1401.

von der Maase, H., Giwercman, A. & Skakkebæk, N. E. (1986b) Radiation treatment of carcinoma-in-situ of testis. *Lancet*, **i**, 624–625.

Waxman, M. (1976) Malignant germ cell tumor in situ in a cryptorchid testis. *Cancer*, **38**, 1452–1456.

Williams, T. R. & Brendler, H. (1977) Carcinoma in situ of the ectopic testis. *Journal of Urology*, **117**, 610–612.

Discussion

Hargreave If a testicular cancer patient is in any case going to be treated with chemotherapy for his primary tumour do you still advise biopsy of the contralateral testis especially if you think the chemotherapy will cure CIS? Also, have you any biopsy evidence of the effect of chemotherapy on CIS? Have you compared biopsies before and after chemotherapy?

von der Maase Yes we have. The testis may be a sanctuary, but follow-up biopsies have shown that all CIS cells (detected in a pretherapy biopsy) have disappeared after intensive chemotherapy with cisplatin, vinblastine or VP-16, and bleomycin. On the other hand, I suspect that some of these patients may relapse because cases of relapse in the contralateral testis after these same drugs have been reported. This probably indicates that the intensive chemotherapy did not completely eradicate all the CIS.

I suspect that more modest chemotherapy is less effective in the control of CIS. I have seen four cases of contralateral testicular cancer developing after modest doses of adjuvant vincristine and bleomycin in our early Danish studies. I have no evidence from biopsies taken before and after this regimen but I am certain that these lower doses failed to eradicate CIS which presumably was present at the time of treatment.

Skakkebæk I have slides to show CIS in the contralateral testis at the time of removal of the primary testicular tumour, and one year after the Einhorn regimen there is no residual CIS but only Sertoli-cell-only-tubules. This is similar to the effect of irradiation.

von der Maase Even after chemotherapy, however, normal germ cells may persist and give rise to resumed spermatogenesis although CIS cells are no longer visible.

Oliver You state that chemotherapy has cured established CIS in all eight of your patients who had a repeat biopsy. Did any of these patients have spermatogenesis prior to chemotherapy, and did any have resumption of spermatogenesis? A report from Professor Peckham's group indicated that some patients with a low sperm count prior to chemotherapy had higher counts after treatment. These patients, however, were not biopsied to exclude CIS. Perhaps the chemotherapy cured undetected CIS thereby allowing better recovery of germinal epithelium. Your results would substantiate this contention and may also explain why spermatogenesis may recur after chemotherapy but not radiotherapy.

von der Maase We know that spermatogenesis may return to normal some time after chemotherapy for unilateral testicular cancer, however, we have no data concerning spermatogenesis recovering after chemotherapy in patients with proven CIS in the contralateral testis. I do not claim that chemotherapy necessarily *cures* CIS, but only that CIS was not detected in follow-up biopsy whereas some germ cells persisted. I still expect some of these patients to relapse with contralateral cancer.

Berthelsen We have seen improved spermatogenesis following adjuvant chemotherapy with vincristine and bleomycin after a period of 2–4 years. We have no prospective data on spermatogenesis following the Einhorn regimen.

Oliver We are increasingly changing from postoperative radiotherapy to adjuvant chemotherapy. Do you think this is adequate to eradicate CIS?

von der Maase We may get the answer to your question by chance finding, but I do not think it is open to trial.

Einhorn CIS is a condition with low proliferative activity. Why, then, do you expect it to be eradicted by cisplatin combination chemotherapy, which may simply cause temporary testicular atrophy?

von der Maase We did not expect CIS to disappear after chemotherapy. This was a fortuitous observation detected on biopsy.

Einhorn How long have you followed patients who received cisplatin combination chemotherapy for disseminated testicular cancer, and how frequently have you repeated the biopsies of the contralateral testis?

von der Maase The median follow-up time was 25 months with a range of 4–96 months. Recent biopsy was performed every 2–3 years: more frequent follow-up is not required. Stage I patients can be cured by orchidectomy, but follow-up is still necessary.

Skakkebæk We cannot be certain that these patients will never develop a second testicular malignancy. Our length of follow-up is still limited.

Oliver In your group of patients with CIS who are followed prospectively without receiving treatment, 50% developed invasive cancer within 5 years. Did you ever see spontaneous regression of established CIS in the remaining 11 patients who were tumour-free at 5 years?

von der Maase Spontaneous regression of CIS has never been observed in our patients and I do not think it has ever been documented. In two patients with CIS the first follow-up biopsies were free of CIS, but CIS was again detected in subsequent biopsies one year later. We do not know if CIS eventually becomes invasive in all cases, or if it may remain indefinitely within the tubules.

Skakkebæk In our series to which you refer the 50% of CIS patients who had no evidence of invasive tumour at 5 years were not free from danger. When the follow-up period was prolonged, more patients developed frank testicular cancer.

Holstein In our patients who had CIS in their biopsy, we often found in the subsequent orchidectomy solid seminoma in the rete testis region or an invasive tumour growth in a certain testicular region. Does the irradiation you perform also delete solid seminoma in the contralateral testis in addition to the CIS?

von der Maase In the biopsies of the contralateral testis which we have examined, we have only detected CIS and not solid seminoma.

Holstein Perhaps there was solid seminoma near to the rete testis which you did not sample in your biopsy?

von der Maase Seminoma is very sensitive to radiotherapy therefore it should also be eradicated if it is present but undetected.

Bannwart In our patients who had an orchidectomy following biopsy evidence of CIS, we found infiltrating tumour in seven of nine (80%) cases. It was always seminoma. In your orchidectomy specimens, after finding CIS in the biopsy, did you find only seminoma or did you find, in addition, differentiated testicular tumour or other types of nonseminomatous germ cell tumour such as teratocarcinoma? Would the knowledge that nonseminoma may be present influence your therapy?

von der Maase Eight patients with CIS in our study developed invasive tumour and orchidectomy revealed four seminomas, two nonseminomas and two cases of early invasion of malignant germ cells. The nonseminomas contained embryonal carcinoma and yolk sac tumour. All combinations of germ cell tumour except spermatocytic seminoma may be seen in association with CIS.

Hargreave We have heard evidence that some patients who have CIS detected in a biopsy may also have invasive cancer which is missed because of sampling error. You are selecting your patients because of testicular biopsy in high risk patients or because of very careful examination including ultrasound. In other centres, as many as 80% of patients with CIS may have associated invasive tumour at the time of detection and some of these tumours may not be seminomas. Radiotherapy may not cure the occult nonseminomatous tumours. Only long-term follow-up will resolve this uncertainty.

General discussion on CIS

Chairman T. B. HARGREAVE

Willis The three patients described by Dr Pedersen who had CIS postorchidopexy were 8 and 10 years old at the time of surgery. Does earlier orchidopexy prevent the development of CIS, or is it present at birth?

Pedersen The ages of these three patients were close to the mean age for orchidopexy in our whole group of patients and we have no information on the effect of earlier surgery.

Müller Intersex patients with the androgen insensitivity syndrome or gonadal dysgenesis may have CIS present at birth. This possibly indicates that early orchidopexy will not prevent its occurrence.

Hargreave These intersex patients certainly must have a testicular biopsy. I am doubtful if you can extrapolate from your findings in these rather special patients to the suggestion that phenotypically normal males also have CIS changes from a very early age.

Skakkebæk The evidence from the young intersex patients merely suggests that CIS *may* be present from a very young age. We also think that the presence of CIS cells in infancy is further evidence that they are related to very early, immature germ cells, or gonocytes. Also, the case described by Dr Müller and co-workers (*Cancer*, 1984, **54**, 629–634) of the 10-year-old cryptorchid boy who had CIS detected at that time, and in repeat biopsies till invasion was evident when he was 20 years old, indicates that CIS can persist for many years before invasion occurs. We believe that CIS does not develop from degeneration of spermatogonia, but is present even before birth.

Hargreave Do we have any evidence of biopsies from young cryptorchids showing CIS at an early age?

Jackson There is no evidence in the world literature that the age at operation has any effect on the subsequent development of testicular cancer. If CIS is a necessary precondition for the development of a testicular cancer, then this suggests that age at operation is unlikely to have any effect on CIS development.

Bannwart We have examined more than 200 biopsies from undescended testes in young boys less than 3 years old. We have not detected any instances of CIS. Perhaps the age of biopsy or the age of operation for correction of maldescent is very important. We cannot say for sure that CIS cells do not exist in the testis at this age: perhaps they were present but had not reached the region of the testis immediately below the tunica from where the biopsies were taken.

Hargreave May I urge anyone who is going to perform testicular biopsies on young boys with maldescent to differentiate carefully between the patients with a short cord, where the testis lies in the abdomen or inguinal canal, and those patients with a testis that has passed through the external inguinal ring to lie ectopically in the superficial inguinal pouch. These may be two different lesions.

Berthelsen A possible reason for the difficulty in demonstrating CIS in the prepubertal testes may be that CIS cells are rather few at that time and possibly only present in a small focus. Perhaps only in later life do they spread along the seminiferous tubules.

Skakkebæk There is very little activity in the prepubertal testis so that CIS may easily be overlooked. However, there is some activity and I think eventually the CIS cells can spread from an initial focus along the basal compartment of the tubules under the Sertoli cell layer to involve the whole testis. The CIS cells can spread by way of the rete testis from tubule to tubule. In this way, CIS cells can replace the normal germ cells. This, of course, involves proliferation of the CIS cells.

Grigor Dr Giwercman reported a patient who developed a testicular tumour following a biopsy negative for CIS although this only occurred once in 1500 patients. In the orchidectomy specimen was CIS detected in the tubules adjacent to the tumour? If so, was CIS present at the time of biopsy but missed because of sampling error, or did CIS develop after the biopsy was performed?

Skakkebæk The orchidectomy specimen did not come to my laboratory. I shall try to discover if CIS was present in the adjacent 'normal' testicular tissue.

Hartlapp If you are looking for CIS in the testis how do you select the relevant area to biopsy?

Bruun The biopsy site is chosen at random because CIS is a widespread lesion throughout the testicular parenchyma.

Berthelsen CIS is less commonly found in the testis close to the rete. This area should be avoided.

G. K. Jacobsen When an initial biopsy has shown CIS where should the subsequent biopsy be taken from – the same site or elsewhere at random?

Skakkebæk I think a different site should be chosen.

Hargreave When a biopsy is being taken to investigate infertility it is important to make a general scrotal examination including the epididymis, rete and vas, because additional information is required. Such an exploration may reveal unexpected areas of scar tissue in the testis. This more open biopsy technique enables the surgeon to biopsy any specific lesion he may find. If a second biopsy is being performed, exploration reveals the site of the primary biopsy and this region of fibrosis should be avoided. The disadvantage of this is that the second biopsy causes more scarring and by the time a third biopsy is being taken quite a considerable amount of fibrosis is present.

Grigor Azzopardi *et al*. (*American Journal of Pathology*, **38**, 207–225, 1961) originally described atypical cells in tubules close to sites of testicular scarring (perhaps due to regressed tumour – 'burnt-out' lesion). Surely, therefore, a biopsy should be taken close to an obvious scar in order to increase the chances of detecting CIS, rather than avoiding such scarred areas.

Hargreave An initial biopsy should be taken from an area of scarring, and a subsequent biopsy should avoid scars caused by the first biopsy.

Bannwart We studied orchidectomy specimens which had CIS in a previous biopsy. Horizontal slices were cut and embedded in large plastic blocks after fixation in a mixture of buffered 0.2% glutaraldehyde and 2% formalin. At the site of the previous biopsy there was a scar about 4 mm in diameter which contained no tumour cells. The second biopsy should therefore avoid the site of the first biopsy.

Hargreave Such a scar can be detected by open exploration, and this site avoided for the subsequent biopsy.

Dieckmann If CIS is a necessary precursor lesion for all germ cell cancer, and if it is present after puberty, how do you explain the decrease in the overall incidence of testicular cancer over the age of 40 years, and the slightly increased incidence in elderly patients?

Skakkebæk We believe that the CIS cells are present in small numbers in childhood, and that the numbers increase after puberty by intratubular spread of the CIS cells along the inside of the tubular basement membrane, thereby replacing the seminiferous epithelium. We have evidence that CIS can be present for more than 10 years before an invasive tumour occurs. There is probably some other stimulus required to promote frank tumour formation from the CIS cells. I believe that hormonal stimulation is important; this would account for the neonatal and early adult peaks of tumour incidence. In the majority of cases CIS has probaby given rise to tumour formation before the age of 40; therefore the incidence of testicular cancer decreases thereafter.

Concerning the increase in testicular cancer in elderly patients, I wonder if most of these tumours might be spermatocytic seminomas or somatic tumours, especially lymphomas. There is an increased gonadotrophin level in old age, and this also may be a significant stimulus for tumour development especially if the tumours are derived from germ cells.

Weidner Why do you fix the radiation dose for CIS at 20 Gy? Is it possible to use lower doses to avoid infertility?

I have seen a patient who was irradiated for seminoma in one testis and subsequently developed seminoma in the remaining testis 2 years later. In this case, the spreading rays from the primary radiotherapy provided an insufficient dose. Are there any measurements of the required dose?

von der Maase A dose lower that 20 Gy may be sufficient to eradicate CIS, but I am certain that persistent eradication of CIS requires a dose which will necessarily cause Sertoli-cell-only change in the tubules. Therefore, it is probably not possible to avoid infertility.

We wanted to select a dose of irradiation which could eradicate the CIS cells without significantly affecting the Leydig cell function, and our present treatment appears to satisfy this condition. We shall continue to use 20 Gy. However, if a longer observation time reveals a significant influence on Leydig cell function, we may try to use a lower dose.

I agree that in your case, the dose of radiotherapy to the contralateral testis was too low.

Friedman Perhaps the late peak of germinoma (seminoma) and the earlier peak of other types of germ cell tumours in the male may be homologous to the development of germ cell tumours in the female. There is a tendency for ovarian germ cell tumours to differentiate into dermoid cysts and teratoid tumours during the reproductive period, whereas they present as germinomas or embryonal carcinomas prepubertally and postmenopausally. What controls this differentiation in the female?

Grigor Dr Müller, when you detected CIS in gonadal dysgenesis were the malignant cells still within tubules or was there early invasion? Well-defined tubules are often not seen in streak gonads

Müller All the gonads from intersex patients we have investigated to date have had areas of well-defined tubules and the CIS cells were always found within tubules. Dr Skakkebæk has described a case of gonadoblastoma adjacent to which we found CIS cells in streak gonadal tissue. This may represent the equivalent of CIS in a streak gonad.

Prognostic factors in metastatic testicular cancer

N. J. VOGELZANG *Department of Medicine, Section of Hematology/Oncology, University of Chicago, Chicago, Illinois*

Summary

The prognosis for metastatic testicular cancer has been analysed in seven reports using multivariate analysis. Serum hCG is the most important factor. Volume of metastases, serum LDH and serum AFP are also of prognostic value. Bone, liver, nodal or retroperitoneal metastases are not independent prognostic factors. The prognosis for extragonadal nonseminomas remains in dispute. Future studies should categorize poor prognosis patients using one of the several available prognostic formulas. No consensus yet exists on optimal treatment for such patients.

Key words. Metastatic testicular cancer, multivariate analysis, prognosis.

Introduction

The excellent prognosis and long-term survival of most patients with metastatic germ cell testicular cancer has obscured the poor prognosis and short survival of certain subsets of such patients. That patients with a poor prognosis exist is affirmed by all clinical investigators, yet the precise identification of patients with a 'poor prognosis' has been the subject of much debate. The purpose of this report is to summarize the available literature on patients with poor prognosis metastatic germ cell testicular cancer.

Methods

In February 1986 a standardized letter of inquiry was sent to eighteen clinical investigators who had published articles or abstracts relating to poor prognosis metastatic testicular cancer (Table 1). These physicians were asked to submit 'copies of any paper, chapter or manuscript' in which was discussed 'the determination of the "poor prognostic" group of testis cancer patients or their treatment'. Fifteen of eighteen investigators responded and their reports published or unpublished form the basis of this review. In addition, all abstracts and articles dealing with the prognosis of patients with metastatic testicular cancer wherever possible were reviewed. Thus, several prominent investigators who have recently published on prognostic criteria were not queried (German-Lluch, Begent & Bagshawe, 1980; Medical Research Council Working Party on Testicular Tumours, 1985).

Correspondence: Dr Nicholas J. Vogelzang, Joint Section of Hematology/Oncology, University of Chicago Medical Center, 5841 S. Maryland Avenue, Box 420, Chicago, IL 60637, U.S.A.

× 5) and VAB-6 for a total of 6 months (Bosl et al., 1986b). Only five of fourteen (35%) extragonadal germ cell tumour patients remain alive and only eleven of the twenty-seven (41%) testicular cancer patients remain alive. This survival was identical to a historical control group of twenty-nine patients treated with VAB-6 alone. The model therefore allowed precise identification of a poor risk group of patients without the need for a concomitant control group. Unfortunately, the treatment did not improve the patients' overall survival.

Study 2. One hundred and fifty good risk (probablity of CR > 50%) metastatic testicular cancer or extragonadal seminoma patients were randomized to either three cycles of VAB-6 (total cisplatin dose = 360 mg/m^2) or four cycles of etoposide plus cisplatin (total cisplatin dose = 400 mg/m^2) (Bosl et al., 1986a). With a median follow-up of 20+ months, the CR rate with VAB-6 was 95% while with etoposide/cisplatin it was 91%. There is no difference in the CR rate or in survival. Although longer follow-up is needed, it appears that for good risk metastatic testicular cancer patients treatment with two drugs is equivalent to five-drug treatment.

Study 3. Bajorin et al. (1986) analysed the outcome of 118 patients on 'good' and 'poor' risk MSKCC protocols, in comparison to the outcome predicted by three other prognostic models. The MSKCC model assigned the fewest patients to the 'poor' risk category, and accurately predicted good outcomes in patients considered poor risk by the other models. Bajorin et al. concluded that poor risk is overestimated by other prognostic models.

Medical Research Council Working Party on Testicular Tumours (MRC/TT)
The substantial contributions of Drs Peckham and Bagshawe to the understanding of prognostic factors in germ cell cancer have been amply demonstrated (Germa-Lluch et al., 1980; Medical Research Council Working Party on Testicular Tumours, 1985; Peckham et al., 1985). Recently, investigators at six medical centres in Great Britain have pooled and analysed a total of 458 patients, treated with a variety of chemotherapy regimens (Medical Research Council Working Party on Testicular Tumours, 1985). Prognoses could be least estimated using the Royal Marsden Clinical Staging System of small, large and very large volume disease with 3-year survivals of 86%, 76% and 54% for the three groups respectively. Serum hCG > 1000 IU/l and/or AFP > 500 kU/l worsened the prognosis within each volume category. The investigators also demonstrated: (1) improving survivals for yearly intervals since 1976, (2) lack of impact of type of chemotherapy, (3) worsening prognosis for patients > 30 years old, symptoms duration > 3 months, and for the presence of yolk sac histology. Serum LDH was not analysed and extragonadal germ cell tumour patients were excluded by design.

Indiana University (IU) and the Southeastern Cancer Study Group (SECSG)
The prognosis of 180 patients treated at IU on a single SECSG protocol was the subject of a logistic regression analysis (Birch et al., 1986). Six models were derived which fit the observed results. All models were able to predict complete response with 96–100% accuracy. The model which best predicted failure to achieve com-

plete response was as follows:

$$h_i = 6.729 - 1.830 \times \text{Indiana} - 0.170 \log(\text{hCG}+1)$$

with h_i as previously defined. 'Indiana' refers to the Indiana staging classification (minimal, moderate, advanced).

A second model which also predicted for failure to obtain a CR was:

$$h_i = 10.087 - 1.142 \log(\text{LDH}+1) - 0.204 \log(\text{AFP}+1) - 0.140 \log(\text{hCG}+1)$$

These two models were also able to predict correctly CR and non-CR in a subsequent SECGS study of PVB versus PEB. Note that both models contain hCG and that the second model is very similar to the Bosl et al. model except that AFP becomes of prognostic value.

These models have not yet been used to design prospective treatments for good and poor risk patients.

European Organization for Research and Treatment of Cancer (EORTC)
A complete report on the EORTC multivariate logistic regression analysis will be presented at this meeting by Stoter et al. (1987). With kind permission from Dr Stoter, I have previewed that report.

One hundred and sixty-three patients with non-seminomatous testicular cancer were treated with PVB (two dose levels of vinblastine) by EORTC members. Patients with central nervous system (CNS) metastases were excluded. Fifteen significant clinical variables were found in a univariate analysis. The variables of bone metastases, liver metastases, age, size of or presence of mediastinal metastases and eight other variables were insignificant. Twenty-six variables were then studied in a logistic regression model. The single most important factor was the logarithm of the serum level of hCG, but a final model composed of four variables best described the data. This model correctly predicted 81% of complete remissions. The variables achieving statistical significance were the presence or absence of choriocarcinomatous elements in the primary tumour (trophoblastic — TROPH, 0 = no or possible, 1 = yes), the serum concentration of AFP (0 = 0–999 ng/ml, 1 = ⩾1000 ng/ml), the presence or absence of lung metastases (LUNG, 0 = no, 1 = yes), and the size and number of lung metastases (SIXNB, 0 = none, 1 = 1–3 and ⩽3 cm, 2 = 4–19 and ⩽3 cm or 1–3 and >3 cm, 3 = ⩾20 or 4–19 and >3 cm).

The prognostic equation is as follows:

$$h_i = 1.9381 - 2.1327 \times \text{TROPH} - 2.2723\ \text{ALPH} \\ + 4.878 \times \text{LUNG} - 2.3212 \times \text{SIXNB}$$

The presence or absence of an abdominal mass was not of prognostic value, although five of twelve patients (42%) who relapsed from CR had an abdominal mass ⩾ 10 cm in size.

One hundred and fifty-four of the 163 patients had available data on all four variables. The 154 patients could be divided into three prognostic groups; those with a 89–100% CR rate ($N = 97$), those with a 41% CR rate ($N = 46$) and those with an 18% CR rate ($N = 11$). Ongoing EORTC studies in testicular cancer will be used to validate the model (Stoter et al., 1986).

M. D. Anderson Hospital (MDA)

Samuels *et al.* were among the first investigators to stratify testicular cancer patients by prognostic category (Samuels, Johnson & Holoye, 1975). Although the Samuels staging system has been widely used, recently its predictive ability has been questioned (Logothetis *et al.*, 1985, 1986; Birch *et al.*, 1986). Logothetis *et al.*, using the CISCA/VB$_{IV}$ regimen (Logothetis *et al.*, 1985, 1986), have achieved a 92% (84/91) disease-free survival in patients with testicular cancer and a 56% (5/9) disease-free survival in patients with extragonadal germ cell cancer. In a stepwise logistic regression analysis of 'recognized prognostic variables', a serum β hCG level above 50,000 mIU/ml was of prognostic value to the exclusion of all other variables. With exclusion of the hCG, the modified Samuels staging system became prognostically significant ($P = 0.001$) but the worst of the five Samuels stages (Stage III — B$_5$ Visceral disease, liver, GI, CNS, etc.) was not prognostically significant ($P = 0.422$). Choriocarcinoma histology ($P = 0.078$) and extragonadal origin of the tumour ($P = 0.086$) achieved borderline significance. Serum AFP, obstructive uropathy, and liver metastases were not of prognostic significance. Serum LDH was not analysed.

This regression analysis is difficult to apply broadly to patients with metastatic testicular cancer because of the unique type of chemotherapy regimen used and because there has been no validation of the analysis against an independent data set or in a prospective study.

Institut Gustave-Roussy (IGR)

This institution has completed a multivariate logistic regression analysis of fifty-nine patients treated at IGR from January 1978 to December 1981, on three different protocols, PVB ($N = 6$), VAB-3 ($N = 12$), T79 ($N = 41$) (Droz *et al.*, 1986). The T79 protocol was similar to VAB-4 but administered cisplatin at a dose of 90 mg/m^2. At 4 years, the survival of all patients was 50%. A mathematical model was derived which correctly predicted 84% of complete remissions. The variables achieving statistical significance were the square root of the serum levels of hCG and AFP. The prognostic evaluation is:

$$h_i = 2.10 - 0.0137 \sqrt{hCG} - 0.0385 \sqrt{AFP}$$

Importantly, the presence or absence of choriocarcinoma histology was not significant, nor was the presence or absence of an abdominal mass. The serum LDH level was not considered. The model correctly predicted 82% of complete remissions in twenty-one patients treated at IGR from January 1982 to December 1983.

This model is being validated in two ongoing protocols: good risk patients (probability of CR > 70%) are being treated with VAB-6 × 4 courses while poor risk patients are receiving 2-monthly cycles of etoposide 100 mg/m^2 days 1–5, cisplatin 40 mg/m^2 days 1–5, bleomycin 15 mg i.m. days 8, 15, 21, and vinblastine 0.2 mg/kg day 1. The third cycle of chemotherapy, etoposide 350 mg/m^2 days 1–5, cisplatin 40 mg/m^2 days 1–5, cyclosphosphamide 1.6 g/m^2 days 2–5 with uromitoxan 350 mg/m^2 q. 4 h is followed by autologous bone marrow reinfusion 72 h after completion of last dose. The innovative approach to poor risk patients is of considerable interest. Of concern is the fact that the model was derived from a study in which many patients were treated with < 100 mg/m² cisplatin per course. Additionally, it was able to predict prospectively only 50% of non-responders, implying that severe toxicity may be incurred by some patients with relatively good prognosis.

National Cancer Institute (NCI)
Ozols *et al.* (1984) were the first group to initiate a prospective randomized trial in poor prognosis patients. That study was begun after pilot studies revealed that ultra-high dose cisplatin (40 mg/m²/day × 5) with 6 l/day of normal saline diuresis could induce responses in patients clinically refractory to cisplatin (Ozols *et al.*, 1984), and that the combination of PVBV (cisplatin 40 mg/m²/day × 5, vinblastine 0.2 mg/kg day 1, bleomycin 30 u weekly and VP-16 100 mg/m²/day × 5) was tolerable and effective in patients with 'bulky' stage III disease (Ozols *et al.*, 1983).

The criteria for poor prognosis stage III disease were determined without the use of a multivariate analysis. They include:

1. Advanced abdominal disease (palpable mass or obstructive uropathy or liver involvement or mass > 10 cm).
2. Advanced lung disease (single mass or nodule > 5 cm or ≥ 5 nodules and at least one ≥ 2 cm or > 10 nodules all > 1 cm or cytologically positive pleural effusion or hypoxia (pO_2 < 75) due to metastases).
3. AFP > 1000 ng/ml or hCG > 10,000 mIU/ml.
4. Brain metastases.
5. Bone marrow metastases.
6. Pure choriocarcinoma (Stage II or III).
7. Extragonadal primary.

All patients with pure seminoma are excluded. Poor risk patients are stratified by CNS involvement and the presence of an extragonadal primary, then randomized using a 2:1 randomization to either PVBV or PVB.

With forty-six patients analysed, the survival is 50% with PVB, and 88% with PVBV (Ozols, personal communication, February 1986). The study remains open. The completion of this important study will allow definitive assessment of the role of ultra-high dose cisplatin in poor prognosis germ cell cancer. The study should be analysed using the published prognostic models.

West German Tumour Centre (WGTC)
Scheulen *et al.* (1981) have performed an analysis of prognostic factors in seventy-one patients treated with vinblastine/bleomycin plus cisplatin/doxorubicin between 1977 and 1979. Ten clinical variables were examined and eight were of prognostic value in a univariate analysis. In a multivariate analysis, however, serum LDH was the most important variable (chi-square = 31.3). In the abstract, other significant variables were not mentioned, the model was not tested against an independent data set, nor has any prospective study, employing the model, been reported.

Instituto Nazionale Tumori (INT)

Pizzocaro et al. (1985a) described only a 41% long-term complete remission rate in twenty-seven patients with 'far advanced disease', treated between February 1980 and February 1982 with PVB and cytoreductive surgery. Far advanced disease was clinically defined as: (1) invasion of more than 50% of pulmonary fields or at least one lung metastasis between 2 and 5 cm, (2) a lymph node metastasis larger than 10 cm, and (3) metastases outside of lymph nodes and lung ('extra pulmonary' disease).

This utilitarian clinical model was then prospectively tested from August 1981 to November 1983 in forty patients with the same definition of far advanced disease plus the addition of AFP > 1000 ng/ml and hCG > 50,000 mIU/ml. Therapy with etoposide 100 mg/m^2 days 1–5, cisplatin 20 mg/m^2 days 1–5, and bleomycin 18 mg/m^2 days 2, 9, 16 induced complete remissions in thirty-seven (92.5%) patients with thirty-three patients (82.5%) remaining in CR. Compared to the historical controls (prolonged CR rate of 41%), there was a statistically significant improvement ($P < 0.01$) (Pizzocaro et al., 1985b).

Pizzocaro et al. (1986) have defined good prognosis as all those patients without 'far advanced' disease. From March 1982 to December 1983 they have prospectively treated forty-two such patients with cisplatin 20 mg/m^2 days 1–5, bleomycin 18 mg/m^2 days 2, 9, 16 and reduced dose vinblastine 0.1 mg/kg days 1 and 2. 97.6% (41/42) patients entered CR and forty patients (95%) are alive, free of disease, and off therapy. The patients with the 'worst' prognosis in this good risk group were those with an AFP > 400 ng/ml and an hCG > 1000 mIU/ml.

Pizzocaro et al. have thus apparently identified two groups of patients with differing prognosis (82% versus 95% survival) who require different therapy. Given the large data base and the suggestion that serum AFP, hCG and LDH are continuous (linear) variables for prognosis and survival (i.e. CR rate decreases as hCG and AFP increases), a multivariate logistic regression analysis would be most valuable.

The Finsen Institute (FI)

Daugaard & Rørth (1986) have treated twenty-six poor risk patients with a high-dose cisplatin (40 mg/m^2 days 1–5), etoposide (200 mg/m^2 days 1–5) and bleomycin (15 mg/m^2 weekly). Seventeen of the twenty-six patients had testicular cancer with at least one of the following variables: abdominal disease ⩾ 10 cm, liver metastases, supradiaphragmatic lymph node metastases ⩾ 5 cm, multiple lung metastases (at least one ⩾ 5 cm), or hCG > 100,000 U/l (normal level < 8 U/l).

They achieved CRs in thirteen of the seventeen patients (76%) with a median duration of CR of 18 months (range 3–26 months). In a re-analysis of the patients by this reviewer, using the Bosl et al. model, fourteen of fifteen analysable patients were 'poor risk' with a median probability of CR of 25%. These excellent results are striking and require prospective confirmation. However, the toxicity was substantial with six drug related deaths in twenty-six patients; over 90% of patients experienced neutropenic fevers and required red cell transfusions.

Dana-Farber Cancer Institute (DFCI)
Garnick & Richie (1986) have defined poor prognosis factors as: bone or central nervous system metastases, hCG titre > 2000 ng/ml (10,000 mIU/ml) or pure choriocarcinoma histology, or extragonadal (EG) non-seminomatous (especially yolk sac) tumours. A multivariate analysis has not been done; a full report is in preparation. Using alternating cycles of PVB and PEB (doses not given) only one of six (17%) testicular patients achieved a CR; however six of nine EG patients achieved a CR.

Medizinische Hochschule Hannover (MHH)
Schmoll et al. (1986) have defined the following poor prognosis factors, based on an unpublished multivariate analysis of 200 patients treated in a randomized trial of PVB versus PVB plus ifosfamide: abdominal mass > 10 cm; mediastinal mass > 5 cm; more than five lung metastases ≥ 2 cm; liver, bone, CNS metastases. 'Tumour bulk' was the major prognostic factor but unfortunately AFP and hCG were not included in the analysis since a third of the patients did not have marker levels titred.

Although the addition of ifosfamide had 'no substantial impact' on the prognosis of advanced disease patients, a second study of cisplatin 35 mg/m^2 days 1–5, VP-16 120 mg/m^2 days –15 and bleomycin 15 mg/m^2 i.v. weekly in poor prognosis patients has resulted in a 70% CR rate. This study is difficult to compare with other studies since marker values are not reported.

Others
Other investigators have reported on other prognostic factors or that a variety of chemotherapy regimens have improved the outcome of 'poor prognosis' patients (Von Eyben et al., 1982; Taylor et al., 1984; Chacon et al., 1985; Richardson et al., 1985; Blayney et al., 1986; Levi et al., 1986; Picozzi et al., 1984). However, information on the criteria by which poor prognosis patients were selected, and how such criteria were selected is generally lacking from the preliminary reports. Thus, these studies cannot be further analysed until publication of the completed work. Other studies suffer from small patient numbers.

Discussion
It is clear from the seven multivariate analyses currently completed (Bosl et al., 1983; Medical Research Council Working Party on Testicular Tumours, 1985; Birch et al., 1986; Droz et al., 1986; Logothetis et al., 1986; Stoter et al., 1986), and from the other clinical analyses, that the level of serum hCG is the most important prognostic factor in metastatic testicular cancer (Table 2). This is particularly striking in the EORTC and MDA studies in which hCG excluded all other variables.

The apparent utility of the serum LDH to prognosticate must be confirmed. Three studies have specifically addressed the MSKCC finding (Scheulen et al., 1984; Birch et al., 1986; Stoter et al., 1986) but more data are needed.

Serum AFP levels are of less prognostic significance than hCG levels but in only two of the seven multivariate analyses was AFP level not prognostically significant.

Although the presence or absence of an abdominal/retroperitoneal mass was felt to be a poor prognostic sign in the 1976–82 era, there is a consensus emerging that such 'bulky' disease is not an independent prognostic variable.

The volume of lung metastases continues to enter into many prognostic models (eight of twelve studies). The MRC/TT study emphasized the importance of lung metastases. A continuum of prognosis may exist as was elegantly demonstrated by Stoter *et al.* Other studies should attempt a similar quantitation of the volume of lung metastases.

It is clear that bone and liver metastases alone are not independent prognostic factors. Central nervous system metastases at diagnosis are rare but probably indicate a poor prognosis.

The clinical variable of size of lymph nodes is not an *independent* prognostic factor.

Sharp differences of opinion exist regarding extra-gonadal nonseminomatous primary tumours. This problem will be difficult to resolve due to the rarity of the cancers. These patients should be reported separately, but the available models should be used to characterize their prognosis.

In conclusion, prognosis is not well estimated using only a single clinical marker (i.e. presence or absence of an abdominal mass) but can be accurately estimated using the serum tumour marker levels and an index of tumour volume. Prognosis is a continuum from 0% to 100% survival. An acceptable prognostic system should reflect such a continuum. Prospective evaluations suggest a decreasing incidence of 'poor' prognosis patients. Even with identification of 'poor prognosis' groups, no consensus yet exists as to the optimal chemotherapeutic or surgical programme to be used.

Acknowledgements

The author wishes to thank Deborah Gifford for secretarial help. This work was supported in part by the Jazz and Blues Fund.

References

Bajorin, D., Katz, A., Bosl, G. J. *et al.* (1986) Comparison of eligibility criteria of studies assigning germ cell tumor patients to good risk and poor risk categories. *Proceedings ASCO*, **5**, 106.

Birch, R., Williams, S., Cone, A., *et al.* (1986) Prognostic factors for favorable outcome in disseminated germ cell tumors. *Journal of Clinical Oncology*, **4**, 400-407.

Blayney, D. W., Goldberg, D. A., Leong, L. A. *et al.* (1986) High risk germ cell tumors: Severe toxicity with high dose platinum, vinblastine, bleomycin and VP-16 (PVeBV). *Proceedings ASCO*, **5**, 101.

Bosl, G. J., Geller, N. L., Cirrincione, C. *et al.* (1983) Multivariate analysis of prognostic variables in patients with metastatic testicular cancer. *Cancer Research*, **43**, 3403–3407.

Bosl, G. J., Bajorin, D., Leitner, S. *et al.* (1986a) A randomized trial of etoposide and cisplatin and VAB-6 in the treatment of 'good risk' patients with germ cell tumors. *Proceedings ASCO*, **5**, 104.

Bosl, G. J., Geller, N. L., Vogelzang, N. J. *et al.* (1986b) Alternating cycles of Etoposide and cisplatin and VAB-6 in the treatment of poor risk patients with germ cell tumors. (Submitted.)

Chacon, P. R. D., Estevey, R. A., Cedaro, L. *et al.* (1985) Treatment of poor prognosis germ cell tumors with alternating cycles of cisplatin, bleomycin, vinblastine and VP-16. *Proceedings ASCO*, **4**, 111.

Daugaard, G. & Rørth, M. (1986) High dose cisplatin and VP-16 with bleomycin in the management of advanced metastatic germ cell tumors. *European Journal of Cancer and Clinical Oncology* (in press).

Droz, J. P., Kramar, A., Piot, G., et al. (1986) Multivariate logistic regression analysis of prognostic factors in patients with advanced stage non-seminomatous germ cell tumors of the testis. *Proceedings ASCO*, **5**, 98.

Garnick, M. B. & Richie, J. P. (1986) Intensive alternating chemotherapy with cisplatin (P) – vinblastine (V) – bleomycin (B) (PVB) with P – etoposide – B (PEB) for poor prognosis germ cell and undifferentiated cancers. *Proceedings ASCO*, **5**, 101.

Germa-Lluch, J. R., Begent, R. H. J. & Bagshawe, K. D. (1980) Tumor-marker levels and prognosis in malignant teratoma of the testis. *British Journal of Cancer*, **42**, 850–855.

Levi, J., Raghavan, D., Harvey, V. et al. (1986) Deletion of bleomycin from therapy for good prognosis advanced testicular cancer: a prospective randomized study. *Proceedings ASCO*, **5**, 97.

Logothetis, C., Samuels, M. L., Selig, D. et al. (1985) Improved survival with cyclic chemotherapy for nonseminomatous germ cell tumors of the testis. *Journal of Clinical Oncology*, **3**, 326–335.

Logothetis, C. L., Samuels, M. L., Selig, D. E. et al. (1986) Cyclic chemotherapy with Cytoxan, Adriamycin and cisplatin (CISCA) and Velban-bleomycin (VB$_{IV}$) in advanced germinal tumors. Results with 100 patients. *American Journal of Medicine* (in press).

Medical Research Council Working Party on Testicular Tumours (1985) Prognostic factors in advanced non-seminomatous germ-cell testicular tumours: results of a multicentre study. *Lancet*, **i**, 8–11.

Ozols, R. F., Ihde, D., Jacob, J. et al. (1984) Randomized trial of PVeBV [High dose cisplatin (P), vinblastine (Ve), bleomycin (B), VP-16 (V)] versus PVeB in poor prognosis non-seminomatous testicular cancer. *Proceedings ASCO*, **3**, 155.

Ozols, R. F., Corden, B. J., Jacob, J. et al. (1984) High-dose cisplatin in hypertonic saline. *Annals of Internal Medicine*, **100**, 19–24.

Ozols, R. F., Deisseroth, A. B., Javadpour, N. et al. (1983) Treatment of poor prognosis nonseminomatous testicular cancer with 'high-dose' platinum combination chemotherapy regimen. *Cancer*, **51**, 1803–1807.

Peckham, M. J., Horwich, A., Blackmore, C. et al. (1985) Etoposide and cisplatin with or without bleomycin as first-line chemotherapy for patients with small-volume metastases of testicular nonseminoma. *Cancer Treatment Reports*, **69**, 483–488.

Picozzi, V. J. Jr, Fuad, F. S., Hannigan, J. F. et al. (1984) Prognostic significance of a decline in serum human chorionic gonadotropin levels after initial chemotherapy for advanced germ-cell carcinoma. *Annals of Internal Medicine*, **100**, 183–186.

Pizzocaro, G., Piva, L., Salvoni, R. et al. (1985a) Cisplatin, etoposide, bleomycin: first line therapy and early resection of residual tumor in far-advanced germinal testis cancer. *Cancer*, **56**, 2411–2415.

Pizzocaro, G., Salvioni, R., Pasi, M. et al. (1985b) Early resection of residual tumor during cisplatin, vinblastine, bleomycin combination chemotherapy in stage III and bulky stage II nonseminomatous testicular cancer. *Cancer*, **56**, 249–255.

Pizzocaro, G., Salvioni, R., Zanoni, F. et al. (1986) Successful treatment of good risk disseminated testicular cancer with cisplatin, bleomycin and reduced dose vinblastine. *Cancer* (in press).

Richardson, R. L., Hahn, R. C., Kvols, L. K. et al. (1985) Bleomycin (B), Etoposide (E), and continuous infusion cisplatin (P) BECIP in metastatic testicular cancer. *Proceedings ASCO*, **4**, 105.

Samuels, M. L., Johnson, D. E. & Holoye, A. (1975) Continuous intravenous bleomycin (NSC-125066) therapy with vinblastine (NSC-49842) in Stage III testicular neoplasia. *Cancer Chemotherapy Reports*, **59**, 563–570.

Scheulen, M. E., Pfeiffer, R., Hoffken, K. et al. (1984) Long-term survival (LTS) and prognostic factor (PF) in patients with disseminated non-seminomatous testicular cancer. *Proceedings ASCO*, **3**, 163.

Schmoll, H. J., Arnold, A., Bergmann, L. et al. (1986) Effective chemotherapy in testicular cancer with bulky disease: platinum ultra high dose/VP-16/bleomycin. *Proceedings ASCO*, **5**, 102.

Stoter, G., Sylvester, R., Sleijfer, D. Th. et al. (1987) Multivariate analysis of prognostic variables in patients with disseminated non-seminomatous testicular cancer; results from an EORTC multi-institutional phase III study. *International Journal of Andrology*, **10**, 239–246.

Stoter, G., Kaye, S., Sleijfer, D. et al. (1986) Preliminary results of BEP (bleomycin, etoposide, cisplatin) versus an alternating regimen of BEP and PVB (cisplatin, vinblastine, bleomycin) in high volume metastatic testicular non-seminomas. An EORTC study. *Proceedings ASCO*, **5**, 106.

Taylor, G., Perry, D., Knight, P. *et al.* (1984) Poor prognosis germ cell tumors treated with cyclophosphamide, dactinomycin, vinblastine, bleomycin, cisplatin (VAB) alternating with VP-16, vincristine (VV). *Proceedings ASCO*, **3**, 158.

Von Eyben, F. E., Jacobsen, G. K., Pedersen, H. *et al.* (1982) Multivariate analysis of risk factors in patients with metastatic testicular germ cell tumours treated with vinblastine and bleomycin. *Invasion Metastases*, **2**, 125–135.

Discussion

Hargreave It is important to remember that different prognostic factors may be involved in the prediction of complete response (CR) as opposed to survival. The current prognostic factors which are used as models to predict CR must be re-evaluated when we have sufficiently long follow-up studies to be able to use survival as the end-point.

Prognostic factors are important in the stratification of patients who are going to receive different treatment according to a randomized scheme. If these prognostic models are not used there is always a danger that the groups of patients being treated may not be truly comparable, and that differences in response may be wrongly ascribed to the therapy.

Oliver I would like to pose two questions. Firstly, serum level of lactate dehydrogenase (LDH) is being increasingly recognized as an important prognostic factor. From your review data it is unclear if LDH is a variable which is independent of hCG levels in the serum. Our data support yours that LDH and hCG are the two most important prognostic factors, but our numbers are small and we cannot distinguish between the two variables. There is a piece of evidence suggesting that LDH levels may be more significant than hCG levels. In patients with terminal drug-resistant disease, the ratio of LDH to hCG levels changes and the LDH-producing disease is present in a greater proportion than in the pretreatment sample. Has this been observed by any other groups who monitor serum LDH levels?

Secondly, as the MRC prognostic factor analysis indicated, there was a more substantial improvement with time, reflecting experience, than was demonstrable as being due to actual changes in drugs used. We must not, therefore, assume that increasing survival is necessarily an effect of changing therapy.

Vogelzang Perhaps we are seeing 'learning curves' as our patient management improves. Since 1982 we have been using chemotherapy at an *earlier* stage and this probably has a bearing on survival.

H. H. Hansen When we are starting a new randomized trial, must we stratify the patients into different prognostic groups using one of the models we have just seen described?

Vogelzang I think that is a very good suggestion.

Bosl In our randomized males, since November 1982 we have prospectively assigned patients into different prognosis groups using our model. These studies are now complete. We have had good responses among patients who were predicted to have a good prognosis by our models, achieving 90% complete remission. The durable response rate is much lower at 35% in patients who, according to our model, are in the poor risk group. This indicates the value of applying these risk models prospectively and randomizing patients within the assigned risk categories.

Hansen Results of such trials may be complicated by the phenomenon of stage migration of patients. The factors involved in selecting patients for referral to treatment centres, and the staging procedures used for assessing extended disease, are changing so that similar patients may be staged differently depending on variable factors.

Vogelzang This is a difficult problem. Our refined techniques using CT scans and other staging procedures should help to maintain accuracy and uniformity.

Multivariate analysis of prognostic variables in patients with disseminated non-seminomatous testicular cancer: results from an EORTC multi-institutional phase III study

G. STOTER, R. SYLVESTER, D. Th. SLEIJFER,
W. W. TEN BOKKEL HUININK, S. B. KAYE,
W. G. JONES, A. T. VAN OOSTEROM,
C. P. J. VENDRIK, P. SPAANDER and M. DE PAUW
Rotterdam Cancer Institute, Rotterdam, The Netherlands

Key words. Testicular cancer, prognostic factors, multivariate analysis.

Introduction

With standard cisplatin combination chemotherapy the risk of death from disseminated non-seminomatous testicular cancer is approximately 30%, including a 5% toxic death rate from these regimens (Einhorn, 1981; Stoter *et al.*, 1984, 1986; Greist *et al.*, 1985; Williams *et al.*, 1985). This underlines the need to define good risk as well as poor risk patients prior to treatment in order to decrease the toxicity in the first category and to intensify the treatment in the second group. Several factors have been reported as influencing the prognosis such as: extent of disease (Skinner, 1982; Ozols *et al.*, 1983; Stoter *et al.*, 1984, 1986; Williams *et al.*, 1985; Medical Research Council Working Party, 1985), initial serum marker concentrations of ßhCG, AFP and LDH (Von Eyben *et al.*, 1982; Newlands *et al.*, 1983; Bosl *et al.*, 1983; Medical Research Council Working Party, 1985) or their rate of decrease during chemotherapy (Picozzi *et al.*, 1985), histology (Pugh, 1976; Stoter *et al.*, 1979), prior treatment (Stoter *et al.*, 1984; Golbey, Reynolds & Vugrin, 1979), treatment protocol, time from diagnosis to treatment (Medical Research Council Working Party, 1985), performance status (Von Eyben *et al.*, 1982) and age.

Since many of these variables may be interrelated, a multivariate analysis of various factors has been performed in order to determine their relative prognostic importance.

Materials and Methods

From July 1979 until March 1983, eleven institutions collaborating in the EORTC GU-Group entered 214 non-pretreated patients with disseminated non-seminomatous testicular cancer in a randomized prospective study, to receive four cycles of induction chemotherapy with cisplatin, vinblastine and bleomycin (PVB), with a randomization between vinblastine 0.4 mg/kg/cycle (100% VBL) or vinblastine 0.3 mg/kg/cycle (75% VBL).

Correspondence: Dr G. Stoter, Rotterdam Cancer Institute, Groene Hilledijk 301, 3075 EA Rotterdam, The Netherlands.

Of the 214 patients, 162 were eligible and evaluable for response. The reasons for inevaluability have been reported elsewhere (Stoter et al., 1986). CR was defined as the complete disappearance of all clinical, radiographic and biochemical evidence of disease. For patients with evidence of residual tumour after four cycles of induction chemotherapy, in the absence of elevated markers, it was mandatory that they underwent debulking surgery. Patients with fibrosis, necrosis and mature teratoma in their resected specimen were classified as CRs.

Histological diagnosis was based on the British classification (Pugh, 1976). Staging of the disease was according to the Royal Marsden Hospital classification (Medical Research Council Working Party, 1985). However, it was also felt necessary to record the exact number and size of all metastatic lesions.

Serum concentrations of ßhCG $\leq$ 4 ng/ml and AFP $\leq$ 16 ng/ml were considered to be normal. Serum concentrations of LDH were measured by different methods in different institutions where the upper limits of normal varied significantly. For these reasons LDH has been expressed as a numerical factor times the upper limit of normal for each institution.

Statistical techniques

The endpoint used in this study to assess the prognostic importance of the different factors is the CR rate. The duration of survival was not retained as an endpoint since only 32/162 (20%) of the patients have died.

Comparisons of the CR rate for the different levels of a given factor were carried out using the classical chi-square test for the comparison of proportions. For ordered categorical variables, Kendall's Tau B and C were calculated as a nonparametric measure of correlation of 'trend'. Kendall and Spearman rank correlation coefficients were also calculated to determine the degree of correlation between the various prognostic factors (Kendall, 1975).

The relative importance of the prognostic factors with regard to the CR rate was studied using a linear logistic regression model (Lee, 1980). The linear logistic regression model assumes that the relationship between the probability p that a patient achieves a CR and the patient's characteristics X_1, X_2, X_m at entry into the study is given by

$$p = e^y/(1 + e^y) \text{ or } \ln p/(1 - p) = y \qquad (A)$$

where $y = \sum_{i=0}^{m} B_i X_i$ is a linear function of the patient's characteristics, $X_0 = 1$ and the B_i are the unknown regression coefficients that are estimated from the data by the technique of maximum likelihood.

Results

Identification of prognostic factors

In order to identify the variables of potential prognostic importance, continuous variables were discretized and a univariate analysis of each variable was carried out by comparing the CR rate for the different levels of the variable. Variables representing tumour histology, markers and lung metastases were all highly significant.

Multivariate analysis
Since some of the variables described above are correlated with each other, it is necessary to apply multivariate techniques that allow all of the variables to act together so that the relative importance of the variables can be determined.

The variables which were analysed in the logistic regression model, and their coding, are given in Table 1. Both step-up (variables are added to the model one by one) and step-down (variables are deleted from the model one by one) methods are used.

The final model, using a step-down procedure, was composed of the following variables which were all available in 154 patients:
TROPH (trophoblastic elements): 0 = no or possible, 1 = yes;
ALPH (serum concentration of AFP): 0 = 0–999 ng/ml, 1 = ≥ 1000 ng/ml;
LUNG (lung metastases): 0 = no, 1 = yes;
SIXNB (size and number of lung metastases): 0 = none, 1 = 1–3 and ≤ 3 cm, 2 = 4–19 and ≤ 3 cm or 1–3 and > 3 cm, 3 = ≥ 20 or 4–19 and > 3 cm.

Once these values are known for any patient, the probability of a CR can be estimated.

The following model was obtained

$$\hat{p} = \frac{e^{\hat{y}}}{1 + e^{\hat{y}}}$$

where
$$\hat{y} = 1.9381 - 2.1327 \times \text{TROPH} - 2.2723 \times \text{ALPH} + 4.878 \times \text{LUNG} - 2.3212 \times \text{SIXNB} \quad \text{(B)}$$
as an 'optimal' estimate of the CR rate.

Once the values of TROPH, ALPH, LUNG and SIXNB (see Table 2) are known for any given patient, the above formula for $\hat{p}$ gives an estimate of the probability that a patient will have a CR. Risk groups can then be formed based on the value of $\hat{p}$.

Of special note is the fact that the *single* most important variable, LB = $\log_{10}$ (ßhCG+1), was not retained in the final model.

Variables other than the four included in the final model provide no significant additional information with respect to predicting the probability of CR.

Risk groups
Table 2 presents the composition of the risk groups according to the possible values of these four variables, while Table 3 gives the observed and predicted probabilities of CR by patient characteristics within each group. Finally the observed CR rate for all patients within each risk group is given in Table 4. From this last table it is seen that within each group there is excellent agreement between the observed number of CRs and the number of CRs predicted by the model, and that the observed CR rate ranges from 100% in risk group 1 to only 18% in risk group 4.

Discussion
Approximately 70% of all patients with disseminated non-seminomatous testicular cancer achieve a CR with cisplatin based combination chemotherapy. However, patients with bad prognostic characteristics fare worse.

Table 1. Variables analysed in the logistic regression model

*1. RT 19 (reponse to treatment): 0=no CR, 1=CR
2. TROPH (trophoblastic elements in primary tumour): 0=no or possible, 1=yes
3. TROP (trophoblastic elements in primary tumour): 0=no, 1=possible, 2=yes
4. TROPP (trophoblastic elements in primary tumour): 0=no, 1=yes or possible
5. TRT11 (treatment arm): 0=100% VBL, 1=75% VBL
6. PMAR (elevated markers): 0=normal AFP and ßhCG, 1=elevated AFP or ßhCG
7. BURDEN (tumour volume): 0=low volume, 1=high volume
8. BETA (ßhCG): 0=0–49, 1=50–999, 2=10^3–9999, 3=$\geq 10^4$ ng/ml
9. NBETA (ßhCG elevated): 0=no, 1=yes (>4 ng/ml)
10. LB = $\log_{10}$ (ßhCG+1)
11. ALPH (AFP): 0=0–999, 1=$\geq 10^3$ ng/ml
12. NALPHA (AFP elevated): 0=no, 1=yes (>16 ng/ml)
13. LA = $\log_{10}$ (AFP+1)
14. LDH6 (LDH above 2.5 times upper limit of normal): 0=no, 1=yes
15. INFRA (infradiaphragmatic metastases): 0=no, 1=yes
16. SINFRA (size of infradiaphragmatic metastases): 0=none, 1=<5 cm, 2=$\geq$5 cm, 3=$\geq$10 cm
17. MEDIA (mediastinal metastases): 0=no, 1=yes
18. SUPRA (supraventricular metastases): 0=no, 1=yes
19. LUNG (lung metastases): 0=no, 1=yes
20. SIZE (size of lung metastases): 0=none, 1=$\leq$2 cm, 2=$\leq$3 cm, 3=>3 cm
21. NUMB (number of lung metastases): 0=none, 1=1–3, 2=4–19, 3=$\geq$20
22. SIXNB (size by number of lung metastases): 0=none, 1=1–3 and $\leq$ 3 cm, 2=4–19 and $\leq$3 cm or 1–3 and >3 cm, 3=$\geq$20 or 4–19 and >3 cm
23. SIZXNB (size by number of lung metastases): 0=none, 1=1–3, 2=4–19 and $\leq$3 cm, 3=$\geq$20 or 4–19 and >3 cm
24. SITE (number of metastatic sites): 0=0–1, 1=2, 2=3–5
25. AGER (age >45 years): 0=no, 1=yes
26. HP21 (liver metastases): 0=no, 1=yes

*Dependent variable.

Table 2. Composition of risk groups

Risk group	No. of patients	TROPH	ALPH	LUNG	SIXNB
1	24	no	<1000	yes	1
2	3	yes	<1000	yes	1
	1	no	$\geq$1000	yes	1
	20	no	<1000	yes	2
	49	no	<1000	no	0
3	0	yes	$\geq$1000	yes	1
	3	yes	<1000	yes	2
	10	no	$\geq$1000	yes	2
	14	no	<1000	yes	3
	7	yes	<1000	no	0
	12	no	$\geq$1000	no	0
4	0	yes	$\geq$1000	yes	2
	6	yes	<1000	yes	3
	4	no	$\geq$1000	yes	3
	0	yes	$\geq$1000	no	0
	1	yes	$\geq$1000	yes	3

Table 3. Response rate by patient characteristics

Risk group	No. of patients	Observed no. of CR	Predicted no. of CR	Observed P*	Predicted P*
1	24	24	24	1.0	0.989
2	3	2	3	0.667	0.914
	1	1	1	1.0	0.902
	20	20	18	1.0	0.898
	49	42	43	0.857	0.874
3	0	—	—	—	0.522
	3	1	2	0.333	0.510
	10	4	5	0.40	0.475
	14	5	6	0.357	0.463
	7	3	3	0.429	0.452
	12	6	5	0.50	0.417
4	0	—	—	—	0.119
	6	2	1	0.333	0.093
	4	0	0	0	0.082
	0	—	—	—	0.078
	1	0	0	0	0.010

*P = probability of CR.

Table 4. Response rate of risk group

Risk group	Predicted no. of CR	Observed no. of CR	No. of patients	Observed percentage of CR
1 } = I	24	24	24	100
2 }	65	65	73	89
3 = II	21	19	46	41
4 = III	1	2	11	18
Total	111	110	154	71

Obviously, the main goal of clinical research is to decrease the toxicity of treatment regimens in good risk patients and to intensify the treatment of poor risk patients. For that reason it is of utmost importance for physicians to be able to estimate prospectively the probability of CR in each one of their patients. The best tool for such an estimation is the linear logistic regression model since it provides an 'optimal' subset of variables for use in determining a patient's prognostic category.

Applied to the data in this study the model yielded four prognostic variables: TROPH (trophoblastic elements in the primary tumour: yes or no), ALPH (serum level of AFP below or above 1000 ng/ml), LUNG (lung metastases: yes or no) and SIXNB (size and number of lung metastases). On the basis of these four variables we can divide our patient population into four risk groups (Table 2), varying from a very high to a very low probability of achieving CR (Tables 3 and 4). In practice one might define three treatments of differing intensity corresponding to the three risk groups (I, II, III) in Table 4.

We have assessed the degree of correct prediction of CR with the requirement that the probability of achieving CR is $p \geq 0.80$. Both sensitivity (correct prediction of CR) and specificity (correct prediction of no CR) are acceptable; however, the misallocation rate is high (37%).

The results of any multivariate prognostic factor analysis are of course a function of the variables which are analysed, the way in which they are analysed and of the endpoint of the analysis, i.e. CR, disease-free survival or overall survival. For instance, in the initial phase of this analysis, using a step-up procedure, LB = $\log_{10}$ (ßhCG+1) appeared to be the single most important variable (Table 3). When we decided to omit the Royal Marsden classification of lung metastases and let them take on a continuum of values with regard to size and number, LB fell out of the model using a step-down procedure and LUNG and SIXNB remained in the model, with greater predictive power than LB. It became clear that for our patient population the Royal Marsden staging classification of lung metastases had to be modified (Table 1, point 22). This did not hold true for retroperitoneal metastases. Even when we provided a separate category for patients with infradiaphragmatic metastases larger than 10 cm (Table 1, point 16), the variable SINFRA, while significant in a univariate analysis, still was not retained by the model. However, it is striking to observe that 5/12 (42%) patients who relapsed from CR had large infradiaphragmatic metastases ≥ 10 cm (two patients) or ≥ 15 cm (three patients). SINFRA might have been retained if we could have used disease-free survival as an endpoint.

Investigators in the U.S.A. (Bosl et al., 1983; Birch et al., 1986) and in Europe (Medical Research Council Working Party, 1985; Von Eyben et al., 1982) have performed multivariate analyses with slightly different variables and endpoints. All models yield tumour markers and/or tumour volume as significant variables, although it is clear that none of the model results are identical.

The EORTC GU-Group is currently performing randomized studies (protocol 30824) for patients with high and low volume metastases. Applying the results of our model to the very preliminary data from these studies, we find the same trend in CR rates in the various risk groups. However, the CR rate in each category is higher than in the study here described, i.e. approximately 100%, 80% and 50% for risk groups I, II and III, respectively, perhaps due to improved patient treatment.

Once the data of protocol 30824 are complete, a new analysis will be done to determine if we will arrive at the same model. In that case we will use the model in future studies to select the patients prospectively for low or high intensity treatment.

Acknowledgement

The authors are indebted to Mrs A. Sugiarsi for typing the manuscript.

References

Birch, R., Williams, S., Cone, A., Einhorn, L., Roark, P., Turner, S. & Greco, F. (1986) Prognostic factors for favorable outcome in disseminated germ cell tumours. *Journal of Clinical Oncology*, **4**, 400–407.

Bosl, G. J., Geller, N. L., Cirrincione, C., Vogelzang, N. J., Kennedy, B. J., Whitmore, W. F., Jr, Vugrin, D., Scher, H., Nisselbaum, J. & Golbey, R. B. (1983) Multivariate analysis of prognostic variables in patients with metastatic testicular cancer. *Cancer Research*, **43**, 3403–3407.

Einhorn, L. H. (1981) Testicular cancer as a model for a curable neoplasm: The Richard and Hinda Rosenthal foundation award lecture. *Cancer Research*, **41**, 3275–3280.

Golbey, R. B., Reynolds, T. F. & Vugrin, D. (1979) Chemotherapy of metastatic germ cell tumors. *Seminars in Oncology*, **6**, 82–86.

Greist, A., Roth, B., Einhorn, L. & Williams, S. (1985) Cisplatin combination chemotherapy for disseminated germ cell tumors: long term follow-up. *Proceedings of American Society of Clinical Oncology*, **4**, 100.

Kendall, M. (1975) In: *Rank Correlation Methods*, chapters I–IV and IX, pp. 1–66 and 123–131. Charles Griffin, London.

Lee, E. (1980) Identification of risk factors related to dichotomous data. *Statistical Methods for Survival Data Analysis*, pp. 338–365. Lifetime Learning Publications, Belmont, California.

Medical Research Council Working Party on Testicular Tumours (1985) Prognostic factors in advanced non-seminomatous germ-cell testicular tumours: results of a multicentre study. *Lancet*, **i**, 8–11.

Newlands, E. S., Begent, R. H. J., Rustin, G. J. S., Parker, D. & Bagshawe, K. D. (1983) Further advances in the management of malignant teratomas of the testis and other sites. *Lancet*, **i**, 948–951.

Ozols, R. F., Deisseroth, A. B., Javadpour, N., Barlock, A., Messerschmidt, G. L. & Young, R. C. (1983) Treatment of poor prognosis non-seminomatous testicular cancer with a 'high-dose' platinum combination chemotherapy regimen. *Cancer*, **51**, 1803–1807.

Picozzi, V. J., Jr, Hannigan, J. F., Jr, Freiha, F. S., Rogoway, W. M. & Torti, F. M. (1985) Prognostic significance of day 1 and day 22 marker levels in advanced male germ cell cancer. *Proceedings of American Society of Clinical Oncology*, **4**, 102.

Pugh, R. C. B. (1976) Testicular tumours—introduction. *Pathology of the Testis*, pp. 139–162. Blackwell Scientific Publications, Oxford.

Skinner, D. G. (1982) Advanced metastatic testicular cancer: the need for reporting results according to initial extent of disease. *Journal of Urology*, **128**, 312–314.

Stoter, G., Vendrik, C. P. J., Struyvenberg, A., Brouwers, Th. M., Sleijfer, D. Th., Schraffordt-Koops, H., Van Oosterom, A. T. & Pinedo, H. M. (1979) Combination chemotherapy with cis-diamminedichloroplatinum, vinblastine and bleomycin in advanced testicular nonseminoma. *Lancet*, **i**, 941–945.

Stoter, G., Vendrik, C. P. J., Struyvenberg, A., Sleijfer, D. Th., Vriesendorp, R., Schraffordt-Koops, H., Van Oosterom, A. T., Ten Bokkel Huinink, W. W. & Pinedo, H. M. (1984) Five-year survival of patients with disseminated non-seminomatous testicular cancer treated with cisplatin, vinblastine and bleomycin. *Cancer*, **54**, 1521–1524.

Stoter, G., Sleijfer, D. Th., Ten Bokkel Huinink, W. W., Kaye, S. B., Jones, W. G., Van Osterom, A. T., Vendrick, C. P. J., Spaander, P., De Pauw, M. & Sylvester, R. (1986) High dose versus low dose vinblastine in cisplatin–vinblastine–bleomycin (PVB) combination chemotherapy of non-seminomatous testicular cancer: a randomized study of the EORTC Genito-Urinary Tract Cancer Cooperative Group. *Journal of Clinical Oncology* (in press).

Von Eyben, F. E., Jacobsen, G. K., Pedersen, H., Jacobsen, M., Clausen, P. P., Zibrandtsen, P. C. & Gullberg, B. (1982) Multivariate analysis of risk factors in patients with metastatic testicular germ cell tumours treated with vinblastine and bleomycin. *Invasion Metastasis*, **2**, 125–135.

Williams, S., Einhorn, L., Greco, R., Birch, R. & Irwin, L. (1985) Disseminated germ cell tumors: a comparison of cisplatin plus bleomycin plus either vinblastine (PVB) or VP-16 (BEP). *Proceedings of American Society of Clinical Oncology*, **4**, 100.

Discussion

Hargreave It is important to use *multi*variate regression analyses because these will indicate which factors are independently important. They are often difficult to understand and at first the conclusions may seem bizarre; however, we must accept them and see how the results stand up to subsequent analysis when the response rate and ultimate survival of the patients are known.

Rustin Why did you choose complete remission (CR) rate rather than survival as your end-point? A considerable proportion of patients will have necrotic residual tumour masses and will not relapse, yet they are not in CR.

Stoter Only 20% of our patients have died so that the survival curve is inapplicable as an end-point because of the small number of patients who would have reached the end-point. Survival rate is only reliable if many deaths occur.

All our CR patients who relapsed have had surgical and pathological confirmation of their relapse.

Dieckmann Why did you not include extrapulmonary metastases in your studies? In our patients, the presence of liver metastases was found to be a criterion of very bad prognosis even in the absence of pulmonary metastases.

Stoter We did look at extrapulmonary spread, for example to the liver. These were each of prognostic value as univariate factors, but because of correlation with other variables they ceased to be independent variables in the multivariate model.

Levi Have you measured the total volume of tumour metastases rather than just looking at the sites, and how does this correlate with outcome? It is important to recognize that any multivariate statistical analysis must include biological features of importance. As there is a continuum of relevant prognostic factors, selection of only a few factors based on the level of statistical significance may be misleading.

Stoter The outcome of any multivariate analysis is obviously a function of the variables which have been investigated. We have analysed the total number of metastases, the number of sites, and the total sum of the surface areas of lymph node metastases. An accurate assessment of the total volume of tumour in litres could not be obtained. With regard to histology, we have taken into account all different components in the primary tumour.

Oliver Your data suggest that serum hCG level is not an independently variable prognostic factor over the presence of lung metastases. However, clinically and biometrically, the level of serum hCG is a more precise measurement with regard to quantitation. There must surely be very few cases in your series with extensive lung metastases who do not have high serum hCG levels. Would it be possible for you to prove that very high levels of hCG is an independent variable to confirm the findings of Dr Newlands that levels greater than 50,000 IU/l indicate a poor prognosis? You only consider if serum hCG is elevated or not, but if serum hCG is a continuously variable factor, there must be a cut-off value above which it becomes an independent variable. Very high levels of hCG may indicate trophoblastic tumour which in itself carries a poor prognosis as a specific variable in your model.

Stoter We did analyse hCG and AFP as continuous variables. We find that serum hCG is the most important *single* factor in our patient population. Levels of 10,000 ng/ml and above are consistently related to a CR rate below 25%. However, hCG dropped from the model because it was highly correlated with lung metastases.

Surveillance following orchidectomy for Stage I testicular cancer

M. J. PECKHAM and M. BRADA   *Institute of Cancer Research and The Royal Marsden Hospital, Sutton, Surrey*

Summary

Surveillance following orchidectomy was introduced in the management of Stage I testicular nonseminoma in 1979 and Stage I seminoma in 1983. Of 132 nonseminoma patients followed for 12–84 months (median 43 months) the relapse rate is 27%. Relapses were diagnosed 2–44 months after orchidectomy with 90% of relapses appearing within the first year. Of the 132 patients, 131 are alive and disease-free. The pattern of relapse was as follows: 47% of relapses occurred in abdominal nodes, 13% in abdominal nodes and lung, 17% in the lung and 23% with elevated serum markers as the only evidence of disease; 26% of relapsing patients had normal serum AFP and hCG levels. The prognostic significance of thirteen clinical histopathological and biochemical factors has been analysed by multiple regression analysis. Histology and lymphatic invasion within the primary tumour are significant independent prognostic factors.

A total of thirty-six patients had scrotal interference prior to removal of the primary tumour. This was not a contra-indication to surveillance. None has developed scrotal recurrence and the overall relapse rate (11%) is comparable to that observed in the surveillance series as a whole.

Fifty-two patients with Stage I seminoma have been observed from 12–41 months after orchidectomy. Seven (13%) have relapsed and six of the seven relapses have been confined to retroperitoneal lymph nodes. Preliminary data suggests that pre-orchidectomy elevation of serum hCG is not a significant prognostic factor.

Key words: Surveillance, testicular cancer, histology, tumour markers, relapse.

Introduction

Analysis of historical data strongly suggested that 70–80% of men with clinical Stage I nonseminomatous teticular tumours were likely to be cured by orchidectomy alone (Peckham, 1981). Given the effectiveness of chemotherapy in patients with small volume metastases and the feasibility of detecting relapsing Stage I patients with a minimal tumour load it was reasonable to assume that the probability of cure with salvage treatment would be extremely high. Accordingly, in 1979 routine lymph node irradiation was discontinued in favour of close surveillance after orchidectomy for Stage I nonseminomatous tumours (Peckham *et al.*, 1982,

---

Correspondence: Dr M. J. Peckham, Institute of Cancer Research and The Royal Marsden Hospital, Downs Road, Sutton, Surrey SM2 5PT.

1983; Peckham, 1985). It was recognized that excellent treatment results for Stage I disease could be obtained with radical lymph node dissection and deferred chemotherapy (Skinner & Skardino, 1979) and radiotherapy with deferred chemotherapy (Peckham et al., 1979). Hence the issue under investigation was not curability but curability with avoidance of unnecessary therapy.

Before embarking on the surveillance study a detailed analysis was carried out on Stage I patients receiving lymph node irradiation between 1964 and 1979 (Raghavan et al., 1982). The objective was to examine factors predisposing to relapse. Two factors with prognostic significance were identified; the behaviour of serum markers following orchidectomy and involvement by tumour of the spermatic cord. In this study histology was not a significant factor, although in previous studies the relapse rate had been significantly higher in embryonal carcinoma than in teratocarcinoma (Peckham, 1979).

Entry criteria into the surveillance study included normal serum marker levels or rapid normalization of raised serum marker levels following orchidectomy. If tumour was demonstrated in the cut end of the spermatic cord the patient was excluded; in practice only one such example has been encountered. Patients who show persistent elevation of serum alphafetoprotein and/or hCG levels after orchidectomy were designated Stage IM and treated with chemotherapy. Pre-orchidectomy serum marker levels were obtained whenever possible and attempts made to obtain at least twice weekly measurements during the post-orchidectomy period to allow the regression rate to be measured. The histology of the primary tumour was reviewed in all cases and the material processed for the presence of tissue hCG and AFP using the immunoperoxidase method. The primary tumour was examined histologically for evidence of vascular invasion and lymphatic permeation and the local extent of the tumour assessed in terms of involvement of the spermatic cord, epididymis and tunica. Trans-scrotal needle biopsy or aspiration, scrotal orchidectomy, prior orchidopexy or testicular biopsy with delayed orchidectomy were not considered contra-indications to surveillance. The surveillance protocol consisted of monthly visits for the first year, 2-monthly for the second year and 3-monthly for the third year. Initially CT scans were performed on alternate visits for the first 2 years but this practice has been discontinued with no scans during the second year. Serum AFP and hCG levels are measured at each visit.

Results of surveillance for Stage I nonseminomatous germ cell tumours

Between 1979 and 1985, 132 patients with clinical Stage I nonseminomatous germ cell tumours were followed after orchidectomy and managed with chemotherapy in the event of relapse. Of 132 patients followed for 12–84 months (median 43 months) the relapse rate is 27% (Table 1). Relapses were diagnosed 2–44 months after orchidectomy (median 6 months) with 31/35 (90%) of relapses appearing within the first year (Fig. 1). Of the thirty-five relapsing patients, thirty-four (97%) are alive and disease free (Table 2).

The pattern of relapse was as follows: seventeen patients (47%) relapsed in abdominal nodes, four (13%) with abdominal and lung metastases, six (17%) with lung metastases and eight (23%) with elevated serum markers as the only evidence of disease (Table 3). Of thirty-five patients who relapsed twenty-six (74%) had

Table 1. Surveillance after orchidectomy for clinical Stage I testicular germ cell tumours: outcome in patients followed for a minimum of 1 year (The Royal Marsden Hospital, 1979–85)

Histology	No. of patients	Relapses	%	Observation time after orchidectomy in months (median)
MTI (teratocarcinoma	72	13	18	12–84 (43)
MTU (embryonal carcinoma)	47	19	40	14–81 (42)
MTT	5	1	20	17–74 (59)
Seminoma, raised AFP	3	2	67	55, 58, 75
Differentiated teratoma	5	0	–	14–59 (45)
Total	132	35	27	12–84 (43)

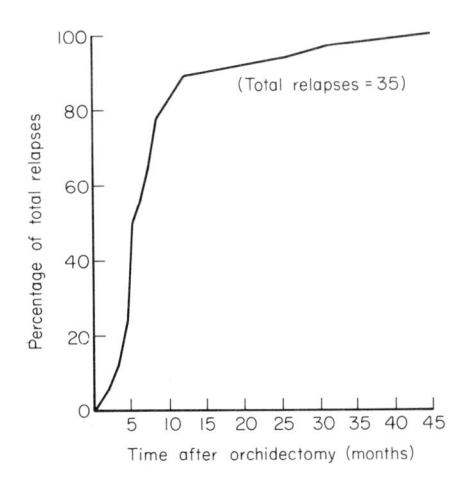

Fig. 1. Surveillance for Stage I testicular non-seminoma: time to relapse after orchidectomy (The Royal Marsden Hospital, 1979–85).

Table 2. Surveillance for clinical Stage I nonseminomatous germ cell testicular tumours: results of treatment for relapse (The Royal Marsden Hospital, 1979–85)

			Time after chemotherapy (months)	
Total relapse	Alive	Alive disease free	Range	Median
35	34	34	11–76	35

Table 3. Surveillance for Stage I nonseminomatous germ cell tumour of the testis: site(s) of relapse (The Royal Marsden Hospital, 1979–85)

	Initial site(s) of relapse			
Total relapses diagnosed, 1979–85	Abdominal nodes	Lung	Abdomen and lung	Markers only
35	17 (47%)	6 (17%)	4 (13%)	8 (23%)

elevated serum levels of either AFP or hCG but nine (26%) had normal serum marker levels. In the latter group relapse was proven histologically in five patients and in four was obvious on sequential scans (Table 4). Overall, of the 132 patients only eight had metastases resected for diagnostic purposes either before or after chemotherapy.

Table 4. Surveillance after orchidectomy for clinical Stage I testicular germ cell tumours: tissue diagnosis in relation to treatment for relapse (The Royal Marsden Hospital, 1979–84)

Total patients	Tissue diagnosis prior to treatment for relapse		Excision of residual masses after chemotherapy
	Fine needle aspirate	Node biopsy	
132	3 (2%)	2 (2%)	6 (5%)

Table 5. Influence of histology and presence or absence of lymphatic invasion in patients observed after orchidectomy for Stage I testicular nonseminoma (data from Hoskin et al., 1986)

Histology	Lymphatic invasion within primary tumour	
	No	Yes
MTI	6/50* (12%)	4/10 (40%)
MTU	11/31 (33%)	7/9 (78%)

*Number relapsing/total patients.

An important eventual aim of the surveillance study is to identify prognostic factors which would permit immediate chemotherapy for high risk patients. Recently an analysis of prognostic facors has been carried out on 126 patients entered into the surveillance study between February 1979 and March 1985 (Hoskin et al., 1986). The prognostic significance of thirteen clinical histopathological and biochemical factors was analysed. Vascular invasion and lymphatic invasion within the primary tumour, histology and involvement of the epididymis and rete testis were significantly associated with an increased risk of relapse. However, multiple regression analysis showed that only histology and lymphatic invasion were significant independent prognostic factors. As shown in Table 5, the relapse rate varied from 6/50 (12%) in MTI patients without lymphatic invasion to 7/9 (78%) in MTU patient with lymphatic invasion. These findings provide the basis for the consideration of adjuvant chemotherapy in patients with apparent clinical Stage I testicular nonseminoma who are at high risk of harbouring occult metastases.

As noted above, we have not regarded scrotal interferences as a contraindication to surveillance. A total of thirty-six patients had scrotal interference prior to the removal of the primary tumour (Kennedy et al., 1985). None of these thirty-six patients developed scrotal recurrence during surveillance and the overall relapse rate (4/36; 11%) is comparable to that observed in the surveillance series as a whole. These observations suggest that the propensity of testicular germ cell tumours to spread locally after scrotal interference is low.

Surveillance for Stage I seminoma

The successful adoption of the surveillance policy in nonseminomatous tumours has raised the possibility that a similar policy may be applicable in Stage I seminoma. In favour is the probable low incidence of occult metastases in retroperitoneal lymph nodes in patients with clinical Stage I disease. Maier, Sulak & Mittemeyer (1968), in a series of Stage I patients submitted to radical lymph node dissection, reported a node positive rate of only 8%. On the other hand, seminomas tend to grow more slowly than teratomas and the time to relapse following orchidectomy may be more protracted rendering a surveillance policy difficult to operate. Furthermore, whereas in teratomas alphafetoprotein and hCG are valuable tumour markers, until recently there has been a lack of a useful marker in seminoma although placental alkaline phosphatase appears to be of some value in this respect.

Table 6. Stage I seminoma: results of treatment by orchidectomy and lymph node irradiation and subsequent complications (The Royal Marsden Hospital, 1964–83)*

Total patients	No. of relapses	Deaths from seminoma	Peptic ulceration
240	5 (2%)	0	15 (6%)

*Data from Hamilton et al. (1986).

Table 7. Surveillance for Stage I seminoma of the testis* (The Royal Marsden Hospital, 1983–85)

No. of patients	No. relapsing	%
52	7	13

*Follow-up 12–41 months (median 23 months).

The results of radiotherapy in Stage I seminoma are excellent. As shown in Table 6, of 240 patients treated at The Royal Marsden Hospital there has been no death from seminoma and the relapse rate is only 2% (Hamilton et al., 1986). However, the morbidity of radiotherapy, although low, is not negligible. Thus 6% of patients developed peptic ulcers following treatment and although it is difficult to be sure of the role of irradiation in aetiology it seems probable the majority were induced or exacerbated by treatment.

In 1983 a prospective study of surveillance following orchidectomy was initiated in clinical Stage I seminoma. Between February 1983 and July 1985 fifty-two patients were entered into the study; these have been observed for 12–41 months (median 23 months) and seven (13.4%) have relapsed (Table 7). It is of interest that six of the seven relapses have been confined to the retroperitoneal lymph nodes, two patients having Stage IIA disease and four Stage IIB disease. One patient relapsed with small volume abdominal disease and limited lung metastases (Stage IVAL$_1$). The time to relapse has ranged from 9 to 23 months following orchidectomy with four relapses appearing within the first year and three during the second year. Five Stage II patients were treated with infradiaphragmatic radiotherapy, three are disease free at 5, 10 and 21 months but two have relapsed, one in the neck and one in the mediastinum. Both have been successfully treated with carboplatin. One Stage IIB patient was treated with carboplatin and is disease free at 10 months and the patient with Stage IV disease is currently receiving carboplatin.

So far no factors have been identified which predict relapse, although tumour volume, local invasiveness and the presence or absence of vascular invasion and lymphatic permeation have not been evaluated. There is no suggestion that raised serum marker levels prior to orchidectomy increase the risk of relapse. Thus, eight patients had raised hCG levels (8–3000 iU/l) and of this group none has relapsed compared with one of fourteen patients with normal pre-orchidectomy titres. Similarly, the demonstration of hCG on immunocytochemical staining of the primary tumour appears to be of no significance in terms of the probability of eventual relapse. There appears to be an excellent correlation, however, between the demonstration of markers in tumour tissue and the presence of raised serum levels prior to orchidectomy.

Discussion

Experience over the past 7 years has demonstrated the feasibility of surveillance in the management of Stage I testicular nonseminomatous tumours. Node dissection and radiation therapy are thus avoided and more than 70% of patients require no further therapy. Approximately a quarter of the patient population subsequently manifest metastases 90% of which are diagnosed within the first year of follow-up. Early detection of relapse and the institution of chemotherapy ensure effective salvage treatment. Multiple regression analysis of prognostic factors suggests that it may be possible, in the relatively near future, to identify high risk patients who would benefit from immediate chemotherapy following orchidectomy. These trends together with the development of less toxic chemotherapy schedules employing etoposide rather than vinblastine, possibly omitting bleomycin and substituting carboplatin for cisplatin, render surveillance an increasingly attractive form of management.

The situation with Stage I seminoma is less clear. So far there is only scanty information on the natural history of Stage I seminoma after orchidectomy. Placental alkaline phosphatase is less satisfactory than alphafetoprotein and hCG as a tumour marker and the tempo of relapse may be somewhat slower than is the case for nonseminoma requiring a more protracted observation period. Furthermore, the risk of occult metastases is lower than is the case for nonseminomatous tumours and the results of low dose radiotherapy are excellent although there is some associated morbidity. Surveillance in seminoma should be regarded as a clinical research investigation to be conducted in situations where regular follow-up can be assured and the appropriate investigation instituted without delay. Until more data are available routine postoperative radiotherapy should be regarded as the treatment of choice.

References

Donohue, J. P., Einhorn, L. H. & Periz, J. M. (1978) Improved management of non-seminomatous testis tumors. *Cancer*, **42**, 2903–2908.

Hamilton, C., Horwich, A., Easton, D. & Peckham, M. J. (1986) Radiotherapy for Stage I seminoma testis; results of treatment and complications *Radiotherapy and Oncology*, **6**, 115–120.

Hoskin, P., Dilly, S., Easton, D., Horwich, A., Hendry, W. & Peckham, M. J. (1986) Prognostic factors in Stage I non-seminomatous germ-cell testicular tumors managed by orchidectomy and surveillance: Implications for adjuvant chemotherapy. *Journal of Clinical Oncology*, **4**, 1031–1036.

Kennedy, C. L., Husband, J. E., Bellamy, E. A. & Peckham, M. J. (1985) The accuracy of CT scanning prior to para-aortic lymphadenectomy in patients with bulky metastases from testicular teratoma. *British Journal of Urology*, **57**, 755–758.

Maier, J. G., Sulak, M. H. & Mittemeyer, B. T. (1968) Seminoma of the testis: Analysis of treatment success and failure. *American Journal of Roentgenology*, **102**, 596–602.

Peckham, M. J. (1979) An appraisal of the role of radiation therapy in the management of non-seminomatous germ-cell tumors of the testis in the era of effective chemotherapy. *Cancer Treatment Reports*, **63**, 1653–1658.

Peckham, M. J. (1981) Investigation and staging: general aspects and staging classification; non-seminomas: current treatment results and future prospects. *The Management of Testicular Tumours* (ed. by M. J. Peckham), pp. 89–101 and 218–239. London.

Peckham, M. J. (1985) Orchidectomy for clinical Stage I testicular cancer: progress report of the Royal Marsden Hospital study. *Journal of the Royal Society of Medicine*, **78**, Suppl. 6, 41–42.

Peckham, M. J., Barrett, A., McElwain, T. J. & Hendry, W. F. (1979) Combined management of malignant teratoma of the testis. *Lancet*, **ii**, 267–270.

Peckham, M. J., Barrett, A., Husband, J. E. & Hendry, W. F. (1982) Orchidectomy alone in testicular Stage I non-seminomatous germ-cell tumours. *Lancet*, **ii**, 678–619.

Peckham, M. J., Barrett, A., Horwich, A. & Hendry, W. F. (1983) Orchidectomy alone for Stage I testicular non-seminoma: a progress report from the Royal Marsden Hospital. *British Journal of Urology*, **55**, 754–759.

Raghavan, D., Peckham, M. J, Heyderman, E. & Tobias, J. S. (1982) Prognostic factors in clinical Stage I non-seminomatous germ-cell tumours of the testis. *British Journal of Cancer*, **45**, 167–173.

Skinner, D. G. & Scardino, P. T. (1979) Relevance of biochemical tumor markers and lymphadenectomy in the management of non-seminomatous testis tumors: current perspective. *Transactions of the American Association for Genitourinary Surgery*, **87**, 293–298.

Discussion

Pizzocaro What were the sites of the latest relapses in your patients, and clinical stage of the patients who had abdominal relapses; that is, how large were the retroperitoneal metastases?

Brada Our experience is similar to the Danish results. The latest relapses were detected in the abdomen and not in the lung. I do not have exact figures as to the size of the metastases but the majority had small volume disease.

Vogelzang What is the latest relapse in your series, and how many have relapsed after an interval of 2 years?

Brada One patients relapsed at 43 months. Four of our 35 patients recurred after 2 years.

Debruyne Were your 132 patients *consecutive* patients and if not how many patients dropped out due to protocol violations?

Brada All patients eligible by the criteria described were included in the study.

Minor violations of protocol such as occasional failure to attend at monthly intervals did not constitute reason for exclusion. All patients entered into the study have been included in the analysis.

Oliver When patients initially present, it may be difficult to make an immediate stage classification because of difficulty in assessing suspicious lymphangiograms or CT scans and the presence of tumour is only revealed after prolonged follow-up. If patients with suspicious radiology who subsequently show progression are excluded, the relapse rate on surveillance will be lower. How many patients are excluded because of borderline abnormality in CT scan or lymphangiogram?

Brada Of course some patients with equivocal CT scan or lymphangiogram do fit into this category. Patients with evidence of progression and/or elevation of serum markers on repeat investigations were treated with chemotherapy and not included in the surveillance study. Borderline radiographic abnormality alone was not a reason for exclusion. Patients with no evidence of lymphangiographic or CT scan progression were entered into the study.

Scardino What was the overall relapse rate in the abdomen in your series? Although the first sign of relapse was in the abdomen in 17/35 (49%) of your patients, an additional four patients relapsed in the abdomen and lung simultaneously giving a total of 60% who relapsed in the abdomen initially. Were there any *late* relapses in the abdomen, that is, among the remaining 14 patients who relapsed with disease elsewhere, and in your whole group of patients how many *ever* developed evidence of disease in the abdomen?

Brada The abdomen was the site of relapse in 21 patients, 17 of whom suffered recurrence in the abdomen alone. The latest recurrence after orchidectomy was confined to the retroperitoneal lymph nodes.

Scardino We have seen late relapse of embryonal carcinoma in the abdomen 14 years after initial treatment and we are aware that this has also been observed at other major centres around the world. In surveillance surveys it is possible to see relapses 5, 10 or even 15 years later.

Skakkebæk I wonder if some of the very late recurrences could be due to small non-palpable tumours or CIS in the contralateral testes? Have you any information on the results of contralateral testicular biopsies?

Brada We do not perform contralateral biopsies and so far we have not detected any contralateral tumours.

Orchidectomy alone versus orchidectomy plus radiotherapy in stage I nonseminomatous testicular cancer: a randomized study by the Danish Testicular Carcinoma Study Group

M. RØRTH, H. VON DER MAASE, E. S. NIELSEN, M. PEDERSEN and H. SCHULTZ *Department of Oncology ONB, Finseninstitutet, Copenhagen*

Summary

All Danish patients with stage I nonseminomatous testicular cancer diagnosed between December 1980 and January 1984 entered a randomized study comparing irradiation of retroperitoneal lymph nodes with surveillance only after orchidectomy. Twenty-four of the seventy-nine patients in the observation-only group have relapsed, three patients relapsing more than 2 years after orchidectomy. Ten of the seventy-three patients receiving irradiation have relapsed, all within 10 months after orchidectomy. The median time to relapse in both groups was 4.5 months. Irradiation prevented retroperitoneal relapses. Thirty-three of the relapsed patients were rendered disease free with chemotherapy, and one is still being treated. Four deaths have occurred, all unrelated to testicular cancer or antineoplastic treatment. Absence of embryonal carcinoma and presence of teratocarcinoma correlated with improved relapse-free survival. Patients with increased serum concentrations of tumour markers before orchidectomy had an increased risk of relapse. Surveillance-only is a reasonable treatment strategy in clinical stage I nonseminomatous testicular cancer. Preferably control and treatment of relapses should take place in specialized centres.

Key words. Nonseminoma, surveillance, stage I, radiotherapy.

Introduction

Before the era of cisplatin based combination chemotherapy patients with stage I nonseminomatous testicular cancer were treated with radical retroperitoneal lymph node dissection (RPLND) or irradiation of the para-aortic and ipsilateral pelvic lymph nodes (RT). Both these strategies gave reasonable survival rates (Fraley, Lange & Kennedy, 1979). The survival rates improved considerably when it became possible with chemotherapy to cure patients who subsequently relapsed.

Correspondence: Dr Mikael Rørth, Department of Oncology ONB, Finseninstitutet, DK-2100 Copenhagen Ø.

The use of RT and RPLND in the treatment of stage I patients has varied in different countries, reflecting the fact that the final outcome in terms of survival was fairly similar for both treatments.

Extensive surgery like RPLND carries a certain operative mortality, albeit very low in experienced hands (Whitmore, 1982). A major complication has been retrograde ejaculation and consequent infertility.

RT can be complicated by radiation enteritis and carries a certain risk of secondary neoplasms in the irradiated field (Glatstein, 1982).

Both these treatment modalities thus have finite complication rates which, if possible, should be minimized or avoided.

Some of the stage I patients should be curable with orchidectomy alone. The actual percentage of these patients being cured is conceivably variable with time due to the sophistication of diagnostic procedures (CT-scan, tumour markers) and better experience of the clinicians. Peckham et al. (1982) argued that the proportion of patients curable with orchidectomy alone should be 60–80%.

With the advent of modern techniques for follow-up and of curative chemotherapy regimens it became possible to apply a 'wait and see' strategy for patients with stage I nonseminomas. Such a strategy has to prove itself in carefully monitored studies before being an acceptable practice.

In Denmark RT was formerly the standard treatment after orchidectomy for stage I patients. In December 1980, therefore, the Danish Testicular Carcinoma Study Group (DATECA) embarked on a study comparing RT with surveillance only. The main objectives of the study were to define the proportion of patients curable with orchidectomy alone and to define a group of patients with high risk of relapse. A preliminary analysis of the trial has been published earlier (Rørth et al., 1985).

Material and Methods

Virtually all patients with testicular cancer in Denmark are referred to one of five oncological centres for staging and treatment after orchidectomy.

All patients in this study were subjected to standard staging procedures as described by Schultz et al. (1984). These included bipedal lymphangiography, CT-scan and measurements of the tumour markers AFP and hCG in serum. Clinicoradiological stage I was defined as no evidence of residual disease demonstrable by these procedures. Histology was reviewed by the pathologists at the oncological centres. The tumours were classified according to WHO with slight modifications (Jacobsen et al., 1984). In mixed tumours each tumour component was recorded separately.

Patients were stratified according to the presence or absence of tumour markers in serum before orchidectomy. Randomization was carried out at each centre using a closed envelope system.

Patients allocated to RT received 40 Gy in twenty-three fractions, five fractions per week, to the para-aortic and ipsilateral pelvic lymph nodes.

All patients were followed with monthly examinations for the first year, bi- or trimonthly for the second year and thereafter at increasing intervals. The controls included X-ray of the thorax and serum tumour markers. CT-scan was repeated every 4 months during the first year.

Results

From December 1980 to January 1984, 156 patients entered the trial. Seventy-nine patients were allocated to observation only and seventy-seven to RT. Four patients refused RT and they are not included in the analysis (one relapsed 3 months after orchidectomy, and all four are currently without evidence of disease).

With median observation times of 39 months (irradiated group) and 41 months (observation only group) ten patients in the irradiated group and twenty-four patients in the observation group have relapsed (Fig. 1). The difference in relapse rates is significant ($P < 0.05$).

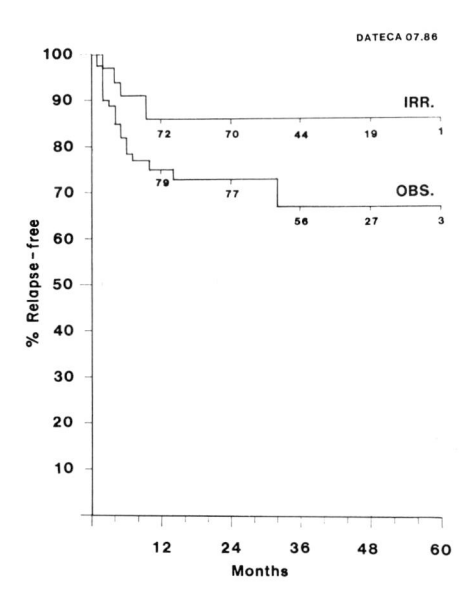

Fig. 1. Life table analysis of relapse-free survival in patients with stage I nonseminoma. IRR: irradiated group. OBS: observation only group. Small numbers indicate patients observed.

The median time to relapse was 4.5 months in both groups. All relapses in the irradiated group occurred within 10 months after orchidectomy. In the observation group there has been three late relapses at 24, 32 and 63 months after orchidectomy. The relapse after 63 months occurred in one of the two patients who, at the time of analysis, had been followed for more than 5 years.

As noted in Table 1, most relapses in the observation group were found in the retroperitoneal area. All the late relapses were in this area. No such relapses were seen in the irradiated group.

All the thirty-four relapsing patients were treated with cisplatin, vinblastine (or VP-16) and bleomycin essentially according to the schedule of Einhorn & Donohue (1977). One patient is still being treated, and all the others achieved complete response and are continuously free of disease. Four patients have died of medical diseases unrelated to testicular cancer, two in each randomization group. All four patients were without residual germ cell tumour.

Table 1. Site of relapses in patients with stage I nonseminoma

	IRR.	OBS.
Lungs	8	6
Retroperitoneum		16
Other		5
Markers only	2	2
n	10	24

IRR.: Irradiated group.
OBS.: Observation only group.

The influence of histology on relapse rates was analysed with the chi square test for each individual histological subtype. In the observation group the absence of embryonal carcinoma and the presence of teratocarcinoma was significantly correlated to the increased relapse-free survival ($P < 0.05$). In the irradiated group no such correlation was found.

Relapse rates were higher in patients with increased tumour markers in the serum before orchidectomy in both the observation group (Fig. 2a) and the irradiated group (Fig. 2b).

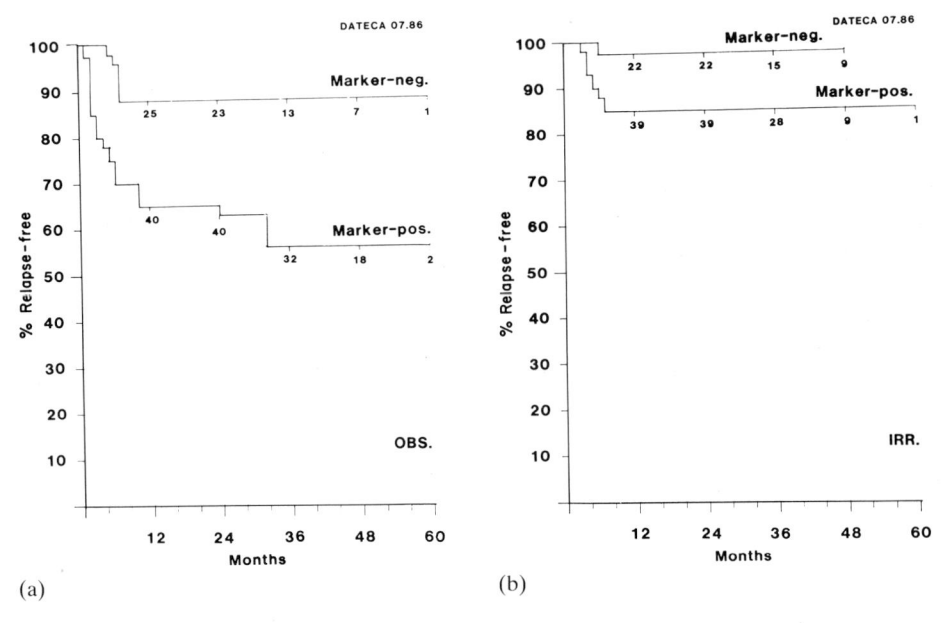

Fig. 2. (a) Life table analysis of relapse-free survival with regard to tumour marker status before orchidectomy in the observation only group. Small numbers indicate patients observed. (b) Life table analysis of relapse-free survival with regard to tumour marker status before orchidectomy in the irradiated group. Small numbers indicate patients observed.

Discussion

This study has confirmed that the 'wait and see' management strategy can be carried out in a consecutive series of unselected patients with stage I nonseminomatous testicular cancer. It has also shown that RT effectively prevented relapses in the retroperitoneal area.

Most relapses occurred early after orchidectomy, but it is important to stress that late relapses do occur, apparently always in the retroperitoneal area. Improved diagnostic methods in this area are therefore still very much needed.

CT-scan can only be interpreted in terms of size of lymph nodes and with the present technology the overall accuracy is not higher than 70% (Lien *et al.*, 1986). Combination of lymphangiography and CT-scan increases the accuracy (Tesoro-Tess *et al.*, 1985). The relatively high relapse rates found in the present study indicate that alternative techniques are needed (NMR-scanning, radio-imaging).

All patients with relapses have been successfully treated with chemotherapy (one patient is currently being treated). This is in accordance with the results of others (Read *et al.*, 1983; Peckham, Horwich & Hendry, 1986; Schraffordt Koops *et al.*, 1986). It thus seems likely that *a priori* resistance to chemotherapy in germ cell tumours only becomes a problem when the tumour load is large.

It is still too early to define a high risk group in which adjuvant systemic treatment should be contemplated. With regard to histology of the primary tumour, embryonal carcinoma of the WHO classification and malignant teratoma undifferentiated of the British classification seem to be correlated to increased risk of relapse. Our finding of an increased risk in patients with increased concentrations of tumour markers in serum before orchidectomy has not been corroborated in the above mentioned studies.

The occurrence of late relapses in the retroperitoneum reported here and by Pizzocaro *et al.* (1986) stresses the need for careful and long term control of these patients. The surveillance strategy is certainly feasible and has been successfully applied in several centres. It should still be considered an experimental strategy to be carried out in specialized centres. Careful evaluation of the ongoing studies for a further period of some years is necessary before final conclusions can be drawn.

References

Einhorn, L. H. & Donohue, J. P. (1977) Cis-diaminodichloroplatinum, vinblastin and bleomycin combination chemotherapy in disseminated testicular cancer. *Annals of Internal Medicine*, **87**, 293–298.

Fraley, E. E., Lange, P. H. & Kennedy, B. J. (1979) Germ-cell testicular cancer in adults. *New England Journal of Medicine*, **301**, 1370–1375.

Glatstein, E. (1982) Optimal management of clinical stage I non-seminomatous testicular carcinoma: One oncologist's view. *Cancer Treatment Reports*, **66**, 11–14.

Jacobsen, G. K., Barlebo, H., Olsen, J., Schultz, H., Starklint, H., Søgaard, H. & Væth, M. (1984) Testicular germ cell tumors in Denmark 1976–1980. Pathology of 1058 consecutive cases. *Acta Radiologica Oncologica* **23**, 239–247.

Lien, H. H., Stenwig, A. E., Ous, S. & Fosså, S. D. (1986) Influence of different criteria for abnormal lymph node size on reliability of computed tomography in patients with non-seminomatous testicular tumor. *Acta Radiologica Diagnostica*, **27**, 199–203.

Peckham, M. J., Barrett, A., Husband, J. E. & Hendry, J. E. (1982) Orchidectomy alone in testicular stage I non-seminomatous germ cell tumours. *Lancet*, **ii**, 678–680.

Peckham, M. J., Horwich, A. & Hendry, W. F. (1986) Surveillance following orchidectomy for clinical stage I germ cell malignancy. *Germ Cell Tumours II* (ed. by W. G. Jones, A. M. Ward and C. K. Anderson), pp. 441–449. Pergamon Press, Oxford.

Pizzocaro, G., Zanoni, F., Milani, A., Salvioni, R., Piva, L., Pilotti, S., Bombardieri, E., Tesoro-Tess, J. D. & Musumeci, R. (1986) Orchidectomy alone in clinical stage I nonseminomatous testicular cancer: A critical appraisal. *Journal of Clinical Oncology*, **4**, 35–41.

Read, G., Johnson, R. J., Wilkinson, P. M. & Eddleston, B. (1983) Prospective study of follow up alone in stage I teratoma of the testis. *British Medical Journal*, **287**, 1503–1505.

Rørth, M., von der Maase, H., Nielsen, E. S., Schultz, H. & Pedersen, M. (1985) Treatment of non seminomatous testicular germ cell tumors in Denmark since 1979. *Progress in Clinical and Biological Research*, **203**, 539–551.

Schraffordt Koops, H., Sleijfer, D. T., Oosterhuis, J. W., de Bruijn, H. W. A., Marrink, J. & Oldhoff, J. (1986) Orchidectomy alone in clinical stage I non-seminomatous testicular tumours. *Germ Cell Tumours II* (ed. by W. G. Jones, A. M. Ward and C. K. Anderson), pp. 425–430. Pergamon Press, Oxford.

Schultz, H. & The Danish Testicular Carcinoma Study Group (1984) Testicular carcinoma in Denmark 1976–1980. Stage and selected clinical parameters at presentation. *Acta Radiologica Oncologica*, **23**, 249–253.

Tesoro-Tess, J. D., Pizzocaro, G., Zanoni, F. & Musumeci, R. (1985) Lymphangiography and computerized tomography in testicular carcinoma: How accurate in early stage disease? *Journal of Urology*, **133**, 967–975.

Whitmore, W. F. (1982) Surgical treatment of clinical stage I non-seminomatous germ cell tumors of the testis. *Cancer Treatment Reports*, **66**, 5–10.

Discussion

Pizzocaro What was the clinical stage, and in particular how large were the retroperitoneal metastases of the patients who had abdominal relapses?

Rørth All relapses after more than 12 months were in the retroperitoneum and the majority were small. The relapse after 63 months was a large retroperitoneal mass.

Einhorn In your 152 patients you had four deaths due to causes unrelated to their tumour. What were these causes and had any of these required chemotherapy?

Rørth In the observation-only group one patient aged 65 died of pulmonary emboli 33 months after orchidectomy. One patient aged 53 died of cerebral disease due to alcoholism 20 months after orchidectomy. In the irradiated group one patient aged 27 died from Romano–Wards syndrome (cardiac arrythmia) 34 months after orchidectomy. One patient aged 70 died of a myocardial infarction 44 months after orchidectomy. None of these four patients had relapsed and none had received chemotherapy.

Einhorn When dealing with small numbers it is difficult to assess the toxic effects of chemotherapy. Such reports may falsely attribute cardiovascular toxicity to cisplatin treatment, whereas such effects may have occurred independently of therapy.

I believe the surveillance policy is being opened up in the MRC in England. Has this study started yet?

Oliver The MRC surveillance study has recruited more than 300 cases and is due to close. Analyses will begin in October 1986.

Bannwart Concerning the histology of late relapses in stage I nonseminomatous tumours, do you ever see sarcomatous metastases?

Rørth We have seen three relapses after more than 12 months. Residual teratoma may be found in recurrences but we have never seen recurrence with sarcoma in stage I patients.

Brada Our results are similar in the Royal Marsden patients.

Rørth In the Danish group, approximately half of the patients have been biopsied from the contralateral testis. None of the very late relapses belongs to this group.

Debruyne What is the message from your study with regard to radiation therapy in NSGCT stage I?

Rørth Radiotherapy *does* effectively eradicate retroperitoneal disease; however, relapses outside the retroperitoneum do occur.

Approximately 70% of patients with stage I tumour will be cured by orchidectomy alone. As all relapsing patients can be salvaged with chemotherapy, the message is that radiotherapy may be left out of the management of stage I nonseminoma patients. But we must be sure that we can diagnose stage I disease accurately and we must determine what features are associated with risk of recurrence. We need more time before we can reach a conclusion as it will take a few more years of observation before all relapses have been diagnosed. Until then we recommend a surveillance policy carried out by specialized centres with frequent follow-ups.

Pizzocaro What do you think of *nerve-sparing* lymph node dissection for stage I nonseminoma? This makes follow-up much easier as only the chest and serum markers need to be examined after properly executed retroperitoneal lymph node dissection (RPLND). It is very difficult to follow the retroperitoneal nodes for 3-5 years with repeated lymphangiography and CT scans in the surveillance policy.

Rørth In good hands, this is an excellent policy but a very careful and extensive operation is required. Follow-up after RPLND should still be careful as relapses especially in the lung *do* occur. We have no experience with primary RPLND in Denmark but I suspect that RPLND *must* cause some degree of morbidity and reduced fertility. RPLND is overtreatment in 70% of patients. Our diagnostic procedures are steadily improving and I therefore anticipate improving staging and thereby reduced incidence of relapse in the surveillance group.

Einhorn I suspect that these arguments about the management of stage I disease will not be resolved till the turn of the century. Studying available data I see that nearly half of the MTU or embryonal carcinoma patients are going to relapse.

Brada Adjuvant chemotherapy may be advisable in such (MTU) cases. Although surveillance has the advantage of avoiding unnecessary chemotherapy and 97% cure rate for recurrent disease.

Einhorn In the US we would perform RPLND rather than give chemotherapy for these patients. The philosophy of surveillance is to decrease morbidity but chemotherapy is much more morbid than RPLND.

Brada RPLND does not prevent recurrence in all patients. The tumour may bypass the retroperitoneal nodes and go directly to the lungs (see our Table 3, page 249). Chemotherapy is curative with minimal long-term toxicity.

Limitations to the use of surveillance as an option in the management of stage I seminoma

R. T. D. OLIVER   *The London and St Bartholomew's Medical Colleges and The Institute of Urology*

Summary

Improved definition of seminoma using step sections and tumour markers makes such patients a more selected group than when radiotherapy was first introduced. This and the improvements in radiological staging and the exquisite sensitivity of metastatic seminoma to chemotherapy justifies reappraisal of the role of prophylactic radiotherapy. To investigate this, twenty-six patients have been entered onto a programme of prospective biochemical and radiological surveillance. Though only four (15%) have relapsed, and all easily salvaged by chemotherapy, the relative difficulty and lateness of establishing the diagnosis makes this approach unsuitable for service use. Whether given the chemosensitivity of seminomas, radiotherapy would remain the treatment of choice compared to short courses of adjuvant carboplatin requires testing in a randomized trial.

Key words.   Seminoma, radiotherapy, chemotherapy.

Introduction

The high cure rate of patients with seminoma using prophylactic or therapeutic radiotherapy makes it difficult to justify changes in treatment. However, considering that more than 80% of the rare group of patients with advanced bulky seminoma achieve durable disease-free survival after platinum-based cytotoxic chemotherapy compared to 50–70% seen after radiotherapy (Oliver, Blandy & Hope-Stone, 1984) it is probable that for patients with an equivalent stage of disease chemotherapy is more effective than radiotherapy. Additional evidence that seminoma is even more sensitive to chemotherapy than is malignant teratoma, is the observation that the cure rate of seminoma patients using cisplatin alone is virtually the same as that seen after combination treatment (Oliver *et al.*, 1984). This exquisite sensitivity, the success of surveillance as an option for patients with stage I malignant teratoma (Peckham *et al.*, 1983; Oliver, Hope-Stone & Blandy, 1983), and the observation that lymph node dissection in patients with clinical stage I seminoma performed more than 20 years ago (before the advent of lymphangiography or CT scans) only demonstrated a 10% incidence of occult metastases (Whitmore, 1970), has led this unit to undertake a pilot study of surveillance in

Correspondence: Dr R. T. D. Oliver, Department of Medical Oncology, The London Hospital Medical College, Whitechapel, London E1 1BB.

such patients. This report reviews the results of this study and updates our previous experience with chemotherapy for metastatic seminoma.

Patients and Methods
Prophylactic radiotherapy with 3000 cGy in 3 weeks was standard treatment until January 1982 when all stage I seminoma patients with a negative CT scan and lymphangiogram were entered into surveillance. In this study, CT scans were performed at 2, 6, 12, 24 and 48 months after orchidectomy. Tumour markers (AFP, hCG, placental alkaline phosphatase (PlAP) and hydroxybutryic dehydrogenase (HBD)), and chest X-ray were performed at monthly intervals for the first 6 months, 2-monthly for the second 6 months, 3-monthly for the second year, 4-monthly for the third year, 6-monthly for the fourth year and annually thereafter.

Chemotherapy regimens
Since 1978 patients with large volume (diameter greater than 5 cm) stage II, III and IV seminoma have been treated with platinum-based chemotherapy. This was initially bleomycin, vinblastine and cisplatin, though since 1980 selected patients, predominantly previously untreated patients with negative tumour markers, have received cisplatin 50 mg/m^2 on days 1 and 2 every 3 weeks. Patients with elevated hCG or AFP, or recurrent tumour after previous radiotherapy, received bleomycin, etoposide and cisplatin. All patients received four courses of chemotherapy.

Tumour markers
Details of methodology and interpretation of results have been presented in detail elsewhere (Tucker *et al.*, 1985).

Results
Twenty-six patients with stage I seminoma have been entered into surveillance and all except three have been followed for more than 12 months. There have been four (15%) relapses compared to five of eighteen (28%) of a similar group of patients with nonseminoma (Table 1). All of the nonseminoma relapses occurred at or before 12 months following orchidectomy, while all except one of the patients with seminoma who relapsed did so after 12 months. Despite regular monitoring with placental alkaline phosphatase, three of the four relapses proved difficult to diagnose (Table 2). All three had a negative fine needle aspiration biopsy of a

Table 1. The London Hospital, St Bartholomew's Hospital and Institute of Urology surveillance studies for stage I testicular cancer

Tumour histology	No. of cases	Median duration of follow-up (years)	No. of relapses (%)	Time to relapse (months)
Seminoma (1983–86)	26	1.5	4 (15%)	3, 18, 18, 22
Non-seminoma (1980–83)	18	4	5 (28%)	3, 3, 6, 6, 12

Table 2. Clinical features of stage I seminoma patients who relapsed

Time relapse established (months after orchidectomy)	Months of uncertainty before relapse established	Site of nodal relapse	Disease-free survival post chemotherapy (months)
3	NIL	Neck	48+
8	6	Para-aortic	9+
22	18	Common iliac	3+
18	9	Para-aortic	*

*On treatment

Table 3. Marker status at relapse of seminoma in stage I patients

Patient	AFP (ng/ml)	hCG (mIU/ml)	PlAP	Smoking status
1	< 10	< 15	0.23	S
2	< 10	< 15	0.65	S
3	< 10	< 15	0.48	N
4	< 10	115	0.52	ES

S = Smoker; N = Non-smoker; ES = Ex-smoker.

suspicious lesion, two of which subsequently regressed for periods of 6 and 12 months, both in association with a decline of a borderline elevation of PlAP. At relapse one of four had elevated serum hCG and three of four had elevated serum PlAP (Table 3). Although population-based statistical analysis of patients before and after treatment demonstrates that it is possible to use the PlAP assay to discriminate patients with active disease from those without, even if they are smokers (Table 4), making decisions on the basis of borderline elevations of serum PlAP in patients on surveillance who are smokers is not easy and severely limits its value (Table 5).

Though the simplicity and reduced toxicity of using single agent cisplatin rather than combination chemotherapy makes it very attractive for treating the older seminoma patient, the latest analysis does suggest that the continuous

Table 4. Serum PlAP before and after treatment of metastatic seminoma

	PlAP level (OD units)		
	< 0.4	0.4–1.00	> 1.0
Seminoma (smoker, n = 11)			
Before treatment	36%	18%	46%
After treatment	73%	9%	18%
Seminoma (non-smoker, n = 14)			
Before treatment	29%	21%	50%
After treatment	100%	0	0
Normal control (n = 136)	96%	4%	–

Table 5. PlAP levels in patients on surveillance

	N	No. of assays	No. positive*
Smokers who relapsed	3	15	2
Smokers who did not relapse	9	45	27
Non-smokers who relapsed	1	15	4
Non-smokers who did not relapse	12	69	0

* >0.5 OD for smoker, >0.3 OD for non-smoker.

Table 6. Chemotherapy for metastatic seminoma

	Single agent platinum			BVP/BEP		
	All cases ($n = 20$)	Previously untreated ($n = 16$)	Relapse post radio-therapy ($n = 4$)	All cases ($n = 20$)	Previously untreated ($n = 9$)	Relapse after previous treatment ($n = 11$)
Complete response	11	8	3	15	7	8
NAD post-surgery*	6	6	–	2	1	1
Relapse	3	1	2	–	–	–
Continuously NAD	13 (65%)	12	1	15 (75%)	7	8
Currently NAD	17 (85%)	14	3	15 (75%)†	7	8
	Median follow-up 36 months			Median follow-up 44 months		

NAD = No actual disease.
*Two persistent seminoma; one mature teratoma; five necrotic.
†Two patients died in complete remission of drug toxicity.

Table 7. Continuous disease-free survival following single agent platinum chemotherapy for relapsed seminoma

	N	Continuously disease free
HCG-negative seminoma	12	11
HCG-positive seminoma	8	2

disease-free survival may be somewhat less (65% v. 75% (Table 6)). Two of the failures were only microscopic deposits discovered at surgery and three of the remaining five failures were salvaged by combination chemotherapy. The higher failure rate seen in hCG-positive cases (Table 7) suggests that exclusion of these cases may reduce the difference in response rate.

Discussion

Given that 97% of all newly diagnosed patients with seminoma treated by a policy using predominantly radiotherapy are cured (Thomas, 1985) it is extremely difficult to justify making any changes to first-line management policy. However, there are two factors which need to be taken into consideration. Even in the era before modern staging procedures reduced the incidence of metastatic seminoma from 15% to 7% (Thomas, 1985), those surgeons who were doing lymph node dissections were reporting positive nodes in only 10% of clinical stage I seminoma patients (Whitmore, 1970), while in patients with stage I nonseminoma the same surgeons were reporting 40% of cases having pathological evidence of spread. It is now well established that the relapse rate of modern stage I patients with malignant teratoma on surveillance is in the region of 20–25% (Peckham et al., 1983; Oliver et al., 1983). On this basis one might suspect that the relapse rate of stage I seminoma today would be less than 10%. Even though our numbers are small, combined with those of Peckham (these proceedings) they do suggest that the relapse rate may well be in excess of 10%. This taken with the relative difficulty of proving relapse in three of the four cases and the late stage at which they present suggests that as a service option surveillance is not as good as radiotherapy which has a less than 1% risk of relapse.

Though radiotherapy is not entirely without risk in respect of late toxicity (Blandy, Oliver & Hope-Stone, 1983), such as the incidence of peptic ulceration and cardiovascular disease, it is clearly less toxic than four courses of platinum-based combination treatment.

However, given the results from the use of single agent platinum in the hCG-negative patients it is possible that using two courses of the less toxic analogue carboplatin which Peckham, Horwich & Hendry (1985) have shown to be as good as cisplatin might be sufficient to eliminate all risk of relapse and make a very good option for a randomized comparison with radiotherapy.

References

Blandy, J. P., Oliver, R. T. D. & Hope-Stone, H. F. (1983) A British approach to the management of patients with testicular tumours. *International Perspectives in Urology*, 7, 207–223.

Oliver, R. T. D., Hope-Stone, H. F. & Blandy, J. P. (1983) Justification of the use of surveillance in the management of Stage I germ cell tumours of the testis. *British Journal of Urology*, 55, 760–763.

Oliver, R. T. D., Blandy, J. P. & Hope-Stone, H. F. (1984) Possible new approaches to the management of seminoma of the testis. *British Journal of Urology*, 56, 729–733.

Peckham, M. J., Barrett, A., Horwich, A. & Hendry, W. F. (1983) Orchidectomy alone for Stage I testicular non-seminoma: a progress report. *British Journal of Urology*, 55, 754–757.

Peckham, M. J., Horwich, A. & Hendry, W. F. (1985) Advanced seminoma: treatment with cisplatinum based combination chemotherapy or carboplatin (JM8). *British Journal of Cancer*, 52, 7–13.

Tucker, D. F., Oliver, R. T. D., Travers, P. & Bodmer, W. F. (1985) Serum marker potential of placental alkaline phosphatase-like activity in germ cell tumours. *British Journal of Cancer*, 51, 631–639.

Thomas, G. M. (1985) The role of radiation therapy in all stages and extents of seminoma. *Germ Cell Tumours II* (ed. by W. G. Jones, A. Milford Ward and C. K. Anderson), pp. 219–227. Pergamon Press, Oxford.

Whitmore, W. F. (1970) Germinal tumours of the testis. *Proc. 6th Nat. Cancer Conference*, p. 219. J. P. Lippincott, Philadelphia.

Discussion

von der Maase Beginning early 1985, 140 stage I seminoma patients entered a study in Denmark and we now have a median follow-up period of 12 months. Ten patients have relapsed, eight being treated with radiotherapy and two with chemotherapy. All are presently without evidence of disease.

Oliver Your data taken with ours and that of Peckham is probably sufficient to establish that surveillance is not a viable service option compared to radiotherapy which has a virtual 0% relapse rate particularly as one has a permanent fear in such patients of paraplegia being the first sign of relapse. However, the issue for the future is, given the relative low toxicity of carboplatin, can adjuvant chemotherapy with two courses of carboplatin do as well as radiotherapy?

Retroperitoneal lymph node dissection in clinical stage IIA and IIB nonseminomatous germ cell tumours of the testis

G. PIZZOCARO   *Section of Urologic Oncology, Istituto Nazionale Tumori, Milano*

Summary

From 1980 to 1984 inclusive, ninety-one consecutive evaluable patients underwent primary retroperitoneal lymphadenectomy for clinical stage IIA or IIB nonseminomatous germinal testicular cancer. Nodes were negative in twenty cases (22%), and forty-seven patients (52%) were treated with chemotherapy either postoperatively (thirty clinically understaged patients) or at relapse (seventeen cases). After a median follow-up period of nearly 5 years (range 18–78 months) the disease-free survival was 98%. None of thirty patients with radiographic abnormalities ⩾ 3 cm in the retroperitoneal nodes had negative histology, and twenty-two (73%) were treated with chemotherapy. Preoperative serum levels of AFP and hCG were not useful in selecting patients with positive nodes. Primary chemotherapy is now used in patients with radiographic evidence of retroperitoneal metastases ⩾ 3 cm.

Key words.   Retroperitoneal lymphadenectomy, stage II, testis cancer.

Introduction

Clinical stages IIA and IIB nonseminomatous germ cell tumours of the testis can be primarily treated with either surgery or chemotherapy. The advantages of retroperitoneal lymphadenectomy are pathological staging and the possibility of curing approximately 50% of patients without the use of aggressive chemotherapy (Pizzocaro *et al.*, 1984b). The advantage of the primary use of cisplatin combination chemotherapy is to avoid major surgery in complete responders to chemotherapy (Peckham & Hendry, 1985). The long-term survival after both forms of treatment is in the range of 96–98%. We reviewed our series of patients consecutively submitted to primary retroperitoneal lymphadenectomy for clinical stage IIA and IIB nonseminomatous testicular cancer from 1980 to 1984 inclusive, and tried to find out selective criteria for either primary surgery or primary chemotherapy.

Patients and Methods

Ninety-four consecutive patients underwent primary retroperitoneal lymphadenectomy for clinical stage IIA or IIB nonseminomatous testicular cancer in the 5-year period considered. Most patients had orchidectomy performed elsewhere and their

Correspondence: Dr Giorgio Pizzocaro, Istituto Nazionale Tumori, Via G. Venezian 1, 20133 Milano, Italy.

Relapse and disease-free survival
Of the seventy-one patients assigned to observation for pathological stage I, IIA or IIB disease, seventeen (28%) developed relapse, versus none of the thirty patients treated with postoperative chemotherapy for either pathological stage IIC or postoperative stage III disease. Relapses occurred from 1 to 33 months after lymphadenectomy. The median time to relapse was 7 months. Serum markers were elevated at relapse in eleven cases (65%) and in six they were the only sign of tumour progression.

The lung was affected in six cases, the mediastinum in two, and the liver in one. One patient had a recurrence in the inguinal scar after orchidectomy performed elsewhere. All patients with relapse had repeated lymphangiography and CT of the abdomen. In only one case was a retroperitoneal recurrence documented. It was in the contralateral iliac nodes which were not usually removed during lymphadenectomy.

Fifteen (88%) of seventeen patients with relapse entered continuous complete remission from 12 to 57 months (median 32 months) after starting cisplatin combination chemotherapy. One patient died of cancer 8 months after relapse, and another one is alive with disease which has been present for 19 months. The overall disease-free survival of the ninety-one clinical stage IIA and IIB nonseminomatous germ cell tumours treated with primary retroperitoneal lymphadenectomy was 98% after a median follow-up period of nearly 5 years (range from 18 to 78 months). In particular, cisplatin combination chemotherapy was employed in forty-seven patients (52%) and forty-four (48%) were cured with surgery alone. Chemotherapy was used in 32% of forty patients in clinical stage IIA and in 67% of those in clinical stage IIB.

Treatment side effects
Operative mortality was nil. Only two patients suffered major complications (one ischaemic ureteral necrosis and one bowel obstruction) which required further surgery. Another nine patients had minor complications. The major side effect of retroperitoneal lymphadenectomy was loss of antegrade ejaculation. It occurred in fifty-six (83%) of sixty-seven patients who underwent a bilateral paraortic dissection and in only four (16%) of twenty-four patients who had a unilateral lymphadenectomy. Overall, antegrade ejaculation was postoperatively lost by 66% of cases, and it recovered spontaneously in five patients only. All of the forty-seven patients who were treated with chemotherapy were hospitalized during treatment and suffered from severe to moderate toxicity. Granulocytopenic infections developed in ten (21%) of forty-seven patients. In these cases the vinblastine dosage was either reduced from 0.3 to 0.2 mg/kg or the interval between cycles was prolonged to 4 weeks. Seven patients (15%) had documented lung fibrosis, and bleomycin was immediately withheld in all of them. Vigorous hydration prevented renal toxicity in all cases. Other toxic signs have been reported elsewhere (Pizzocaro *et al.*, 1985a, b, 1986).

Discussion
The major controversy in the management of clinical stage IIA and IIB testicular nonseminoma centres on the choice of surgery or chemotherapy as the primary

Table 5. Management by primary surgery or chemotherapy for clinical stage IIA and IIB testicular cancer

Authors	No. of cases	Retroperitoneal lymphadenectomy	Chemotherapy	Disease-free survival
Present study	91	91 (100%)	47 (52%)	89 (98%)
Peckham et al. (1985)	54	12 (22%)	54 (100%)	52 (96%)

treatment. Unfortunately, there are few data allowing direct comparison between the two procedures (Table 5). In our surgical series 52% of patients required either immediate chemotherapy or chemotherapy at relapse. In Peckham & Hendry's (1985) series only 22% of patients required postchemotherapy lymph node dissection, but three other patients relapsed in the retroperitoneal nodes. The disease-free survival was closely similar in the two groups. Two-thirds of cases lost antegrade ejaculation in our series, and an unknown percentage of patients were treated with unnecessary chemotherapy in the Peckham & Hendry's (1985) study. In our opinion surgery is to be preferred when the probability of negative nodes is relatively high and the chance of advanced disease is very low. This is the case for clinical stage IIA tumours where 40% of cases had negative nodes and only 32% of patients were treated with chemotherapy. Conversely, primary chemotherapy may be indicated in clinical stage IIB tumours where only 8% of patients had negative nodes and 67% were treated with chemotherapy. The indication for primary chemotherapy is even more striking in patients with radiographic abnormalities larger than 3 cm. In these cases there was no false positive clinical staging and 73% of cases had to be treated with chemotherapy.

Acknowledgement

Supported in part by grant n. 85.02308.44. Project 'Oncology', Italian National Research Council (C.N.R.), Rome.

References

Peckham, M. J. & Hendry, W. F. (1985) Clincal stage II nonseminomatous germ cell testicular tumours. Results of management by primary chemotherapy. *British Journal of Urology*, 57, 763–768.
Pizzocaro, G., Piva, L., Salvioni, R., et al. (1984a) Adjuvant chemotherapy in resected stage II nonseminomatous germ cell tumors of testis. In which cases is it necessary? *European Urology*, 10, 151–158.
Pizzocaro, G., Zanoni, F., Milani, A., et al. (1984b) Retroperitoneal lymphadenectomy and aggressive chemotherapy in nonbulky clinical stage II nonseminomatous germinal testis tumors. *Cancer*, 53, 1363–1368.
Pizzocaro, G., Piva, L., Salvioni, R., et al. (1985a) Cisplatin, etoposide, bleomicyn first-line therapy and early resection of residual tumor in far-advanced germinal testis cancer. *Cancer*, 56, 2411–2415.
Pizzocaro, G., Salvioni, R., Pasi, M., et al. (1985b) Early resection of residual tumor during cisplatin, vinblastine, bleomicyn chemotherapy in stage III and bulky stage II nonseminomatous testicular cancer. *Cancer*, 56, 249–255.
Pizzocaro, G., Salvioni, R. & Zanoni, F. (1985c) Unilateral lymphadenectomy in intraoperative stage I nonseminomatous germinal testis cancer. *Journal of Urology*, 135, 485–489.
Pizzocaro, G., Salvioni, R., Zanoni, F., et al. (1986) Successful treatment of good-risk disseminated testicular cancer with cisplatin, bleomycin and reduced-dose vinblastine. *Cancer*, 57, 2114–2118.

Discussion

Ozols Is there any difference in relapse rate between patients who had unilateral, and those who had bilateral, lymphadenectomy?

Pizzocaro No. Unilateral and bilateral lymphadenectomy are not comparable in this series because they were performed in different categories of patients.

Unilateral lymphadenectomy was performed in 24 patients who had no clinical evidence of retroperitoneal metastases and 20 of these were confirmed to be negative histologically whereas four had microscopic deposits. Only three of these 24 patients relapsed but there was no evidence of nodal recurrence.

Bilateral lymphadenectomy was performed in the remaining 67 patients with intra-operative evidence of metastases. Postoperative chemotherapy was given to 30 of these patients either because they had postoperative pathological stage IIC disease or because persistent tumour markers put them into stage III. None of these patients receiving postoperative chemotherapy relapsed. The other 37 patients had pathologically confirmed stage IIA or IIB disease and 14 relapsed.

Vogelzang Our results are similar to yours. The results of the Testicular Intergroup Study (TIS) indicate that there is no difference in relapse between their stage IIA and IIB disease. How does your data compare to the TIS data? Some centres indicate a continuum of relapse between stage IIA and stage IIB.

Pizzocaro We also had the same relapse rate (approximately 35%) in our pathological stages IIA and IIB patients. However, in patients with pathological stage IIC disease receiving no postoperative chemotherapy, we had an 86% relapse rate (Pizzocaro *et al.*, 1984, *European Journal of Urology*, **10**, 151–158).

Einhorn I can comment on the Intergroup Study. In the two centres there were 204 patients who had pathological (not clinical) stage IIA or IIB disease. Stage IIA is defined as the number of lymph nodes involved being less than 5, and the largest lymph node being less than 2 cm in size. In stage IIB patients, the largest lymph node is greater than 2 cm in size or there are more than five positive lymph nodes. The relapse rates of the two different stages were within 10% of each other and the difference was not statistically significant.

Another interesting result from this study is the significance of vascular invasion at the time of lymphadenectomy. In the US Intergroup adjuvant study, vascular invasion had zero implication as far as eventual relapse is concerned.

Debruyne We apply a slightly different approach in that we give all patients postoperative chemotherapy. For IIA disease we give two cycles of platinum-based chemotherapy. Stage IIB patients receive three cycles after RPLND. So far we have obtained a 100% survival rate in our series which is smaller than Dr Pizzocaro's series. Can you comment on the systematic administration of chemotherapy after resection of retroperitoneal lymph nodes in these patients?

Pizzocaro Our two patients who were not cured had pulmonary disease at relapse which was unresponsive to chemotherapy. One of them had negative nodes. On the other hand, in the American Intergroup Study there are also one or two cancer-related deaths in the patients receiving adjuvant chemotherapy.

The advantage of performing primary RPLND in clinical stage IIA and IIB patients is the avoidance of unnecessary chemotherapy in patients who can be cured with surgery alone.

If a long careful follow-up can be guaranteed, almost all patients who relapse after radical surgery alone can be salvaged with deferred chemotherapy and only an occasional patient with a chemo-resistant tumour will be lost. Such unresponsive patients, however, would also be lost following adjuvant chemotherapy or primary chemotherapy.

Furthermore, I think that the systemic use of adjuvant chemotherapy in patients with positive nodes after RPLND makes the use of primary surgery less attractive than the use of primary systemic chemotherapy in patients with clinical stage IIA and IIB disease.

Adjuvant chemotherapy in nonseminomatous testicular tumour stage II

J. H. HARTLAPP, L. WEISSBACH* *and* R. BUSSAR-MAATZ* (for Testicular Tumor Study Group, Bonn), *Medizinische Universitätsklinik, Bonn, and *Krankenhaus Am Urban, Berlin, West Germany*

Summary
Preliminary results of a random prospective trial to investigate the necessary extent of adjuvant chemotherapy are presented. Two hundred and sixty-three patients entered the study, of whom 210 (forty-eight stage IIA patients, 162 stage IIB patients) could be evaluated. Two hundred and eight patients are currently free of disease, since three of the five patients with relapses (one stage IIA patient, four stage IIB patients) achieved a complete remission. One IIB patient who had relapsed achieved a partial remission, whereas the final IIB patient who progressed is presently undergoing chemotherapy. One patient died of pneumonia after the first course of VBP. Toxicity consisted mainly of nausea, vomiting and loss of hair, 17% of the patients suffered infection, and 7% experienced sepsis.

Key words. Nonseminomatous testicular germ cell tumour, chemotherapy, toxicity, prognosis.

Introduction
With the advent of polychemotherapy, virtually all patients with early stage testicular cancer can expect to be cured. One point in question is the need for cytostatic treatment for all stages of lymph node metastases and the necessary extent and continuance of such treatment. Efforts must be made to decrease the morbidity of current treatment regimens. Reducing the dosage while maintaining the same excellent therapeutic results might be one solution.

The results of a random multicentre prospective and nationwide study, which investigated the necessity and extent of adjuvant chemotherapy in stage IIA and stage IIB patients, are presented.

Materials and Methods
Forty-eight clinics in the Federal Republic of Germany, West Berlin and Austria are co-operating in this study (see appendix).

For the purpose of our trials, all patients were staged by extended retroperitoneal lymphadenectomy, and the early stages have been defined as shown in Table 1 (Hartlapp & Weissbach, 1982).

Correspondence: Priv.-Doz. Dr med. J. H. Hartlapp, Medizinische Universitätsklinik, Sigmund-Freud-Strasse 25, D-5300 Bonn 1, W. Germany.

Table 1. Definition of early stages of testicular cancer

Stage	TNM classification	Definition
I	$T_{1-4a}N_0M_0$	Tumour confined to within scrotum (possibly involving tunica albuginea/rete testis/epididymis/spermatic cord)
IIA	$T_{1-4a}N_{1,4}M_0$	Nodal involvement confined to *solitary* retroperitoneal metastasis < 2 cm, completely resectable
IIB	$T_{1-4a}N_{1-2,4}M_0$	Nodal involvement: multiple metastases < 5 cm, or single metastasis > 2 cm ≤ 5 cm, completely resectable

Patients were treated with vinblastine (V), bleomycin (B) and cisplatin (P) according to Einhorn & Donohue (1977). The dosage schedule is given in Table 2.

Table 2. Dosage schedule used in the treatment of early stage testicular cancer

Vinblastine	6 mg/m^2/day*	days 1 and 2
Bleomycin	12 mg/m^2/day†	days 1 to 5‡
Cisplatin	20 mg/m^2/day	days 1 to 5§

* Approx. 0.16 mg/kg/day.
† Approx. 0.3 mg/kg/day, total dose per course 120 mg.
‡ Drug given by continuous infusion with rigorous hydration.
§ Drug given with rigorous hydration.

Patients were divided into two groups, stage IIA and stage IIB, according to the extent of their disease. The stage IIA participants were then subdivided into an observation (no treatment) group, or a treatment group who received two courses of VBP (Fig. 1). In consideration of small retroperitoneal tumour mass (solitary metastasis < 2 cm), we believe it to be justifiable to compare a treatment with an observation group. The second group, stage IIB, was subdivided into one or two treatments, receiving either two or four courses of VBP (Fig. 2).

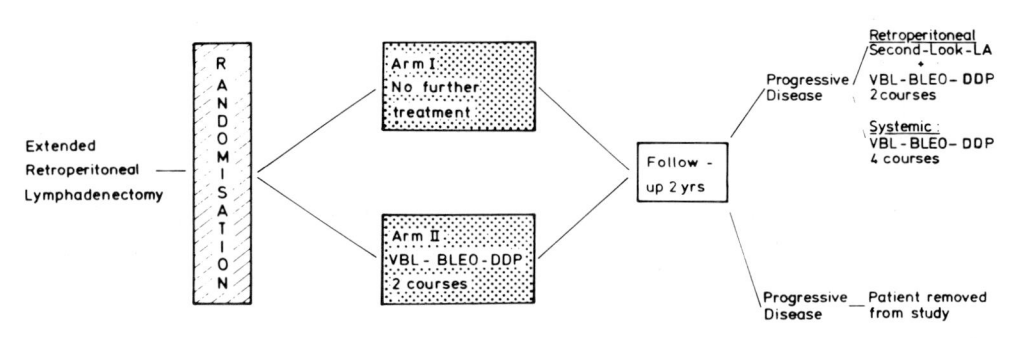

Fig. 1. Randomized phase III clinical trial nonseminomatous, nonchoriocarcinomatous metastatic testicular germ cell tumours stage IIA.

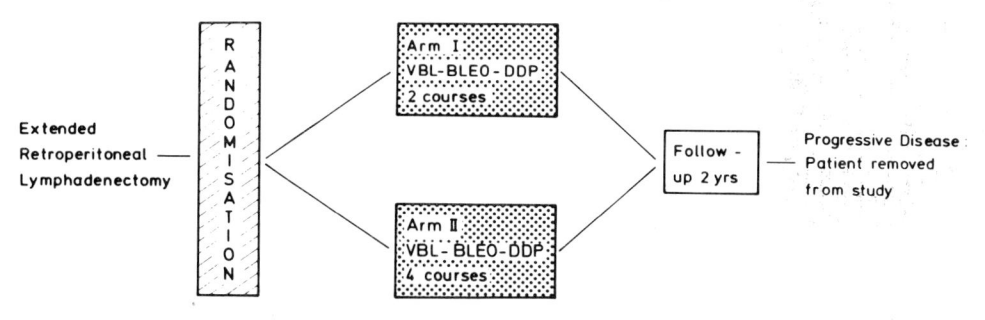

Fig. 2. Randomized phase III clinical trial nonseminomatous, nonchoriocarcinomatous metastatic testicular germ cell tumours stage IIB.

To date, fifty-eight patients have entered group IIA of whom forty-eight could be evaluated. Two hundred and five patients have entered the IIB group of whom 162 were evaluated. We believe that the prognosis of stage IIB patients is not as good as that of IIA patients. Therefore the aim of this study group was to evaluate the respective merits of two as opposed to four courses of treatment with regard to curativity and morbidity.

Results

So far, five relapses have been observed following retroperitoneal lymphadenectomy with the median follow-up period being 17–18 months (Table 3).

Table 3. Frequency of relapse and median follow-up after RLND* for stages IIA and IIB testicular cancer

Stage of disease	Number of relapses	Median follow-up (months)
IIA		
Control	1/16	18 (1–24)
2 × VBP	0/32	18 (1–24)
IIB		
2 × VBP	3/87	17 (1–24)
4 × VBP	1/75	18 (1–24)

* RNLD = retroperitoneal lymph node dissection.

Only one stage IIA patient, randomized to the observation group, suffered a pulmonary progression 10 months after treatment. He then received two courses of VBP and two courses of PEI (cisplatin, etoposide, ifosfamide) and has been in complete remission for 1 year.

Three stage IIB patients, randomized to be treated with two courses of VBP, showed progession. The patterns of relapse were as follows.

One patient revealed metastases in the supraclavicular zone immediately following the second course of VBP. Following surgical removal of histologically defined metastases, and two further courses of VBP, he has been in complete remission for 1 year. The second patient, showing more than twenty retroperitoneal lymph node metastases at primary diagnosis, received only one-third of the platinum dose during the second course of primary therapy. He suffered lung metastases 7 months after chemotherapy. Following two courses each of VBP and PEI, he achieved complete remission which has been stable for 2 years.

The last patient suffered a pulmonary progression 7 months after chemotherapy: he is in partial remission at the present time having achieved this after four courses of chemotherapy.

Three months after therapy, one stage IIB patient having been randomized to be treated with four courses of VBP revealed lung metastases. This patient is presently undergoing chemotherapy.

Twenty-eight stage IIA patients and eighty-four stage IIB patients were randomized to receive two courses of therapy, and 85.7% of stage IIA and 82.2% of stage IIB patients completed their treatment schedule without deviation from the study protocol (Table 4). On the contrary, only 55% of patients randomized to the treatment group with four courses finished the programme, 5% refusing chemotherapy: he is in partial remission at the present time having achieved this after four courses of chemotherapy.

Table 4. Toxicity related deviations from adjuvant chemotherapy protocol

	Stratification group		
	IIA 2 courses VBP	IIB 2 courses VBP	IIB 4 courses VBP
Number of patients in treatment groups (with minimum follow-up 3 months)	28	84	76
Without problem	24 (85.7%)	69 (82.2%)	42 (55.0%)
Dosage reduction	3 (10.7%)	11 (13.0%)	14 (18.0%)
Therapy discontinued	1 (3.6%)	3 (3.6%)	9 (11.0%)
Therapy refused	0	1 (1.2%)	11 (16.0%)

Amongst all the stage II patients, three patients were unable to complete their treatment because of bone marrow toxicity, and nine patients were discontinued because of other toxicities. The dosage also had to be reduced in the groups receiving two courses of therapy because of bone marrow toxicity (nine patients) and other toxicities (five patients).

Patients had to be removed from trial or have been given lower dosages because of toxicities mostly during the third and fourth course. Only one patient died of penumonia after the first course, pulmonary fibrosis being previously identified. The toxicity of treatment, affecting 82–94% of patients, mainly consisted of nausea, vomiting and loss of hair (alopecia) (Table 5). Fewer patients experienced fluid retention, stomatitis, intestinal obstruction, infection, paraesthesia, pigmentation or sepsis.

Table 5. Toxicity of chemotherapy

	n = 198	%
Nausea	187	94
Vomiting (≤ 3 occasions)	170	86
Alopecia	163	82
Vomiting (> 3 occasions)	139	70
Fluid retention	63	32
Stomatitis	43	22
Intestinal obstruction	39	20
Infection	34	17
Paraesthesia	20	10
Pigmentation	20	10
Sepsis	14	7
Haemorrhage	6	3
Gastrospasm	6	3
Diarrhoea	4	2
Paresis	3	2
Nose bleeding	3	2
Gastritis	3	2
(Thrombo)phlebitis	2	1
Phlebitis (arm)	2	1
Pneumonia	2	1
Tonsillitis	2	1
Hyperbilirubinaemia	2	1
Circulatory collapse	2	1
Backache	2	1

Discussion

Given the high curability of early stage tumours being achieved today by modern polychemotherapy, we initiated a random prospective multicentre study to investigate the necessary extent of cytostatic chemotherapy and the possibility of decreasing its side effects by reducing dosages with regard to the stages. A trial of the Testicular Intergroup Study investigated the overall need for chemotherapy following radical retroperitoneal lymph node dissection.

Following treatment with two courses of chemotherapy, the relapse rate was 6%, compared with a relapse rate of 49% for the observation (control — no adjuvant chemotherapy) group (Williams et al., 1986). These results emphasize the requirement for adjuvant chemotherapy. We subdivided stage II patients depending on retroperitoneal tumour mass. Taking into account the still low number of recruited patients, our stage IIA results suggest that a small tumour mass does not require adjuvant therapy since only one patient in the control group relapsed. All patients receiving two chemotherapeutic courses entered complete remission.

We consider patients with either more than one metastasis, or a metastasis greater than 2 cm as patients at higher risk, and therefore an overall renunciation of adjuvant therapy was not justified. This is confirmed by the results of the Intergroup Study. Four of our stage IIB patients showed recurrence: one was in the treatment group with four courses of VBP and three were in the group with two courses. The follow-up is being continued and the results will be described.

The toxicity of the chemotherapeutic regimen was tolerable. Most of the side effects were observed during the first course of treatment.

The patients' willingness to tolerate the side effects declined with each course. The therapy either had to be stopped or the dosage was reduced mainly during the third or fourth course of treatment.

Conclusions

For stage II testicular cancer, therapy with only two courses of adjuvant chemotherapy following radical RLND is sufficient. The relapse rate (3.5%) is low compared to the results of the Intergroup Study. A final conclusion regarding the prognosis of stage IIA patients must await examination of a larger number of patients. However, bearing in mind this reservation, a renunciation of adjuvant therapy seems justifiable for this subgroup.

Acknowledgements

The study on which this work was based was supported by the Federal Ministry of Research and Technology, West Germany.

References

Einhorn, L. H. & Donohue, J. P. (1977) Cis-diamminedichloroplatinum, vinblastine, bleomycin combination chemotherapy in disseminated testicular cancer. *Annals of Internal Medicine*, **87**, 293–298.

Hartlapp, J. H. & Weissbach, L. (1982) Zur Notwendigkeit der Unterteilung des Stadium II bei Hodentumoren. *Nicht-seminomatöse Hodentumoren* (ed. by H. J. Illiger, H. Sack, S. Seeber and L. Weissbach), pp. 72–75. S. Karger Verlag, Basel.

Williams, S., Muggia, F., Einhorn, L., Hahn, R., Donohue, J., Brunner, K., Stablein, D., Dewys, W., Crawford, D. & Spaulding, J. (1986) Resected stage II testicular cancer: Immediate adjuvant chemotherapy versus observation. *Proceedings of the American Society of Clinical Oncology*, **5**, 98 (Nr. 380).

Appendix: Members of the Testicular Tumour Study Group Bonn

Aachen	RWTH Aachen	H. Rübben
Arnsberg	Karolinen-Hospital	R. Vannahme
Bad Münder	Klinik Deisterhort	J. Borghardt
Berlin	Krankenhaus Am Urban	L. Weissbach
Berlin	Rudolf-Virchow-KH	A. C. Mayr
Berlin	Krankenhaus Moabit	H. H. Fülle
Bielefeld	St. Franziskus-Hosp.	P. Utsch
Bonn	Med. Univ.-Klinik	J. H. Hartlapp
	Urol. Univ.-Klinik	R. Schaefer
Bremen	Zentral-Krankenhaus	G. Glaser
Darmstadt	Städt. Kliniken	
	Med. Klinik	R. Katz
	Urol. Klinik	Ch. Lönne
Erwitte	von Hoerde'sches Marienhospital	M. Walczak
Frankf.-Höchst	Städt. Krankenhaus	J. Haselberger
Freiburg	Med. Univ.-Klinik	T. Hecht
	Urol. Univ.-Klinik	W. Vahlensieck
Fulda	Städt. Kliniken	M. Droller

Gelsenkirchen	Marienhospital	K. Oelbracht
Gelsenk.-Horst	St. Josephs-Hospital	K. Rieche
Giessen	Urol. Univ.-Klinik	W. Weidner
Göttingen	Med. Univ.-Klinik	C. Unger
	Urol. Univ.-Klinik	M. Blech
Gö.-Weende	Ev. Krankenhaus	B. Brüggeboes
Hagen	Allg. Krankenhaus	M. Hakemi
Hamburg	Bundeswehrkrankenhaus	M. Hartmann
Hamburg	Allg. KH St. Georg	R. Hubmann
Hannover	Med. Hochschule	E. Seidl
Heidelberg	Med. Univ.-Klinik	U. Räth
	Urol. Univ.-Klinik	H. Krüger
Homburg/Saar	Saarl. Krebszentrale	H. Delbrück
	Urol. Univ.-Klinik	K. Niklas
Höxter	St. Ansgar-Krankenhaus	H.-D. Adolphs
Innsbruck	Urol. Univ.-Klinik	K. Scheiber
Kiel	Urol. Univ.-Klinik	R. Schmalz
Klagenfurt	Allg. öff. Krankenhaus	M. Nachtigall
Koblenz	Städt. KH Kemperhof	C. Charvalakis
Krefeld	Städt. Krankenanstalten	
	Med. Klinik II	J. Hoss
	Urol. Klinik	R. Schmalz
Linz	Allg. öff. Krankenhaus	F. Kaufmann
Mainz	Urol. Univ.-Klinik	D. Wilbert
Mannheim	Urol. Univ.-Klinik	J. Metzler
Offenbach	Stadtkrankenhaus	M. Fensterer
Oldenburg	Städt. Kliniken	H. J. Illiger
Osnabrück	Städt. Krankenanstalten	
	Med. Klinik	G. Wimmer
	Urol. Klinik	W. Mayer
Salzburg	Landeskrankenanstalten	H. Joos
Siegen	Kreiskrankenhaus	
	Haus Hüttental	H. Hamann
Stuttgart	Katharinen-Hospital	
	Med. Klinik	U. Rüther
	Urol. Klinik	R. Jenner
Trier	KH d. Barmherz. Brüder	J.-P. Jeannelle
Ulm	Med. Univ.-Klinik	E. D. Kreuser
Ulm	Bundeswehrkrankenhaus	R. Beckert
Wien	II. Med. Univ.-Klinik	R. Kuzmits
	Urol. Univ.-Klinik	C. Kratzik
Wien	Kaiser-Franz-Josef-Spital	J. Pont
Worms	Stadtkrankenhaus	W. Jellinghaus
Würselen	Knappschaftskrankenhaus	R. Ostwald
Wuppertal	Klinikum Barmen	J. Gleissner

Discussion

Rankin You report a 20% incidence of intestinal obstruction in your 198 patients. Can you give more information about these patients and the mechanism of the obstruction whether or not it was mechanical obstruction?

Patients and Methods

One hundred and eighteen patients with nonseminomatous germ cell tumours of testicular and extragonadal origin were treated on Memorial Sloan-Kettering Cancer Center (MSKCC) 'good' and 'poor' studies between November 1982, and February 1985. Eighty-one patients have been considered good risk and thirty-seven patients have been considered poor risk. Of the good risk patients, thirty-nine were treated with VAB-6 (cyclophosphamide + vinblastine + bleomycin + cisplatin + actinomycin) (Bosl *et al.*, 1986) and forty-two with etoposide + cisplatin (EP) (Bosl *et al.*, 1985). The poor risk patients were treated with six alternating months of VAB-6 and EP (Leitner *et al.*, 1985). Patients were considered to be good risk at MSKCC if they had a testicular primary and a calculated probability of complete remission (CR) of greater than 0.5. This probability of CR was determined by the use of a mathematical model using pretreatment values of lactate dehydrogenase (LDH) and human chorionic gonadotrophin (hCG) and the number of sites of metastases (Bosl *et al.*, 1983). Poor risk patients included those patients with testicular primary tumours and a probability of CR < 0.5 and those with nonseminomatous germ cell tumours of extragonadal origin (Israel *et al.*, 1985).

The allocation of these 118 patients as good or poor risk at MSKCC was then compared to the allocation of these same patients according to the published criteria of the Indiana University (IU) (Birch *et al.*, 1986), The National Cancer Institute (NCI) (Physician's Data Query, 1985) and the European Organization for Research in the Treatment of Cancer (EORTC) (Stoter & Dennis, 1985).

Results

Thirty-seven of 118 (31%) patients were considered poor risk at MSKCC. In contrast, poor risk status was assigned to forty-four (37%) by IU criteria, fifty-eight (49%) by NCI criteria, and seventy-two (61%) by EORTC criteria.

The patients considered to be good risk at MSKCC but poor risk by the other three criteria were then evaluated for treatment outcome. Of seventeen patients considered to be good risk by MSKCC but poor risk by IU, fifteen (88%) achieved CR. Similarly, nineteen of twenty-six (73%) considered to be poor risk by the NCI and thirty-one of thirty-seven (84%) considered poor risk by the EORTC achieved CR. Of patients considered to be poor risk by MSKCC but good risk by other criteria, five of nine patients (56%) considered good risk by IU, three of six (50%) considered good risk by NCI criteria, and two of four (50%) considered good risk by EORTC achieved CR.

The survival distribution of patients considered to be poor risk by each of the four criteria were then considered. The median survival of poor risk patients by MSKCC criteria was 11.5 months, by IU criteria was 15 months, by NCI criteria was 15 months, and by EORTC criteria was 23.5 months.

Discussion

This analysis indicates a marked disparity between poor risk criteria. It is evident that as the proportion of patients considered to be poor risk increases, then the proportion of patients achieving CR and overall survival will increase. This is clearly a consequence of capturing more patients with a good prognosis in the poor risk trial. These good risk patients are then exposed to unnecessary risks. The differences between various poor risk eligibility criteria are probably the result of different emphasis given to serum tumour markers and bulk of disease. In the MSKCC mathematical model, the pretreatment values of LDH and hCG are considered as continuous variables and are of greater significance than the actual bulk of disease. Tumour markers are not considered by the IU criteria although a recent publication from the Southeastern Cancer Study Group indicates that the pretreatment value of hCG does improve the predictive ability of the IU model (Birch et al., 1986). In the NCI and EORTC models, single sites of metastases are considered to be poor risk: examples include retroperitoneal masses which are either palpable or are of specific size, and hepatic metastases. In the logistic regression analysis by which the MSKCC mathematical model was developed, neither palpable retroperitoneal disease nor hepatic metastases were independent variables which improved the predictive ability.

The outcome of trials designed for poor risk patients will, therefore, be dependent upon the criteria used to choose the patients. A high CR rate in a poor risk trial does not necessarily mean that the treatment is better than standard treatment. In a recently reported trial conducted by the EORTC, 77% of patients receiving a standard course of vinblastine + bleomycin + cisplatin, and 78% of patients receiving alternating cycles of etoposide + cisplatin and vinblastine + bleomycin + cisplatin, achieved a CR (Stoter et al., 1986). These high CR rates are similar to the 84% CR rate in those patients considered to be good risk by MSKCC but poor risk by the EORTC.

In summary, eligibility criteria for poor risk trials in patients with germ cell tumours should be as restrictive as possible in order to prevent good risk patients from experiencing unnecessary toxicity from a more intensive treatment programme. Tumour markers do provide information about a patient's prognosis that cannot be derived from an analysis of extent of tumour alone. Given the diversity of poor risk definitions, only randomized trials will enable new treatment strategies to be defined which might be an improvement over standard treatment.

Acknowledgement
This work was supported by NCI grant #CA-05826 and Contract CM-07337.

References
Birch, R., Williams, S., Cone, A., Einhorn, L., Roark, P., Turner, S. & Greco, F. R. (1986) Prognostic factors for favorable outcome in disseminated germ cell tumors. *Journal of Clinical Oncology*, **4**, 400–407.
Bosl, G. J., Bajorin, D., Leitner, S. P., and participating investigators. (1986) A randomized trial of etoposide (E) + cisplatin (P) and VAB-6 in the treatment (Rx) of 'good risk' patients (Pts) with germ cell tumors (GCT). *Proceedings of the American Society of Clinical Oncology*, **5**, 104.
Bosl, G. J., Geller, N. L., Cirrincione, C., Vogelzang, N. J., Kennedy, B. J., Whitmore, W. F., Vugrin, D., Scher, H., Nisselbaum, J. & Golbey, R. B. (1983) Multivariate analysis of prognostic variables in patients with metastatic testicular cancer. *Cancer Research*, **43**, 3403–3407.
Bosl, G. J., Gluckman, R., Geller, N. J., Golbey, R. B., Whitmore, W. F., Herr, H., Sogani, P., Morse, M., Martini, N., Bains, M. & McCormack, P. (1986) VAB-6: An effective chemotherapy regimen for patients with germ cell tumors. *Journal of Clinical Oncology*, **4**, 1493–1499.

Bosl, G. J., Yagoda, A., Golbey, R. B., Whitmore, W., Herr, H., Sogani, P., Morse, M., Vogelzang, N. & MacDonald, G. (1985) Role of etoposide-based chemotherapy in the treatment of patients with refractory or relapsing germ cell tumors. *American Journal of Medicine*, **78**, 423–428.

Israel, A., Bosl, G. J., Golbey, R. B., Whitmore, W. Jr, & Martini, N. (1985) The results of chemotherapy for extragonadal germ-cell tumors inthe cisplatin era: the Memorial Sloan-Kettering Cancer Center experience. *Journal of Clinical Oncology*, **3**, 1073–1078.

Leitner, S. P., Israel, A. M., Bosl, G. J., Schneider, R. S., & participating investigators. (1985) Treatment of poor prognosis germ cell tumors (GCT) with alternating cycles of VP-16/cisplatin (DDP) and VAB-6: an update. *Proceedings of the American Society of Clinical Oncology*, **4**, 104.

Levi, J., Raghavan, D., Harvey, V., Thomsen, D., Gill G., Byrne, M., Burns, I. & Woods, R. (1986) Deletion of bleomycin from therapy for good prognosis advanced testicular cancer: A prospective randomized study. *Proceedings of the American Society of Clinical Oncology*, **4**, 97.

Stoter, G. & Denis, L. (1985) The chemotherapy of disseminated testicular nonseminomatous germ cell tumors and the clinical research of the EORTC Genitourinary Group. *Acta Urologica Belgica*, **53**, 428–435.

Stoter, G., Kaye, S., Sleijfer, D., ten Bokkel Huinink, W., Jones, W., van Oosterom, A., Splinter, T., Pinedo, H., Sylvester, R. & Keizer, J. (1986) Preliminary results of BEP (Bleomycin, etoposide, cisplatin) versus an alternating regimen of BEP and PVB (cisplatin, vinblastine, bleomycin) in high volume metastatic (HVM) testicular non-seminomas. An EORTC study. *Proceedings of the American Society of Clinical Oncology*, **5**, 106.

Discussion

Hansen On the issue of prognostic factors and stage of disease could you give me information on the staging procedures for lymph node, liver, brain metastases, etc? Is there agreement among the various investigators on the staging procedures used?

Bosl At MSKCC we use the usual procedures including chest X-ray, serum markers and CT scan of the abdomen but very little else unless indicated. CT scan of the brain is used if there are cerebral symptoms, and CT scan of the thorax is only used if there is a suggestion of hilar disease. I think staging is fairly consistent comparing our procedures with those done at Indiana University. Invasive procedures are not performed unless indicated.

There is an important point concerning marker levels, especially hCG. The level of serum hCG is helpful but the assay used is extremely important. Many of the assays available cannot relate international units with amount in nanograms, and the correction factors are widely variable. It is therefore difficult to compare levels between different centres when different assays are in use.

Levi Please speculate on why serum levels of LDH, a very nonspecific marker of prognosis in other tumour types, should be so predictive of outcome in testicular cancer.

Bosl I believe that serum LDH is an indirect measurement of cell turnover and possibly also a measure of extent of disease. It is a very valuable, although admittedly nonspecific, marker in this disease. It should be noted that most patients with advanced seminoma will have increased serum LDH making it useful in *all* types of germ cell tumours.

Our most recent statistical analysis indicates that LDH is also a very good marker for prediction of relapse.

Oliver It appears paradoxical that serum LDH is very high in association with seminoma, but these high values are not as predictive of failure in seminoma as for nonseminoma.

Bosl There are very few seminoma patients who fail to be put in the good prognosis group by our model. In fact, in our trial of over 30 seminoma patients in the good risk group, we have had only two patients who failed.

Treatment of poor prognosis germ cell tumours with high dose cisplatin regimens

R. F. OZOLS *Medicine Branch, National Cancer Institute, U.S.A.*

Summary

We have developed an intensive combination chemotherapy regimen for the treatment of patients with poor risk nonseminomatous testicular cancer. This regimen (termed PVeBV) consists of cisplatin [P] (at twice the dose used in previous combination chemotherapy regimens), vinblastine [Ve], bleomycin [B], and VP-16 [V]. Cisplatin was administered in hypertonic saline with vigorous chlorouresis. In a pilot study we demonstrated that PVeBV was an active regimen in high risk patients but associated with severe myelosuppression. Consequently, a clinical trial of PVeBV *vs* standard PVeB chemotherapy in high risk patients is currently in progress at the Medicine Branch of the National Cancer Institute. Patients eligible for this trial must be previously untreated and have bulky disease either in the abdomen or lungs as well as other poor prognostic features. A preliminary analysis of this trial demonstrates a higher complete remission rate (87%) for PVeBV compared to (62%) for PVeB. There has only been one relapse (4%) in patients randomized to receive PVeBV compared to a 20% relapse rate in patients receiving PVeB. There is no statistically significant increase in survival for patients randomized to PVeBV; however, there is a statistically significant prolongation of disease-free survival in patients receiving the intensive four-drug regimen. The increased toxicity of PVeBV was due primarily to more severe myelosuppression. These results demonstrate that PVeBV chemotherapy can be administered to high risk testicular cancer patients with acceptable toxicity and that the preliminary analysis of a randomized trial suggests that PVeBV may be superior to PVeB in the treatment of these high risk patients.

Key words. Poor prognosis, autologous bone marrow, high dose cisplatin, PVeBV.

Introduction

During the last decade there have been dramatic improvements in the treatment of patients with testicular cancer. However, there is a subset of patients with disseminated testicular cancer in whom standard cisplatin therapy has been markedly less successful. The overall complete response rate in this group of patients with poor prognostic features is approximately 40–60%. These results are in marked contrast to the 85–95% complete remission rate achieved for patients with advanced stage disease without any of these poor prognostic features. Approximately one-third of all patients with advanced stage testicular cancer will present with poor prognostic features and thus the development of more effective treatment for this subset of patients remains an important clinical goal in the management of advanced stage testicular cancer.

Correspondence: Dr Robert F. Ozols, Medicine Branch, NCI, Bldg 10, Rm 12N226, 9000 Rockville Pike, Bethesda, MD 20892, U.S.A.

Identification of high risk (poor prognosis) testicular cancer patients

Table 1 summarizes the different classification systems which have been proposed to identify prospectively testicular cancer patients with poor prognostic features. It is apparent that there is considerable variation among the individual classification systems as to the specific clinical criteria used to define high risk patients, although all the classifications include bulky disease in the lung and/or abdomen as the major prognostic factor which predicts for a decreased complete response rate.

Table 1. Criteria for advanced poor prognosis testicular cancer

Reference	Advanced abdominal disease	Advanced pulmonary disease
Samuels et al., 1975	Palpable mass, liver metastases, ureteral displacement, obstructive uropathy	Mediastinal mass, hilar mass, pulmonary nodule > 2 cm, pleural effusion
Vugrin et al., 1984	Same as Samuels and any mass > 5 cm	Same as Samuels and more than 5 metastases per lung field
Skinner, 1982	Palpable mass	More than 10 nodules or any nodule > 3.5 cm
Pontes et al., 1984	> 6–10 nodes, palpable mass, residual disease after RLND*	6–10 nodules/lung field, > 3.5 cm nodule, hilar or mediastinal involvement
Samson et al., 1980	'Large retroperitoneal masses', liver metastases	> 5 nodules each > 2.0 cm
Einhorn & Williams, 1985	Palpable mass,† hepatic metastases	Mediastinal mass > 50% intrathoracic diameter, > 10 metastases per lung field, multiple masses > 3 cm

* RLND = retroperitoneal lymph node dissection.
† Palpable abdominal mass without pulmonary disease is not advanced disease in this system.

Certain histological subtypes of germ cell tumours are also associated with a decreased response to chemotherapy. In particular, endodermal sinus tumours clearly have a worse prognosis which appears to be independent of the fact that they frequently present as bulky mediastinal tumours (Kuzur et al., 1982; Logothetis et al., 1985). On the other hand, it is not clear whether the reported decreased complete remission rate in some series of extragonadal tumours is due to an intrinsically different response rate or is the result of the large tumour burden with which these patients usually present (Hainsworth et al., 1982; Logothetis et al., 1985).

Development of a new intensive combination chemotherapy regimen for patients with bulky testicular cancer

In order to determine the effect of more intensive induction chemotherapy in poor prognosis testicular cancer patients, a new drug combination, PVeBV (Table 2), consisting of cisplatin (at twice the dose used in previous combination chemotherapy regimens), vinblastine, bleomycin, and the epidodophyllotoxin VP-16-213 was

Table 2. PVeBV chemotherapy

Cisplatin (P)	40 mg/m^2 i.v. q.d. × 5	
Vinblastine (Ve)	0.2 mg/kg i.v. day 1	every 21 days
VP-16 (V)	100 mg/m^2 i.v. q.d. × 5	
Bleomycin (B)	30 u i.v. q. wk	

* Administered in 250 ml 3% saline with 6 litres per day normal saline hydration.

administered to ten patients in a pilot protocol at the Medicine Branch (Ozols et al., 1983). Previously untreated patients underwent collections of their bone marrows prior to chemotherapy after which they received three 21-day cycles of PVeBV without dose modification for haematological toxicity. Patients who had either elevated markers after three cycles of PVeBV or residual carcinoma in a resected mass underwent an additional cycle of chemotherapy with more intensive doses of VP-16 (200 mg/m^2 q.d. × 5) followed by re-infusion of autologous bone marrow. The rationale for this new drug regimen was as follows:

(a) The importance of cisplatin dose in the treatment of testicular cancer was previously established (Hayes et al., 1977; Samson et al., 1984). Doses of cisplatin > 120 mg/m^2 have not routinely been used because of the increased incidence of renal toxicity. However, recent studies (Litterst, 1981; Earhart et al., 1983) demonstrated that cisplatin nephrotoxicity, but not the anti-tumour effect, could be reduced in animals if cisplatin was administered in hypertonic sodium chloride solution. A likely explanation for this protective effect relates to the aquation equilibria of cisplatin and the formation of reactive and cytotoxic intermediates. Thus, from thermodynamic considerations and from animal toxicity studies, it was considered likely that the cisplatin dose could be escalated by maintenance of a brisk chlorouresis and concomitant administration of cisplatin in hypertonic saline.

(b) VP-16 has significant activity in testicular cancer patients who have relapsed after primary cisplatin based chemotherapy (Williams & Einhorn, 1982; Hainsworth et al., 1985).

(c) Vinblastine and bleomycin were included in the induction regimen since previous studies have demonstrated clinical synergy for this combination in the treatment of advanced stage testicular cancer patients.

(d) The use of high dose ablative therapy early in the treatment course of a patient theoretically would be advantageous since the number of drug-resistant clones may increase as a function of time and extent of previous therapy.

Ten patients with bulky nonseminomatous testicular cancer were treated with the PVeBV regimen as outlined (Ozols et al., 1983). Six patients were previously untreated and four had failed cisplatin based chemotherapy regimens. All six previously untreated patients achieved a complete remission. Four of these patients achieved a complete remission with three cycles of PVeBV while the other two patients achieved a complete remission with an additional cycle of high dose cisplatin plus VP16 (200 mg/m^2 i.v. q.d. × 5) followed by autologous bone marrow infusion. There have been no relapses in the group achieving complete remission with all patients followed for longer than 4 years.

Peripheral neuropathy (primarily numbness and tingling in the distal extremities) was similar with PVeBV and PVeB.

Although all patients on PVeB or PVeBV developed audiogram abnormalities following therapy, clinically significant ototoxicity was observed only with PVeBV.

Myelosuppression was more severe with PVeBV than PVeB. 87% of patients on PVeBV had a white blood cell count of < 1000 per μl compared to 50% for PVeB. Neutropenic fevers requiring antibiotic therapy occurred in 80% of PVeBV patients compared to 56% of PVeB patients. Bacterial infections (sepsis or other documented source) occurred in 23% of patients on PVeBV while there were no documented bacterial infections with PVeB. Platelet suppression was also more severe with PVeBV (60% of patients with a platelet count of < 20,000 per μl) compared to PVeB (19%).

The major disturbing toxicity in this study has been the 6% incidence of fatal pulmonary fibrosis seen equally in both arms of this trial. This toxicity developed even with careful monitoring of the patients (physical examination, chest X-rays, pulmonary function tests). Bleomycin was discontinued at the earliest sign of pulmonary toxicity and no patient received more than 360 units total dose.

Discussion

While the randomized study at the Medicine Branch, NCI, is continuing to accrue patients, several interim conclusions can be made:
(a) The selection criteria for entry into this trial have correctly identified a group of patients in whom standard therapy is not satisfactory. The 45% projected actuarial survival in patients treated with PVeB is markedly inferior to the 85–95% survival reported for patients with small volume disseminated disease.
(b) Those patients who do not achieve a complete remission with PVeB therapy are not salvaged by treatment with high dose cisplatin and VP-16.
(c) It is not necessary to store bone marrow prior to randomization. Only one patient required an additional cycle of high dose chemotherapy plus autologous marrow to achieve a complete remission.
(d) Respiratory failure due to massive lung disease is the primary characteristic associated with the inability to achieve a complete remission with PVeBV.
(e) While PVeBV is more myelotoxic than PVeB, the duration of the nadirs is short and the effects of the low white count are manageable.
(f) The major toxicity of both PVeBV and PVeB has been the development of pulmonary fibrosis associated with bleomycin therapy.

Furthermore, high-dose cisplatin can be safely administered even in the face of tumour-produced renal obstruction (Ozols et al., 1984). Eight patients treated with PVeBV had evidence of obstructive uropathy including one patient with a non-functioning kidney and a creatinine clearance of 35 ml/min. All patients with obstructive uropathy were treated with PVeBV without dose modification or alterations of the hydration regimen. The post treatment creatinine clearances of these patients were all greater than 93 ml/min.

If the preliminary results on the superiority of PVeBV compared to PVeB are confirmed by additional patient entry and longer follow-up, then this will represent an important change in the treatment of patients with poor prognosis testicular cancer. However, even if PVeBV proves to be superior to PVeB, there will remain additional questions as to the optimum treatment for patients with poor prognosis testicular cancer. While the complete remission rate with PVeBV is impressive (87%), nevertheless a significant minority of patients do not achieve a complete remission with PVeBV therapy. In addition, the toxicity of the PVeBV regimen is substantial, particularly the pulmonary toxicity.

We plan to evaluate a new regimen consisting of high-dose cisplatin, high-dose VP-16, and ifosfamide in patients with poor prognosis germ cell tumours. High-dose cisplatin will be continued in the new regimen due to the increased efficacy observed with the double dose of cisplatin in PVeBV. Since our initial observation of the therapeutic activity of high-dose cispatin in PVeBV, there have been three other reports (Schmoll et al., 1984; Daugaard et al., 1985; Trump et al., 1985) of high-dose cisplatin regimens in the treatment of poor prognosis germ cell tumour patients. In these studies, similar therapeutic results were obtained (Table 4).

Table 4. High dose cisplatin regimens in testicular cancer patients

Reference	Regimen	Patients	Results
Schmoll et al., 1984	DPP 40 mg/m^2 i.v. q.d. × 5 VP-16 140 mg/m^2 i.v. q.d. × 5 Bleo 15 mg/m^2 i.v. q.wk	15 (previously untreated)	13/15 (87%) CR
Daugaard et al., 1986	DPP 40 mg/m^2 i.v. q.d. × 5 VP-16 200 mg/m^2 i.v. q.d. × 5 Bleo 15 mg/m^2 q.wk	23:15 previously untreated and 8 previously treated	15/23 (65%) CR
Trump et al., 1985	DDP mg/m^2 i.v. q.d. × 5 VP-16 100 mg/m^2 i.v. q.d. × 5	12 previously treated	2/16 (17%) CR

The activity of VP-16 in previously untreated patients as well as in refractory germ cell tumour patients has been confirmed (Hainsworth et al., 1985). Of particular note from these studies has been the clear demonstration that testicular cancer has a steep dose–response relationship with VP-16 (Wolff et al., 1984) and that doses can be escalated significantly higher than were used in the PVeBV combination. Accordingly, we propose to use VP-16 at a dose of 150 mg/m^2 on each day that cisplatin is administered. If the toxicity of this dose of VP-16 is acceptable, then the dose will be further escalated. In addition to VP-16 and high dose cisplatin, patients will also receive ifosfamide. The group at Indiana University has demonstrated that a combination of VP-16, cisplatin, and ifosfamide (VIP) is an active regimen in the treatment of refractory germ cell tumour patients (Loehrer, Einhorn & Williams, 1985). In their study, cisplatin was administered at 20 mg/m^2 on days 1–5, VP-16 was at 75 mg/m^2 days 1–5, and ifosfamide was given at 1.2 g/m^2 on days 1–5. N-acetyl cysteine, 2 g was given every 6 h orally to prevent haemorrhagic cystitis. Courses were repeated every 21 days for four to six cycles. Objective responses were observed in 17/51 (34%) patients. In our study, we will initially use the same dose of ifosfamide but double the dose of both VP-16 and cisplatin.

single agent cisplatin and hypertonic saline in patients previously treated with cisplatin. We produced a 32% response rate and also saw toxic effects, and clearly we are dealing with an active drug as well as a very toxic drug. Hypertonic saline does not protect against any of the other toxic effects and only protects from nephrotoxicity. The response rate indicates that clinically the hypertonic saline does not decrease the cytotoxic effect of cisplatin.

Pizzocaro Have you any experience with the use of glutathione to prevent cisplatin-induced renal toxicity?

Ozols Glutathione (GSH) is important in modulating the antitumour effects of cisplatin, and depletion of glutathione enzymes in the kidney may play a part in platinum-induced nephrotoxicity. However, I am unaware of any reduction in renal toxicity caused by glutathione in an experimental system.

Levi To comment on the question of bleomycin pulmonary toxicity with platinum-based regimens, our data show that there are transient disturbances in creatinine clearances after each dose of cisplatin. As bleomycin is excreted largely by the renal route, the transient disturbances of creatinine clearance have been shown by our studies to increase the incidence of pulmonary toxicity. Serial measurements of creatinine clearances between doses of cisplatin and adjustments of doses of bleomycin accordingly is advised.

Ozols I think that platinum may alter the excretion of bleomycin thereby potentiating its pulmonary toxicity. However, we are seeing the same incidence of pulmonary toxicity with either the low dose (PVeB) or the high dose (PVePV) cisplatin regimen.

Vogelzang Does retinal toxicity occur in the males as it does in the females?

Ozols This is an interesting effect in women which was first suspected when they reported that tomatoes did not look quite as red. They had a different colour perception as well as blurring of vision during treatment. We found that platinum does have toxicity on the rods and cones of the retina affecting red perception. The blurring of the vision does improve with time but the colour perception does not revert to normal. The visual changes have not been identified in men.

Treatment of patients with poor prognosis anaplastic germ cell tumours (AGCT) of the testis and other sites

E. S. NEWLANDS, K. D. BAGSHAWE, R. H. J. BEGENT, G. J. S. RUSTIN, S. M. CRAWFORD and L. HOLDEN *CRC Laboratories, Department of Medical Oncology, Charing Cross Hospital, Fulham Palace Road, London W6 8RF*

Summary

Between 1977 and 1986, 170 male patients with anaplastic germ cell tumours (AGCT) completed chemotherapy with POMB/ACE (platinum, vincristine (oncovin), methotrexate, bleomycin, actinomycin D, cyclophosphamide and etoposide). By increasing the number of courses of POMB in 1979 we have been able to compensate for adverse prognostic factors. Since then each patient has received a minimum of three courses of POMB and 139 patients have completed therapy with an overall survival of 89%, and for those patients who had not received prior radiotherapy the survival is 92%. By increasing the number of courses of POMB, the initial serum concentrations of human chorionic gonadotrophin (hCG greater than 50,000 IU/l) and/or alpha-fetoprotein (AFP greater than 500 kU/l) have ceased to be poor prognostic variables. Neither stage at presentation nor the volume of metastatic disease is a major adverse prognostic variable using this chemotherapy.

Key words. POMB/ACE chemotherapy, anaplastic germ cell tumours.

Introduction

'Anaplastic germ cell tumour' (AGCT) is a term proposed by us to describe the most aggressive histological variants of germ cell tumours and includes embryonal carcinoma, yolk sac and choriocarcinoma, and mixed tumours including any of these elements (Paradinas, 1983). It excludes mature teratomas and pure seminomas. We think that this is a preferable term to the currently widely used 'non-seminomatous germ cell tumours'.

The survival of patients with metastatic testicular germ cell tumours is now good provided that the disease is treated before it becomes very advanced. Einhorn & Donohue (1977) reported the initial results using cisplatin, vinblastine and bleomycin (PVB) and this group had a survival of 64%. Many other centres have used essentially the same combination and in a recent review of the results in the main

Correspondence: Dr E. S. Newlands, Department of Medical Oncology, Charing Cross Hospital, Fulham Palace Road, London W6 8RF.

centres in the U.K. the 3-year survival was 71% of 179 patients using this drug combination (MRC Testicular Tumour Working Party, 1985). This analysis confirmed that (i) the initial volume of the metastatic disease and (ii) the initial concentration of the serum tumour markers, human chorionic gonadotrophin (hCG) and alpha-fetoprotein (AFP) were independent prognostic variables. The survival was worse the larger the volume or the higher the tumour markers at the time of starting treatment. Other drug combinations being used in metastatic germ cell tumours include the VAB/6 combination (cyclophosphamide, vinblastine, actinomycin D, bleomycin and cisplatin) reported by Vugrin, Whitmore & Golbey (1983). However, in this group of thirty-six men, although the complete remission rate was 91%, there were a few patients with the most advanced disease. Peckham et al. (1983) have reported the results of forty-three patients using a combination of bleomycin, etoposide and cisplatin (BEP). In this series, 86% achieved complete remission including fourteen patients with large volume metastatic disease, although in this group of patients none was recorded as having liver or central nervous system metastases.

Ozols et al. (1983) have given high-dose chemotherapy with cisplatin at a total dose of 200 mg/m^2 per course combined with vinblastine, bleomycin and etoposide. However, although the response rate to this approach is high, the toxicity is severe and toxic deaths have occurred. Samson et al. (1984) have performed a randomized study comparing two different doses of cisplatin in the PVB regimen. The most important finding was that patients with large volume metastatic disease had a significantly better survival if they received cisplatin at a dose of 120 mg/m^2 compared to 75 mg/m^2. This confirmed our earlier observation (Newlands et al., 1980) that patients with more advanced disease required a minimum of 360 mg/m^2 of cisplatin in their combination chemotherapy to obtain a high proportion of stable remissions.

POMB/ACE (cisplatin, vincristine, methotrexate, bleomycin, actinomycin D, cyclophosphamide and etoposide) chemotherapy has been developed at the Charing Cross Hospital since 1977. At this time cisplatin had recently been introduced in the PVB regimen by Einhorn & Donohue (1977) and we had identified the activity of etoposide in this disease (Newlands & Bagshawe, 1977). We thought it important to incorporate etoposide as one of the first line agents in the management of AGCT. Between 1977 and 1979 the initial serum concentration of hCG > 50,000 IU/l and/or AFP > 500 kU/l were adverse prognostic factors with a survival of 45%. Since 1979, when we increased the total amount of cisplatin received by each patient to a minimum of three courses of POMB, we have been able to compensate for this adverse prognostic factor. POMB/ACE chemotherapy contains the flexibility of delivering high-dose methotrexate to patients with brain metastases from malignant germ cell tumours, and eight out of ten patients (including one ovarian AGCT) with brain metastases are alive (Rustin et al., 1986). In terms of survival in patients with very advanced disease treated with combination chemotherapy, the only other series which appears to have a comparable survival has used a similar approach of alternating chemotherapy. This series has included cyclophosphamide, adriamycin and cisplatin in an alternating schedule with vinblastine and bleomycin (Logothetis et al., 1985).

Patients and Methods

170 men with metastatic malignant AGCTs have been treated between 1977 and 1 March 1986. The primary sites were: testis, 155; retroperitoneum, 7; mediastinum, 5; unknown, 3. Thirty-one had received prior irradiation to the para-aortic nodes and nine had received some prior chemotherapy.

Staging

The Royal Marsden staging classification (Peckham et al., 1979) has been used to describe tumour extent, site(s) and volume:

- I. Disease limited to testis. No evidence of metastases.
- IM. Disease apparently limited to testis but raised levels of tumour markers hCG and AFP following orchidectomy.
- II. Para-aortic node metastases: A, metastases < 2 cm diameter; B, metastases 2–5 cm diameter; *C, metastases > 5 cm diameter.
- III. Supradiaphragmatic lymph node involvement: abdominal status A, B and *C, as above.
- IV. Extralymphatic metastases: L1, up to three pulmonary metastases < 2 cm diameter; L2, > 3 metastases < 2 cm diameter; *L3, metastases > 2 cm diameter. *H+, liver involvement. *CNS, central nervous system involvement.

*Patients defined as having advanced and bulky disease.

Treatment

The chemotherapy schedules used have been reported previously (Newlands et al., 1980, 1983, 1986).

POMB

Day 1: Vincristine 1 mg/m^2 i.v.; methotrexate 300 mg/m^2 as a 12-h infusion.
Day 2: Bleomycin 15 mg given as a 24-h infusion; folinic acid rescue started 24 h after the start of methotrexate, 15 mg 12-hourly for four doses.
Day 3: Bleomycin 15 mg as a 24-h infusion.
Day 4: Patients are hydrated with 2 litres of saline each containing 20 mmol of KCl per litre and 1 g of magnesium sulphate per litre, which is followed by cisplatin 120 mg/m^2 given with hydration as a 12-h infusion and the hydration continued, including a further gramme of magnesium sulphate (total 3 g) until the vomiting from cisplatin stops.

ACE

Etoposide 100 mg/m^2 i.v. days 1–5; actinomycin D 0.5 mg i.v. days 3, 4 and 5; cyclophosphamide 500 mg/m^2 i.v. day 5.

OMB

Day 1: vincristine 1 mg/m^2 i.v.; methotrexate 300 mg/m^2 as a 12-h infusion.
Day 2: bleomycin 15 mg as a 24-h infusion; folinic acid rescue starts 24-h after the start of methotrexate 15 mg 12-hourly for four doses.
Day 3: bleomycin 15 mg as a 24-h infusion.

The treatment was given in the following sequence: Two courses of POMB followed by ACE, then POMB is alternated with ACE until patients are in biochemical remission as measured by serum hCG and AFP. The usual number of courses of POMB has been three to five. Following biochemical remission, ACE is alternated with OMB until the remission has been maintained for 12 weeks (Fig. 1). No maintenance therapy has been given. The intervals between each course of chemotherapy has been kept to a minimum; usually 9–11 drug-free days.

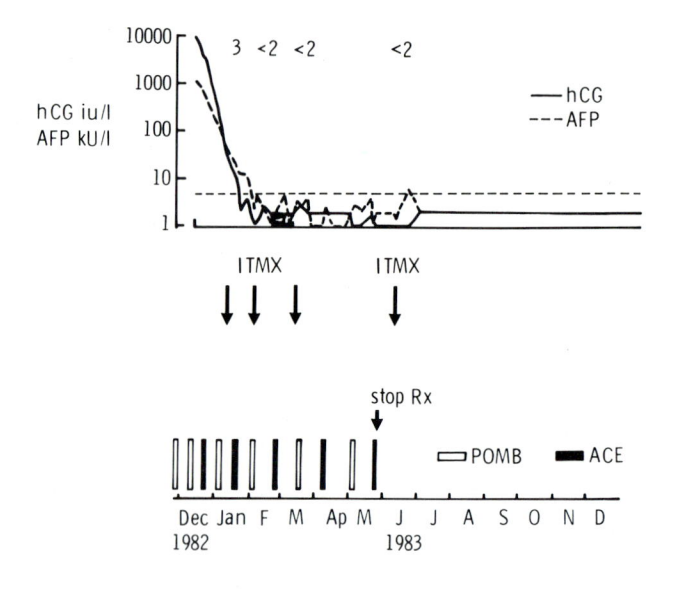

Fig. 1. Testicular anaplastic germ cell tumour with CNS secondaries. Patient presenting with pulmonary metastases (L3) and cerebral secondaries treated with POMB/ACE. The dose of methotrexate i.v. was increased to 1 g/m² and the patient received four lumbar punctures with intrathecal methotrexate. The patient received five courses of POMB and the last but one was OMB.

Central nervous system
Prophylaxis: Three intrathecal injections of methotrexate (12.5 mg) have been given with the first three ACE schedules in patients presenting with pulmonary metastases or a serum hCG greater than 1000 IU/l. CSF hCG estimations have been made routinely.

Established brain metastases: The dose of methotrexate has been increased to 1 g/m² given as a 24-h infusion, and folinic acid starting 6 h after the end of the infusion in a dose of 15 mg 8-hourly for 72 h. Intrathecal methotrexate has been given with the courses of ACE until the brain metastases have completely regressed on CT scanning and CSF hCG concentrations are normal.

Patients presenting with respiratory, liver and renal failure
These very sick patients can be salvaged by initial less intensive therapy with etoposide 100 mg/m² i.v. and cisplatin 20 mg/m² i.v. on days 1 and 2 (sometimes 3 days). This can be repeated at short intervals and normally the full chemotherapy can be started with POMB after two or three of these short courses.

Results

The clinical and radiological stage has not been as major a prognostic variable in patients treated with POMB/ACE chemotherapy as in some other series. In 170 patients treated between 1977 and 1986 the difference in the survival between early metastatic disease (96%) and those with large volume metastatic disease (C and/or L3), the survival was 79% in ninety-three patients ($P = 0.02$). This includes patients who received an inadequate dose (by current standards) of cisplatin between 1977 and 1979. Repeating the analysis in the patients treated since 1979 to 1 March 1986, all patients with minimal metastatic disease (IM, A or L1) were alive. In the most advanced disease (C and/or L3) the survival was 86% in seventy patients ($P = 0.04$).

At the end of chemotherapy it has been our practice to remove residual masses if this is possible. Fifty-nine (35%) of 170 patients have had surgery and the survival for these patients is identical to those who have not received surgery. Obviously this does not mean that the surgery has not been effective in certain patients since a small proportion of the resected masses have contained residual viable tumour and the patients have then received additional chemotherapy. We remain worried about the biological stability of differentiated teratoma and we prefer to remove these masses whenever possible. Metastatic disease to the central nervous system and to the liver have not been adverse prognostic features and the survival of patients with CNS metastases is 80% and for large liver metastases is fourteen (82%) out of seventeen patients.

In 1979 we had identified that an hCG greater than 50,000 IU/l and/or an AFP greater than 500 kU/l was an adverse prognostic factor with a survival of only 45% when patients received only two courses of POMB. By increasing the number of courses of POMB to a minimum of three and increasing this further for those patients with particularly large volume metastatic disease, the presence of high markers has ceased to be a prognostic variable provided the patient has not received prior radiation. Between 1979 and 1986, in the patients who had not received prior radiation there were eighty-two patients presenting with an hCG less than 50,000 and/or an AFP less than 500 kU/l, and the survival was 92%. In those patients presenting with markers at a higher level the survival was 91% in thirty-eight patients. However, an unexpected finding in the analysis was the specific subgroup who continued to have a poor prognosis throughout this series. Patients referred to us having had prior irradiation and who had low concentrations of hCG and/or AFP had good survival throughout this series (Fig. 2) with a survival of 90% in twenty patients. In the patients referred to us having had prior radiation where the hCG is greater than 50,000 IU/l and/or the AFP is greater than 500 kU/l the prognosis continues to be poor, with a survival of 48% in eleven patients ($P = 0.003$). The problem here in this latter group is the early development of drug resistance and inability to get the disease into remission. It would appear that the prior radiotherapy in some way is inducing drug resistance.

During the development of POMB/ACE chemotherapy we have learned how best to use this therapy over the last 9 years. We feel that one of the reasons why the survival has been good despite advanced disease has been the rate of drug delivery, since the POMB combination is only moderately myelosuppressive and

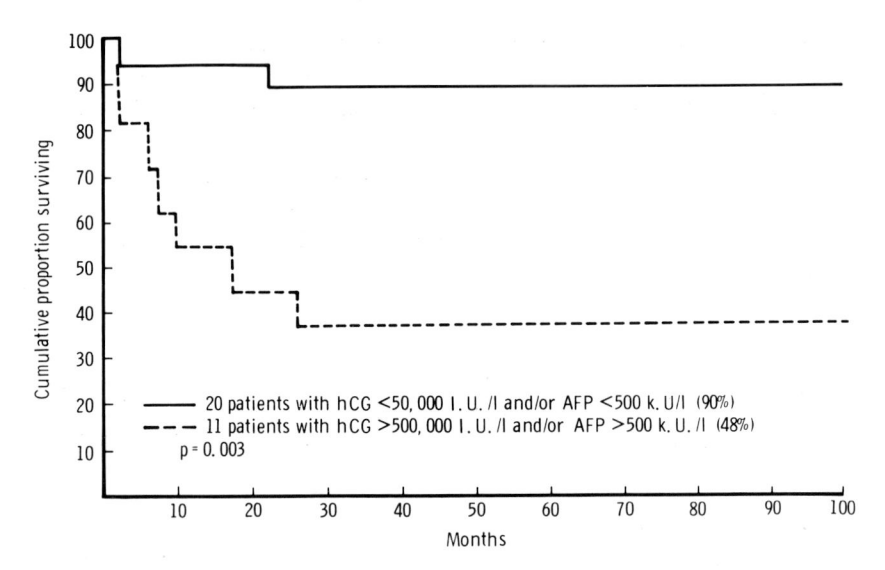

Fig. 2. Life table analyses of patients who had received prior radiotherapy and were treated with POMB/ACE chemotherapy. Throughout 1977–86 patients who had high tumour markers at the time of starting chemotherapy had a poor prognosis.

allows the intervals between therapy to be reduced to between 9 and 11 days in most cases. In Fig. 3 the difference in survival is shown between the patients treated from 1977 to 1979 when they received only two courses of POMB which was clearly inadequate in patients with advanced disease; here the survival is 65% in thirty-one patients. This contrasts with the series since 1979 where in 139 patients the survival

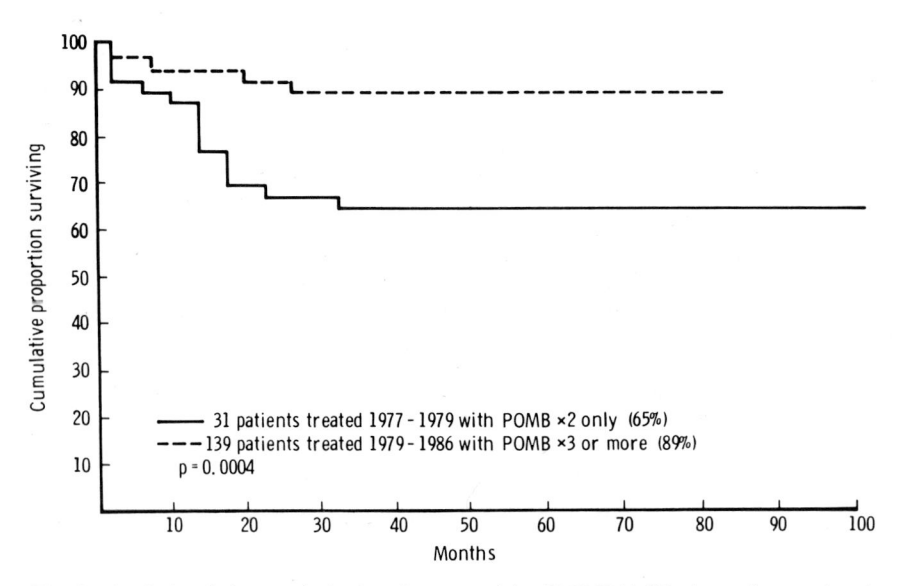

Fig. 3. Analysis of the survival of patients receiving POMB/ACE chemotherapy by time of entry: 1977–79 patients received POMB × 2 only, and after this (1979–86) they have received a minimum of three courses of POMB.

is 89% ($P = 0.0004$). If the patients who had received prior radiation are omitted from analysis, then the survival in patients treated since 1979 rises to 92%. In our series the proportion of patients with advanced disease has declined slightly from two-thirds to just over 60% of the total.

At present we think that POMB/ACE chemotherapy remains the treatment of choice for patients with anaplastic germ cell tumours, particularly in those presenting with factors which in many other series are regarded as adverse prognostic factors.

Acknowledgements
We thank all the surgeons and radiotherapists who have referred patients to us, and the staff at the Charing Cross Hospital for their excellent support. This work was supported in part by the Cancer Research Campaign and the Medical Research Council.

References
Einhorn, L. H. & Donohue, J. (1977) Cis-diamminedichloroplatinum, vinblastine and bleomycin combination chemotherapy in disseminated testicular cancer. *Annals of Internal Medicine*, **87**, 293–298.

Logothetis, C. J., Samuels, M. L., Selig, D., Swanson, D., Johnson, D. E. & Eschenbach, A. C. (1985) Improved survival with cyclic chemotherapy for nonseminomatous germ cell tumours of the testis. *Journal of Clinical Oncology*, **3**, 326–335.

Medical Research Council Working Party on Testicular Tumours (January 1985) Prognostic factors in advanced nonseminomatous germ-cell testicular tumours: results of a multicentre study. *Lancet*, **i**, 8–11.

Newlands, E. S. & Bagshawe, K. D. (1977) Epipodophyllin derivative (VP 16-213) in malignant teratomas and choriocarcinomas. *Lancet*, **ii**, 87.

Newlands, E. S., Begent, R. H. J., Kaye, S. B., Rustin, G. J. S. & Bagshawe, K. D. (1980) Chemotherapy of advanced malignant teratomas. *British Journal of Cancer*, **42**, 378–384.

Newlands, E. S., Begent, R. H. J., Rustin, G. J. S., Parker, D. & Bagshawe, K. D. (1983) Further advances in the management of malignant teratomas of the testis and other sites. *Lancet*, **i**, 948–951.

Newlands, E. S., Bagshawe, K. D., Begent, R. H. J., Rustin, G. J. S., Crawford, S. M. & Holden, L. (1986) Current optimum management of anaplastic germ cell tumours of the testis and other sites. *British Journal of Urology*, **58**, 307–314.

Ozols, R. F., Dreisseroth, A. B., Javadpour, N., Barlock, A., Meisserschmidt, G. L. & Young, R. C. (1983) Treatment of poor prognosis nonseminomatous testicular cancer with a 'high dose' platinum combination chemotherapy regimen. *Cancer*, **51**, 1803–1807.

Paradinas, F. J. (1983) Pathology. In: *Clinics in Oncology*, 2, No. 1, Germ Cell Tumours (ed. by K. D. Bagshawe, E. S. N. Newlands and R. H. J. Begent), pp. 17–50. W. B. Saunders, London.

Peckham, M. J., McElwain, T. J., Barrett, A. & Hendry, W. F. (1979) Combined management of malignant teratoma of the testis. *Lancet*, **ii**, 267–270.

Peckham, M. J., Barrett, A., Liew, K. H., Horwich, A., Robinson, B., Dobbs, H. J., McElwain, T. J. & Hendry, W. F (1983) The treatment of metastatic germ-cell testicular tumours with bleomycin, etoposide and cis-platinum (BEP). *British Journal of Cancer*, **47**, 613–619.

Rustin, G. J. S., Newlands, E. S., Bagshawe, K. D., Begent, R. H. J. & Crawford, S. M. (1986) Successful management of metastatic and primary germ cell tumours in the brain. *Cancer*, **57**, 2108–2113.

Samson, M. K., Rivkin, S. E., Jones, S. E., Constanzi, J. J., Lobuglio, A. F., Stephens, R. L., Gehan, E. A. & Cummings, G. D. (1984) Dose-response and dose-survival advantage for high versus low-dose cisplatin combined with vinblastine and bleomycin in disseminated testicular cancer. *Cancer*, **53**, 1029–1035.

Vugrin, D., Whitmore, W. F. & Golbey, R. B. (1983) VAB-6 combination chemotherapy without maintenance in treatment of disseminated cancer of the testis. *Cancer*, **51**, 211–215.

Discussion

Schraffordt Koops In 59 of your 170 patients a laparotomy was performed after chemotherapy. Why did you not remove the residual tumour in all your patients? Does it depend on histology?

Newlands Most patients had no residual tumour to remove, and some had too many deposits to excise, especially if there were multiple lung deposits. Residual shadow in an X-ray is not synonymous with residual disease and in a number of cases we biopsied the shadow if we were worried. We usually removed a large solitary metastasis in the lung if it did not disappear completely with therapy, or a large retroperitoneal mass. Residual masses were detected in 59/170 patients and these were removed; in most cases these only contained necrotic tissue or differentiated tissue.

The histology of the primary tumour is not a major determining factor as to whether the patient requires surgery. I am not happy about any of the classifications of these tumours; for example, a patient with histological evidence of only seminoma may have serum hCG levels in excess of 1,000,000 IU/l. More detailed examination of a tumour usually reveals more evidence of different cell elements within it so that none of the present classifications help a great deal. We have proposed the term 'anaplastic germ cell tumour' as a term to include the more aggressive histological variants of germ cell tumours including choriocarcinoma, yolk sac tumour, embryonal carcinoma.

Grigor There is much confusion in the literature concerning the terminology of germ cell tumours and it would be useful to have a good name to encompass all the high risk tumour types. However, I think 'anaplastic' is an inappropriate term, using it as you do, because 'anaplastic' has a clearly defined meaning which is different from the meaning that you are giving it. The continued use of 'anaplastic germ cell tumour' for high risk nonseminomatous germ cell tumours can only add to the confusion in terminology and I urge the Charing Cross Group to avoid using this misleading term.

Newlands There is a recognized group of aggressive germ cell tumours and to give this group a *negative* name such as *non*seminomatous germ cell tumour is clearly unsatisfactory. If other pathologists object to our proposed term 'anaplastic germ cell tumour' then we need alternative proposals for an acceptable term.

Rørth Would you please comment on the treatment of brain metastases? We have recently treated a few such patients with systemic chemotherapy alone (without radiotherapy and without intrathecal methotrexate) and obtained complete remission in the brain. Do you think intrathecal methotrexate is necessary in the treatment of these patients?

Newlands Results with gestational choriocarcinoma metastasizing to the brain have shown that it is possible to obtain complete remission with chemotherapy alone without radiotherapy, although we do use intrathecal methotrexate in addition to systemic therapy. In the most recent high risk series, we have about 14 out of 18 long-term survivors. We have used this experience in the treatment of male germ cell tumours giving both high dose systemic methotrexate (1 g/m^2) and intrathecal methotrexate (12.5 mg). The results are also good for males. We have 12 males with brain involvement from germ cell tumours, including two primary brain tumours, followed for a maximum of 6 years, and 10 of the 12 are alive. However, we do not know if it is necessary to include the intrathecal therapy for brain metastases.

Bosl Are you describing 62% of 170 patients with high volume disease, or are your 170 patients 62% of a higher total number of patients? Where were the primary sites of the tumours in these 170 patients and were they all men?

Newlands I refer to 62% of 170 patients with large volume disease or high tumour markers. Most of the patients had testicular primaries but there were also six mediastinal tumours (all in remission) and seven apparently retroperitoneal tumours.

Safirstein I notice that you used mannitol infusion to provide a diuresis prior to administering high dose cisplatin. What was the incidence of severe renal toxicity?

Newlands A proportion of patients have transient elevated levels of serum urea and creatinine and require close monitoring, but major renal toxicity is uncommon. Major renal damage has occured in some cases usually in association with the patient's returning home, continuing to vomit and becoming severely dehydrated. The renal damage can be cumulative and in patients with very advanced disease, dose reduction has been necessary in a few cases near the end of therapy. We have also used prophylactic magnesium supplements.

bulky disease. Since a strong dose–response relationship has been demonstrated for cisplatin in disseminated testicular cancer (Samson et al., 1984), a higher than standard dose of cisplatin might be more useful. Ultra high dose cisplatin can safely be administered without increased renal toxicity using a high i.v. fluid infusion scheme with diuretics and 3% NaCl solution (Ozols et al., 1982; Litterst, 1981). Cisplatin and VP-16 are synergistic in the animal model and are the most active agents in treatment of testicular cancer. As proposed by Ozols et al. (1982), ultra high dose cisplatin (200 mg/m^2 per cycle) could be combined with VP-16 in standard doses and bleomycin, plus velban. Since vinblastine accounts for the high bone marrow toxicity of this four-drug combination the integration of this drug into the combination seems not to be suitable (Blayney et al., 1986).

In this presented trial the combination of ultra high dose cisplatin with high dose VP-16 and standard dose bleomycin was investigated in 116 patients with bulky testicular cancer. This paper describes the data of the preliminary analysis of this cooperative trial of the AIO-Testicular Study Group.

Patients and Methods

One hundred and sixteen patients have been registered in the protocol. The distribution of the patients among the different centres is shown in Table 1, the majority of the patients coming from two centres. The patient characteristics are shown in Table 2. In this preliminary analysis ninety-eight patients are evaluable for response: two have been lost to follow-up, and a further sixteen have been withdrawn from the present study because of early toxicity (three cases), early toxic deaths (two cases), early tumour death (two cases), early progression (one case) or incompletely documented to date (eight cases). Patients have been considered

Table 1. Distribution of 116 testicular tumour patients among the various centres participating in the cooperative trial

Hannover	40
Freiburg	22
Berlin	2
Giessen	1
Bad Sooden-Allendorf	1
Köln	3
Mannheim	3
Heidelberg (Man)	3
Heidelberg (Ho)	1
Hamburg (Barmbeck)	2
Hamburg (Eppendorf)	1
Frankfurt/Main	4
Frankfurt (Höchst)	1
Bremen	3
Karlsruhe	1
Hildesheim	3
Oldenburg	5
München	5

All results expressed as per cent.

eligible for this protocol when they fulfilled the criteria for 'bulky disease', had a Karnofsky status of more than 50%, and had no prior therapy. The definition of bulky disease was: abdominal mass more than 10 cm in diameter; lung metastases more than five in number, with a diameter of more than 2 cm each, or more than twenty metastases with a diameter less than 2 cm; mediastinal mass of more than 5 cm in diameter; or visceral, bone or CNS metastases. The treatment plan was cisplatin 35 mg/m^2 i.v. days 1–5 (2 h infusion), VP-16 120 mg/m^2 i.v. days 1–5 (dose divided into two daily doses), and bleomycin 15 mg/m^2 i.v. days 1, 8, 15. Cycles were repeated on day 22 or when leucocytes reached more than 3000/µl or platelets more than 100,000/µl. A minimum of two cycles was required for evaluation of response. In cases showing response after two cycles, a total of four cycles were administered. If after four cycles residual tumour could be detected and previously elevated markers had been normalized, aggressive surgery was performed as often as possible. If active tumour with the exception of differentiated teratoma could be demonstrated in the resected specimen, two cycles were added for consolidation using 50% of cisplatin dosage, 100% VP-16 dosage and no bleomycin. Patients with only necrosis or fibrosis in the resected specimen have been documented as pathological complete responders. The definition of response was made according to the WHO criteria. Supportive care included a rigid hydration scheme using 2500 ml/m^2 per day of normal saline/glucose 5%/Ringer-lactate, diuretics (frusemide 20–60 mg/day i.v.), and intravenous prophylactic antiemetics (metoclopramide plus dexamethasone). The treatment was given on an inpatient basis with a median of 7 days of hospitalization per cycle.

Table 2. Patient characteristics

Age: mean (range)	28 (17–64) years	
Tumour location:	Lung and mediastinum only	8
	Abdomen only	22
	Mixed	70
Histology		
MTU		35
MTI		17
MTD		6
MTT		17
Seminoma		18
Mixed seminoma + nonseminoma		9
Gonadal tumours		85
Extragonadal tumours		15

All results expressed as per cent.

Results

Of the ninety-eight patients at present evaluable, 41% had a complete remission (CR). In addition 22% could be rendered disease free by surgery with a total of 63% free of disease after completion of induction chemotherapy and surgery. Thirty per cent had a partial remission (PR) and 7% had no change or progression of disease. The median duration of PR is 19+ months (range 4–36+ months). The relapse rate of the CR/NED (complete remission/no evidence of disease) group is only 7% and the median time of remission duration has not yet been reached. The relapse-free survival is identical for CR or NED patients indicating the high quality of the remission. In 70% of patients with residual tumour only differentiated teratoma was found.

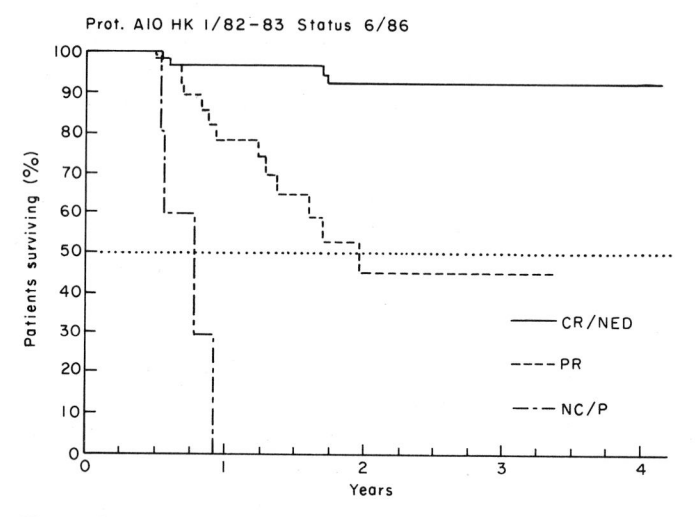

Fig. 1. Overall survival of patients according to response (evaluable patients). CR/NED = Complete response/no evidence of disease. PR = Partial response. NC/P = No change/progressive disease.

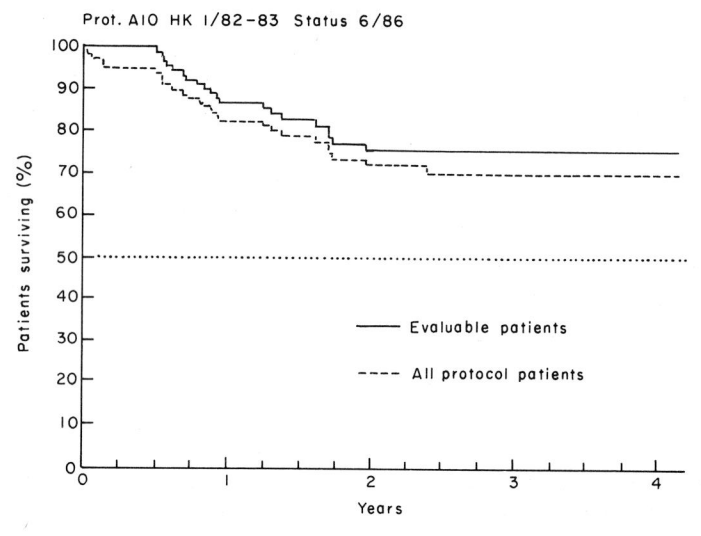

Fig. 2. Overall survival of the total patient population (evaluable patients and all protocol patients).

After a median follow up of 2.2 years (range 4–47 months) 93% of the CR/NED-patients are continuously free of disease and of the entire patient population group 65% are living free of disease. Of the partial responders with a median survival of 24 months (4–38+ months) 46% are living after 2 years. Since patients with no change or progressive disease have a median survival of only 10 months (Fig. 1), the plateau phase of the survival curve of partial responders might indicate a substantial number of long term survivors, for example patients with unresected or unresectable residual differentiated teratoma. The overall survival (Fig. 2) of the patients evaluable for response is 76% and for the entire protocol population 70% (including early toxic or unrelated death). Patients with only abdominal disease responded best with a disease free rate of 83% versus 57% for patients with only lung +/− mediastinal disease and 56% with both lung and abdominal disease.

Toxicity

Toxicity was predominantly related to the bone marrow with a leucocyte nadir of 1300 (range 100–4000)/µl and a platelet nadir of 57,000/µl with a range down to 9000/µl requiring platelet transfusions (Table 3). Fever and/or infections occurred in 35% of all patients and septicaemia in 15%, in two cases lethal: one patient died with pneumonia. The renal toxicity was rather low with grade 1–2 in 10% of all patients and only two lethal renal failures (one patient had an acute renal failure together with septicaemia after the first salvage cycle despite reduction of the cisplatin dosage: one patient with pre-existing renal damage died with acute and chronic renal failure after four cycles). The neurotoxicity was a major problem for 8% of the patients with WHO grade 3: 39% had neurotoxicity grade 1–2. Another major problem was lung toxicity, measured by lung function test and CO diffusion capacity: 32% had grade I–III toxicity and in 2% lethal bleomycin pneumonitis occurred: one patient died of chronic pulmonary failure after achieving complete remission with four cycles; one patient died after acute pneumonitis which might have been induced by an oxygen overload during surgery for pathological documentation of complete response. Five per cent had cardiac toxicity including one patient who died in acute cardio-respiratory failure of undefined origin. Furthermore one patient died of myocardial infarction after three cycles: the autopsy showed severe coronary atherosclerosis and this patient was not documented as having cardiac toxicity.

Table 3. Bone marrow toxicity

	Median	Range
Leucocyte nadir	1,300	100–4,000 per µl
Platelets nadir	57,000	9,000–290,000 per µl

Alopecia and nausea were common: 65% experienced vomiting grade 1–2, 33% grade 3, and 2% grade 4. Raynaud's phenomenon was rarely documented. Ototoxicity was reported in 12% but was never a relevant side effect for the patients.

Besides the eight patients with toxic deaths, two additional deaths occurred for reasons not related to therapy: one patient had an ileus after secondary surgery and one patient died with the above-mentioned myocardial infarction.

Discussion

Patients with disseminated testicular cancer and minimal or moderate extent of disease have an excellent chance of survival, this being 95% if treated with standard chemotherapy such as PVB, PEB or comparable protocols. The 5-year survival rate for patients with bulky disease is 30–60% depending on the definition of 'bulky disease', the chemotherapy used and the number of patients evaluated (Einhorn & Williams, 1980; Logothetis et al., 1985; Bosl et al., 1983). In the published trials the complete response rates achieved and the relapse rates vary considerably. The CR/NED rate in this present trial of 63% with 5% relapse and 65% patients presently without evidence of disease is better than the result achieved in a former AIO-group trial with PVB or PVB + ifosfamide (Schmoll et al., 1984): the survival of the patients with advanced disease in the former trial was 58% after 6 years. However, in this former trial the criteria for bulky disease were less strict than in the present protocol which makes a direct comparison difficult. Furthermore nearly half of the patients with partial response are still without progression and alive after a median follow-up of 2.2 years indicating that a considerable number of these patients will be long-term survivors. These partial responders with stable residual disease as well as the low relapse rate of the CR/NED patients contribute to the 76% overall survival rate. On the other hand, the 7% toxic deaths diminish the apparent advantage of this aggressive protocol. If all patients who entered the protocol are plotted together without exclusion of early treatment related or toxic death the survival of the total patient population is 70% (Fig. 2). This fatal toxicity has to be weighed against the apparent benefit of this aggressive protocol.

The neurotoxicity poses a major problem to many of the patients receiving four or more cycles of ultra high dose cisplatin. In contrast, the renal toxicity was mild except for two patients with renal failure. This study shows that ultra high dose cisplatin can be administered safely when diuretics, hydration and hypertonic saline are used obligatorily. Two of the deaths due to toxicity occurred in the forty-four patients of one treatment centre (4.5%). The other six deaths occurred mainly in the treatment centres with only few patients (8%): this could be a hint that possibly management problems and inexperience with aggressive tumour therapy might have contributed to the fatal toxicity rate of 7% in this high risk patient population.

The results of this study justify a prospective randomized trial comparing this protocol against standard dose platinum in combination with VP-16 and bleomycin. This type of study is ongoing in the South-Eastern Cancer Study Group. The results of the SECSG study and further experience with other regimens (CisCA-VB; POMP-ACE; PVcrB) (Logothetis et al., 1985; Newlands, 1985; Wettlaufer et al., 1984) should be expected before this ultra high dose platinum regimen could be recommended as a standard treatment for patients with bulky testicular cancer. A detailed analysis of this present trial still has to be expected, particularly regarding the response in relation to extent and location of disease.

Acknowledgements

We wish to thank Mrs C. Schwabe and Mr H. Harstrick very much for preparing the manuscript, and Mr Hemelt and Mrs. Lentmann for technical assistance.

References

Blayney, D. W., Goldberg, D. A., Leong, L. A., et al. (1986) High risk germ cell tumors (GCT): Severe toxicity with high dose (HD) platinum (P), Vinblastine (Ve), Bleomycin (B) and VP-16 (V): PVeBV. *Proceedings of the American Society of Clinical Oncology*, **5**, 361.

Bosl, G. J., Geller, N. L., et al. (1983) Multivariate analysis of prognostic variables in patients with metastatic testicular cancer. *Cancer Research*, **43**, 3403–3407.

Einhorn, L. H. & Williams, S. D. (1980) Chemotherapy of disseminated testicular cancer. A random prospective study. *Cancer*, **46**, 1339–1344.

Litterst, C. L. (1981) Alterations in the toxicity of cisdichlorodiammineplatinum and in tissue localization of platinum as a function of NaCl concentration in the vehicle of administration. *Toxicology and Applied Pharmacology*, **61**, 99.

Logothetis, C. J., et al. (1985) Improved survival cyclic chemotherapy for nonseminomatous germ cell tumors of the testis. *Journal of Clinical Oncology*, **3**, 326–335.

Newlands, E. S. (1985) VP-16 in combinations for first-line treatment of malignant germ-cell tumors and gestational choriocarcinoma. *Seminars in Oncology*, **12**, 37–41.

Ozols, F. R., Javadpour, N., Messerschmidt, G. L. & Young, R. C. (1982) Poor prognosis nonseminomatous testicular cancer: an effective high dose cisplatinum regimen without increased renal toxicity. *Proceedings of the American Society of Clinical Oncology*, **1**, 113.

Peckham, M. J., Barrett, A., et al. (1983) The treatment of metastatic germ-cell testicular tumors with bleomycin, etoposide and cis-platin (BEP). *British Journal of Cancer*, **47**, 613–619.

Samson, M. K., Rivken, S. E., Jones, S. E. et al. (1984) Dose response and survival advantage for high versus low-dose cisplatin combined with vinblastine and bleomycin in disseminated testicular cancer. *Cancer*, **53**, 1029–1035.

Schmoll, H. J., Diehl, V., Hartlapp, J., Illiger, J., et al. (1984) Results of a prospective randomized trial: Platinum, vinblastine, bleomycin +/– ifosfamide in advanced testicular cancer. *Controlled Clinical Trials in Urologic Oncology* (ed. by Denis, Murphy, Prout & Schröder), pp. 29–38. Raven Press, New York.

Stoter, G., Kaye, S., Sleyfer, D. et al. (1986) Preliminary results of BEP (Bleomycin, Etoposide, Cisplatin) versus an alternating regimen of BEP and PVB (Cisplatin, Vinblastine, Bleomycin) in high volume metastatic (HVM) testicular non-seminomas. An EORTC-study. *Proceedings of the American Society of Clinical Oncology*, **5**, 413.

Vugrin, D., Herr, H. W., Whitmore, W. F. Jr, et al. (1981) VAB-6 combination chemotherapy in disseminated cancer of the testis. *Annals of Internal Medicine*, **95**, 59–61.

Wettlaufer, J. N., Feiner, A. S. & Robinson, W. A. (1984) Vincristine, cisplatin, and bleomycin with surgery in the management of advanced metastatic nonseminomatous testicular tumors. *Cancer*, **53**, 203–209.

Discussion

Ozols What percentage of your patients had normal levels of serum markers at the completion of therapy?

Schmoll I do not have exact figures but approximately 50% of patients had partial remission with negative markers indicating that they are potentially cured. Some patients with PR were not operated on because they had too many sites of metastases.

Management of advanced metastatic germ cell tumours

GEDSKE DAUGAARD, H. H. HANSEN *and*
M. RØRTH *Department of Oncology ONB, The Finsen Institute, Copenhagen, Denmark*

Summary
Forty patients with poor prognosis germ cell tumours were treated with a combination of cisplatin 40 mg/m^2 and VP-16 200 mg/m^2, both given days 1–5 every 3 weeks, and bleomycin 15 mg/m^2 every week. Of thirty-three previously untreated patients twenty-eight (85%) patients obtained complete remission (CR) and four (12%) patients partial remission (PR). One patient was not evaluable for response. Twenty-four patients are alive 2–32 months after completion of therapy without evidence of disease (median observation 18.5 months). Of seven patients previously treated with cisplatin, five obtained CR (71%), one PR (14%) and one patient had progressive disease. Five patients are still alive, four without evidence of disease after a median follow-up of 22 months (range 16–25 months).

Key words. Germ cell tumours, cisplatin, VP-16, bleomycin.

Introduction
Approximately 70% of patients with testicular cancer treated with cisplatin-based combination chemotherapy regimens will achieve a complete remission (CR). The problem today is to provide studies which in low risk patients will focus on reducing toxicity without loss of efficacy and in high risk patients will lead to the development of more effective drug regimens.

Several approaches directed at improving treatment results in high-risk patients are being explored. We have chosen a schedule in which we use the same drugs as in low risk patients but in higher doses. The rationale behind this is the steep dose response curve for both cisplatin and VP-16 in patients with germ cell tumours.

Material and Methods
Forty patients with poor prognosis germ cell tumours were treated with a combination of cisplatin 40 mg/m^2 and VP-16 200 mg/m^2, both given days 1–5 every 3 weeks, and bleomycin 15 mg/m^2 every week (PEB). At least three courses of this combination were given to all patients. Thirty-nine of the patients had histologically documented germ cell tumours. Histology of the primary tumours were: seminoma, thirteen (one pure seminoma, six seminomas with elevated tumour markers); embryonal carcinoma, twenty-five; choriocarcinoma, four; endodermal sinus tumour, seven; teratocarcinoma, four; unclassified germ cell tumours, four;

Correspondence: Dr Gedske Daugaard, Department of Oncology ONB, The Finsen Institute, Strandboulevarden 49, DK-2100 Copenhagen, Denmark.

tumours with more than one element, thirteen). Thirty-three patients were previously untreated including two patients who were previously treated with radiotherapy and bleomycin in 1974 and 1975, and seven patients had relapsed after prior radio- and/or chemotherapy. Two of these seven patients had previously received radiotherapy, lumboiliac field in two patients, and brain irradiation in one patient.

Seven patients had previously been treated with cisplatin (median 1200 mg accumulated dose, range 900–2060 mg) and three of these patients had also received VP-16 (median accumulated dose 2000 mg, range 1800–5300 mg). All patients without previous cisplatin treatment had at least one of the following prognostic characteristics: (1) advanced abdominal disease ($\geq$ 10 cm in diameter), (2) liver metastases, (3) supradiaphragmatic lymph node metastases ($\geq$ 5 cm in diameter), (4) multiple lung metastases with at least one $\geq$ 5 cm in diameter, (5) serum hCG $\geq$ 100,000 U/l, and (6) extragonadal primary with elevated serum tumour markers (AFP and/or hCG).

Tumour response to therapy was monitored by physical examination, serial serum tumour markers and appropriate radiological studies. After three cycles of chemotherapy a complete re-evaluation was done, including tumour markers and repetition of all previously abnormal roentgenograms. Patients who had residual masses following three series of PEB and negative tumour markers underwent surgical exploration and resection, if possible, of all abnormal tissue. If the resected tissue had any malignant elements or if the patients had elevated markers following three cycles of PEB, the patients were treated with one or more additional series of chemotherapy. Patients who were in complete remission after three cycles of PEB or who had no evidence of residual cancer in the resected specimen received no further treatment.

Results

Previously untreated patients
Characteristics of the thirty-three patients previously untreated with cisplatin are shown in Table 1.

All patients responded to the PEB treatment. Twenty-eight patients obtained CR (85%), where the term CR includes patients who were disease free after secondary surgery, and four patients PR (12%). The term PR has been used for patients who achieved partial regression (> 50%) of measurable disease. Three of these patients died with disease, but mainly from toxicity of treatment, one patient had progressive disease after some months and is now undergoing treatment with other drugs. One patient was not evaluable for assessment of response. He died of respiratory failure within 10 days after start of chemotherapy, but had a marked decrease in serum hCG. Four patients in CR died with thrombo- and leucocytopenia, one of these patients having refused hospitalization. Twenty-four patients are alive 2–32 months after completion of therapy without evidence of disease (median observation 18.5 months). At the completion of three cycles of PEB, fourteen of these twenty-four patients had normal markers, and twelve patients had persistent roentgenographic abnormalities at the site of bulky disease. At surgery eight patients were found to have fibrosis, two a mature teratoma and in two small

Table 1. Tumour load and tumour markers in thirty-three previously untreated germ cell tumour patients

	No. of patients	%	Additional clinical features	No. of patients
Testicular cancer	22	67		
Extragonadal tumour	11	33	With elevated tumour markers	8 (73%)
Liver metastases	5	15		
Abdominal metastases	26	79	≥ 10 cm in diameter	21 (64%)
Supradiaphragmatic glands	11	33	≥ 5 cm in diameter	4 (12%)
Multiple lung metastases	14	42	≥ 5 cm in diameter	4 (12%)
Mediastinal tumour	11	33	≥ 5 cm in diameter	7 (21%)
Elevated serum hCG	21	64	More than 100,000 U/l	5 (15%)
Elevated serum AFP	21	64		
Elevated LDH	27*	90		
Others	4	12		
Brain metastases 2				
Bone metastases 2				

*Not measured in three patients.

elements of malignant tissue were found. The last-mentioned patients received two additional cycles of VP-16 and platinum (at decreased doses) and are now without evidence of disease. Five patients were tumour marker negative after four cycles of PEB. One of these patients had residual disease at CT-scan, but no evidence of disease at surgery, three patients were found to have fibrosis, and the last patient a mature teratoma. Five patients received five cycles of PEB: in three cases a mature teratoma was found at surgery, and in two cases fibrosis.

A total of 111 cycles of PEB have been administered to previously untreated patients. The major toxicity of PEB was myelosuppression. In 77% of the cycles the white blood cell count was below 1.0×10^9/l (for median 7 days, range 1–15 days) and in 76% of the cycles thrombocytes were below 25×10^9/l (for median 7 days, range 1–18 days). In five patients bacteraemia was documented during treatment.

Glomerular filtration rate decreased from 103 ± 4 ml/min to 70 ± 4 ml/min (mean ± standard error of mean) after three cycles. 79% of the patients developed a high frequency hearing loss of more than 30 dB in the 2–8000 Hz area. Two patients had a functional hearing impairment that has required the use of a hearing aid. Thirteen patients developed paraesthesia in distal extremities. All patients had gastrointestinal toxicity with nausea, vomiting and mucositis. Two patients did not receive the last two doses of bleomycin because of decreasing CO diffusion capacity.

Previously treated patients
This group consisted of five patients with testicular cancer, one patient with an extragonadal primary tumour and one patient with an embryonal carcinoma of the ovary. These patients were primarily diagnosed between 1979 and 1983. Six patients had elevated serum tumour markers (hCG in six, AFP in five and both in four patients). One of the patients relapsed 4 years after treatment with the 'Einhorn regimen'.

Six of seven patients responded to the PEB treatment. Five patients obtained CR (71%) and one patient PR (14%). One patient became marker negative but died after one and a half cycles with progression of previously irradiated brain metastases and with decreasing lung and kidney function.

Five patients are still alive, four without evidence of disease after a median follow-up of 22 months (range 16–25 months) after completion of therapy. One patient with CR had a relapse after 12 months with increase in serum hCG and evidence of disease in the liver.

Toxicity was comparable to that seen in previously untreated patients but only 52% of the cycles were given without dose modifications.

Discussion

The platinum–vinblastine–bleomycin (pVB) combination chemotherapy and similar platinum based combination regimens have greatly improved the outlook for patients with disseminated germ cell tumours. However, there is a clinically definable subset of patients in whom current combination chemotherapy regimens have been markedly less effective, and likewise treatment of patients failing front-line chemotherapy has been rather unsuccessful, even though long disease-free survival has been reported in some cases.

In a report from the British Medical Research Council Working Party on Testicular Tumours (1985) a poor prognosis group with a 3-year survival rate of 47% was defined. The prognostic factors concerning liver metastases and supra-diaphragmatic lymph node involvement were similar to the ones applied in the present study. We have used, however, the higher limit for the size of retroperitoneal tumour masses ($\geq$ 10 cm diameter versus $\geq$ 5 cm diameter), for lung metastases (multiple, one or more $\geq$ 5 cm diameter versus multiple, one or more $\geq$ 2 cm diameter) and for the serum hCG level (100,000 U/l versus 1000 U/l). This implies that the patients in our series belong to a group with an even worse prognosis than those in the poor prognosis group of the British study. On this background we have compared the treatment results of PEB with the pVB 'Einhorn regimen'. All patients treated at the Finsen Institute with pVB in the period 1979–83 were reviewed. Patients with one or more of the poor prognostic characteristics listed above were included in the study. Only 15% of these patients were without evidence of disease 18.5 months after treatment, compared with 73% after PEB treatment (median observation time 18.5 months). The treatment results with PEB are apparently superior to the pVB treatment in this group of patients with advanced metastatic germ cell tumours. A strict comparison obviously requires a randomized trial, however.

Pizzocaro et al. (1985) have shown that the same results can be obtained with half the doses of cisplatin and VP-16 used in this study in patients with bulky disease. This is in contrast to the results reported by Williams et al. (1985) who found equivalent therapeutic responses with pVB and cisplatin 20 mg/m^2 for 5 days, VP-16 100 mg/m^2 for 5 days and 30 units of bleomycin every week, but only 34% of the patients with advanced disease obtained a favourable response (CR in our terminology).

In our study 85% of the previously untreated patients obtained CR and 12%

PR. 73% are still alive and without evidence of disease. Of the previously treated patients 71% obtained CR and 14% PR, and 57% are still alive without evidence of disease. In spite of the toxicity, the results obtained in this group of often young patients with very poor prognosis are sufficiently encouraging to indicate further exploration of this aggressive treatment in larger series. Only when the results of such series and longer follow-up of the present series are available, can final conclusions be made.

References

The Medical Research Council Working Party on Testicular Tumours (1985) Prognostic factors in advanced non-seminomatous germ-cell testicular tumours: Results of a multicentre study. *Lancet*, i, 8–11.

Pizzocaro, G., Zanoni, F., Salvioni, R., Piva, L. & Milani, A. (1985) High complete remission (CR) rate with cisplatin, etoposide, bleomycin (PEB) and surgery in poor prognosis germ cell tumours (GCT) of the testis. *Proceedings of the American Society for Clinical Oncology*, 4, 110.

Williams, S., Einhorn, L., Greco, A., Birch, R. & Irwin, L. (1985) A comparison of cisplatin plus bleomycin plus either vinblastine (PVB) or VP-16 (BEP). *Proceedings of the American Society for Clinical Oncology*, 4, 100.

Discussion

Pizzocaro I would like to ask the previous three speakers using high dose cisplatin to compare the results of their series with the results obtained with 'normal' doses of VP-16 and cisplatin. We treated high risk patients with conventional doses of VP-16 and cisplatin and had essentially as good results as you have reported here (Pizzocaro *et al.*, 1985, *Cancer*, **56**, 2411–2415).

Daugaard I do not think we are treating similar patients. Residual tumour is present in 20% of your patients and 91% of our patients after three cycles of high dose cisplatin.

Pizzocaro We consider poor risk patients those with nodal metastases >10 cm, lung metastases >5 cm or with more than 50% of the pulmonary fields involved, extrapulmonary spread, serum AFP >1,000 ng/ml, or serum hCG >50,000 mIU/ml (Pizzocaro *et al.*, 1985, *Cancer*, **56**, 2411–2415). These criteria are very similar to Schmoll's and Daugaard's criteria. I also tried to reclassify my series according to the Indiana criteria: 20 patients fell into Indiana advanced disease, and 17 entered continuous complete remission; 20 patients fell into the moderately advanced disease group and 16 entered continuous complete remission. I could not reclassify my series according to Bosl's criteria, because the methods of determining the serum levels of LDH and hCG were not identical. However, I was not able to identify a bad risk subgroup of patients among those treated with platinum, etoposide and bleomycin, while I was able to identify bad risk subgroups in patients treated with PVB (Pizzocaro *et al.*, 1985, *Cancer*, **56**, 249–255; Pizzocaro *et al.*, 1986, *Cancer*, **57**, 2114–2118). Both extent of the disease and tumour marker titres were the most important prognostic factors in patients treated with PVB.

Ozols Could you give more detailed information concerning the six toxic deaths?

Daugaard Out of six patients who died of toxicity, three were aged >45 years, one of these had liver cirrhosis found at autopsy, and one died with cardio-pulmonary insufficiency. We therefore recommend that patients >45 years should not be treated with this intensive regimen. One of the other patients refused hospitalization and died at home, probably from sepsis.

Einhorn You saw significant myelosuppression. Was there equivalent myelosuppression in previously treated and untreated patients?

Daugaard Only approximately 50% of previously treated patients received the full dose of chemotherapy subsequently, whereas approximately 80% of the previously untreated patients received the full dose. Myelosuppression was greater in both groups when the full dose was given rather than the reduced dose, and in the entire series, the patients receiving full dose therapy had greater myelosuppression if they had been previously treated.

Safirstein First, congratulations for using ^{51}Cr-EDTA clearance instead of creatinine clearance or plasma creatinine to assess GFR. What was the course of plasma creatinine in your patients especially at the terminal end of the period of study?

Daugaard During the first and second cycles of chemotherapy a significant decrease in serum creatinine is seen, perhaps due to decrease in lean body mass. Three months after treatment, the serum creatinine is significantly increased.

Schmoll Do you think that this high VP-16 dose of 200 mg/m^2 ×5 is necessary considering the results obtained with lower doses? The dose you use is highly myelotoxic.

Rørth In order to answer this question exactly, several randomized trials should be carried out. At present we do not know the optimal dose. Our intention has been to *maximize* the doses of VP-16 and cisplatin so that we can be sure that treatment failure would not have been overcome by higher doses.

We must realize that we are getting progressively better at treating these patients so that we are getting better survival without changing the drug regimens. It is difficult to titrate the dose of VP-16 with the number of patients we have available.

Cisplatin nephrotoxicity: insights into mechanism

R. SAFIRSTEIN, J. WINSTON, D. MOEL,* S. DIKMAN and J. GUTTENPLAN† *Division of Nephrology and Department of Medicine, Mount Sinai School of Medicine, *Division of Nephrology, Children's Memorial Hospital, Chicago, Illinois, and †Department of Biochemistry, New York University Dental Center, New York, U. S. A.*

Summary

Cis-dichlorodiammine platinum (II), or cisplatin, is currently among the most widely used agents in the chemotherapy of cancer. The chief limit to its greater efficacy is its nephrotoxicity. Acute and chronic nephrotoxicity of cisplatin occurs in man and animals especially after repeated administration. Morphological damage is restricted to the P3 segment of the proximal tubule. Abnormalities of water and solute reclamation and transglomerular passage of fluid are commonly associated with cisplatin nephrotoxicity. The vulnerability of the kidney to cisplatin may be related to its function as the primary excretory organ for platinum. Platinum binds to multiple cellular organelles and macromolecules, yet the precise mechanism of its cytotoxicity has not been delineated. Because abnormalities in renal function are preceded by a period where gross renal function appears normal, it is an ideal model to study the early physiological and biochemical determinants of metal induced acute renal failure.

Key words. Polyuric renal failure, renal uptake and metabolism, tubule respiration, DNA turnover.

Introduction

Cis-dichlorodiammine platinum (II), or cisplatin, has emerged as a principal chemotherapeutic agent in the treatment of otherwise resistant solid tumours. The chief limit to its greater efficacy, however, is its nephrotoxicity. Reducing the dose of cisplatin in an attempt to limit nephrotoxicity has proven to be only partially successful as acute renal failure occurs even after such low doses and especially after its repeated administration (Meijer et al., 1982; Goldstein & Safirstein, 1981). Use of other means to protect the kidney (Yuhas & Culo, 1980; Borch & Pleasants, 1979; Berry et al., 1984) are only partially successful and of uncertain clinical application. It may not be possible to alter or prevent the renal toxicity of cisplatin, however, until a more basic understanding of that toxicity is obtained. This paper summarizes what is known about the biochemical and physiological aspects of cisplatin nephrotoxicity and gives the results of some recent experiments into its possible mechanism.

Correspondence: Dr Robert Safirstein, Department of Medicine, Renal Division, The Mount Sinai Hospital, 1 Gustave L. Levy Place, New York, N.Y. 10029, U. S. A.

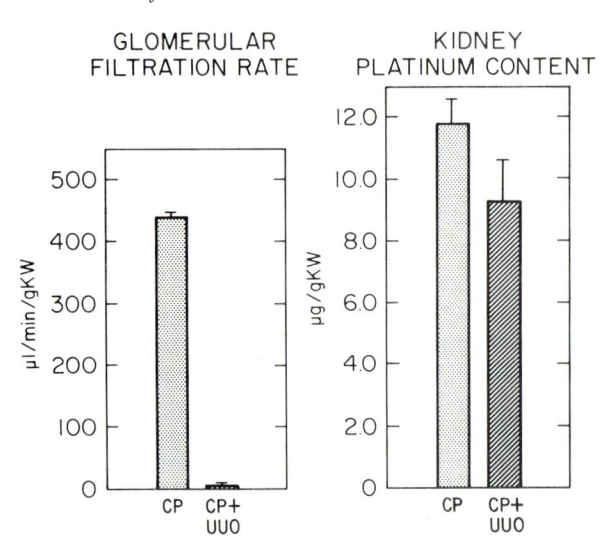

Fig. 1. Platinum content in unilaterally obstructed (UUO) and in normal kidneys 72 h after a 5 mg/kg dose of cisplatin (CP).

determinant of cisplatin nephrotoxicity than has been suggested in the past (see below).

Further evidence linking the kidney's vulnerability to its role in cisplatin transport is provided by autoradiographic studies (Fig. 2). A dark field autoradiograph of a frozen section of kidney from a rat 24 h after an intravenous injection of [^{195m}Pt]cisplatin shows greatest grain density (white grains) at the juxtamedullary and outer stripe region of the kidney with extension into medullary rays. The same pattern was seen at shorter time periods but many more grains could be seen in the outer cortex. A thin (5 μm) section autoradiograph of the outer stripe of the outer medulla at 1 h shows greatest grain density in tubule segments possessing brush borders (Fig. 3). Adjacent thin limbs in this region contain very little platinum. This distribution of grains is consistent with specific localization in the P3 segments of the proximal nephron. Glomeruli and other distal nephron segments contained many fewer grains. As the P3 segment of the proximal tubule is the principal site of cell toxicity of cisplatin and contains the most platinum, these studies provide further evidence that the particular vulnerability of this cell type depends on its ability to accumulate cisplatin.

Cisplatin is excreted largely unchanged in the urine (Fig. 4). Upon entry into the renal cell, however, cisplatin undergoes biotransformation. In addition to binding to cell macromolecules, a large portion (30–50%) of the total cell platinum is in a form whose molecular weight is below 500 Daltons and whose chromatographic behaviour is different from cisplatin (Fig. 4). Another characteristic of this platinum metabolite is the loss of its biological activity as a mutagen. Whereas excreted platinum is mutagenic (Fig. 5), cell platinum is not (Table 3). As the mutagenic activity of platinum coordination complexes is correlated with their cellular toxicity (Lecointe, Macquet & Butour, 1979), the loss of mutagenicity by renal cell platinum suggests that it is less toxic in this form. Confirmation of this will require isolation and identification of this compound. Furthermore, and more

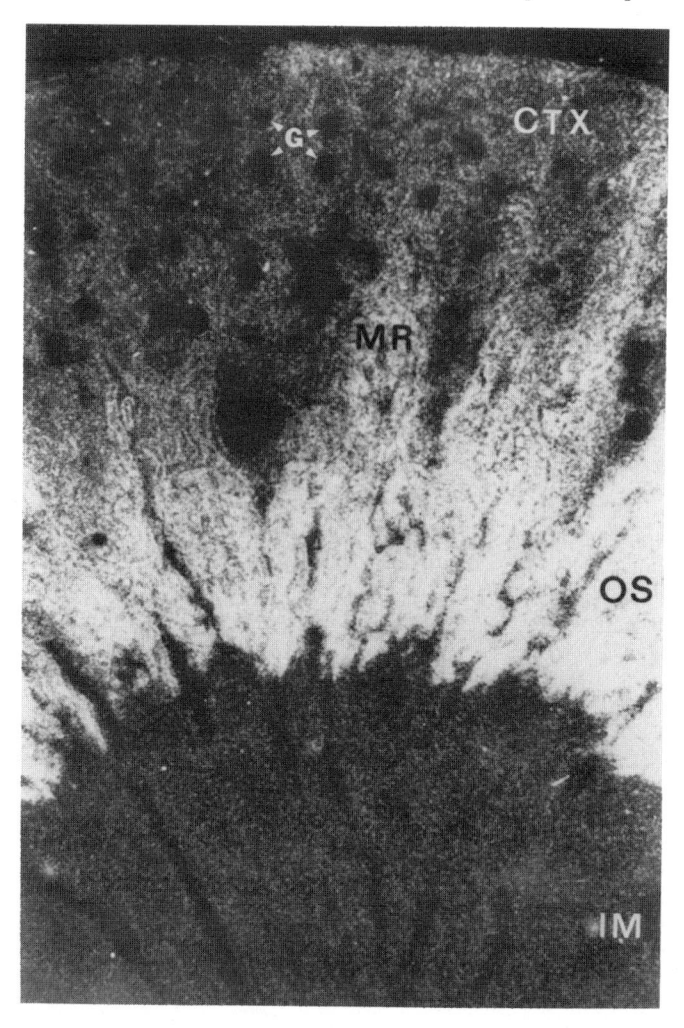

Fig. 2. Dark field illumination autoradiograph of a kidney section prepared from a rat sacrificed 10 min after administration of radiolabelled cisplatin. The kidney was perfusion fixed *in vivo* (2% paraformaldehyde in 0.1 M phosphate, pH 7.4) after the kidneys were flushed with 0.9% NaCl to reduce background activity of cisplatin in vascular and urinary spaces. Autoradiographs were prepared by placing the sections onto glass slices which were previously dipped into a 1:1 solution of Kodak NTB 2 Nuclear Trace Emulsion and 15% glycerol in distilled water. The emulsion was exposed at 5°C for 7–14 days, developed in Kodak D170 (diluted 1:1 with distilled water) and fixed in Kodak Amfix. The greatest accumulation of grains is in the outer stripe region of the outer medulla extending within the medullary rays to the superficial portions of the cortex. CTX = cortex, OS = outer stripe, IM = inner medulla, MR = medullary ray.

speculative, if this inactive compound is formed by an enzyme mediated processs, then the levels of this enzyme might be enhanced by pretreatment with appropriate agents. This approach to reducing cisplatin nephrotoxicity has been reported to be effective in reducing $HgCl_2$ nephrotoxicity (Arias *et al.*, 1976).

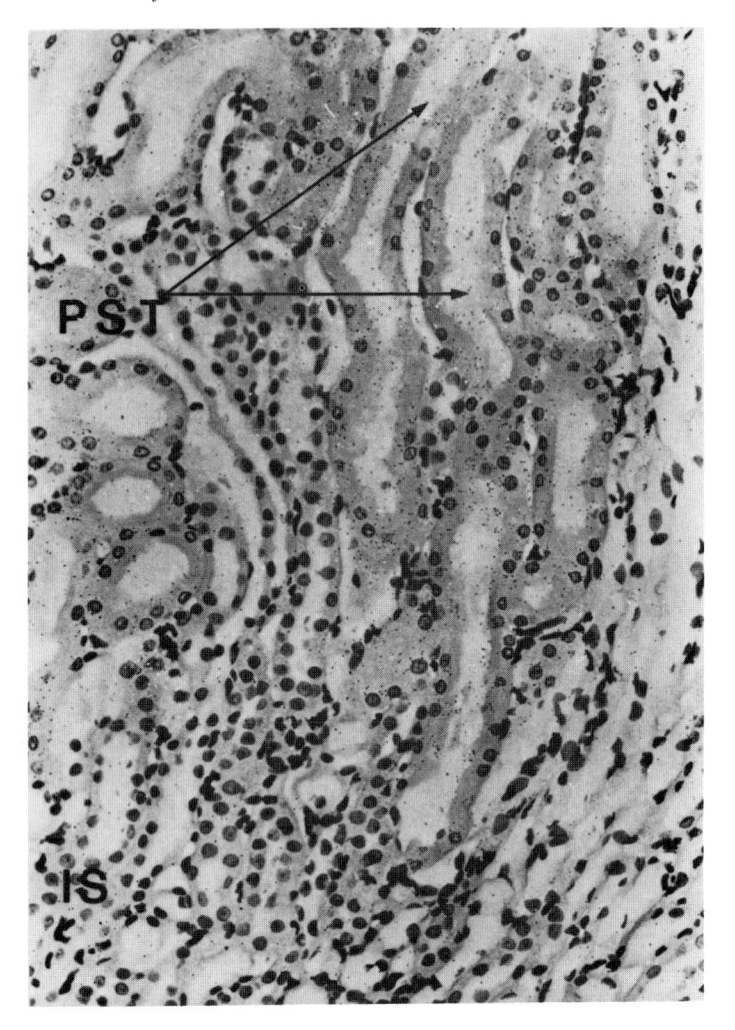

Fig. 3. A high-power photograph of the kidney stained with PAS demonstrating numerous reduced silver grains over the P3 segments but not the thin limbs in the inner medulla. P3: proximal straight tubule (P3 segment), TL: thin limbs.

Table 3. Effects of kidney cytosolic ultrafiltrates from untreated and cisplatin-treated rats on revertant numbers in *Salmonella typhimurium* TA100

Kidney fraction[1]	Treatment[2]	Addition[3]	Revertants[4]
UF	None	None	262
UF	Cisplatin	None	307
UF	None	Cisplatin	1034
None	None	Cisplatin	643

[1]UF, abbreviation for ultrafiltrate of kidney cytosol; [2]refers to treatment of the animals with cisplatin 5 mg/kg BW 24 h prior to isolation of kidneys; [3]refers to addition of an equivalent amount of cisplatin to that seen in the treated animals to the ultrafiltrate of normal animals; [4]refers to number of colonies after spontaneous revertant number have been subtracted. Refer to Safirstein *et al.* (1984) for details.

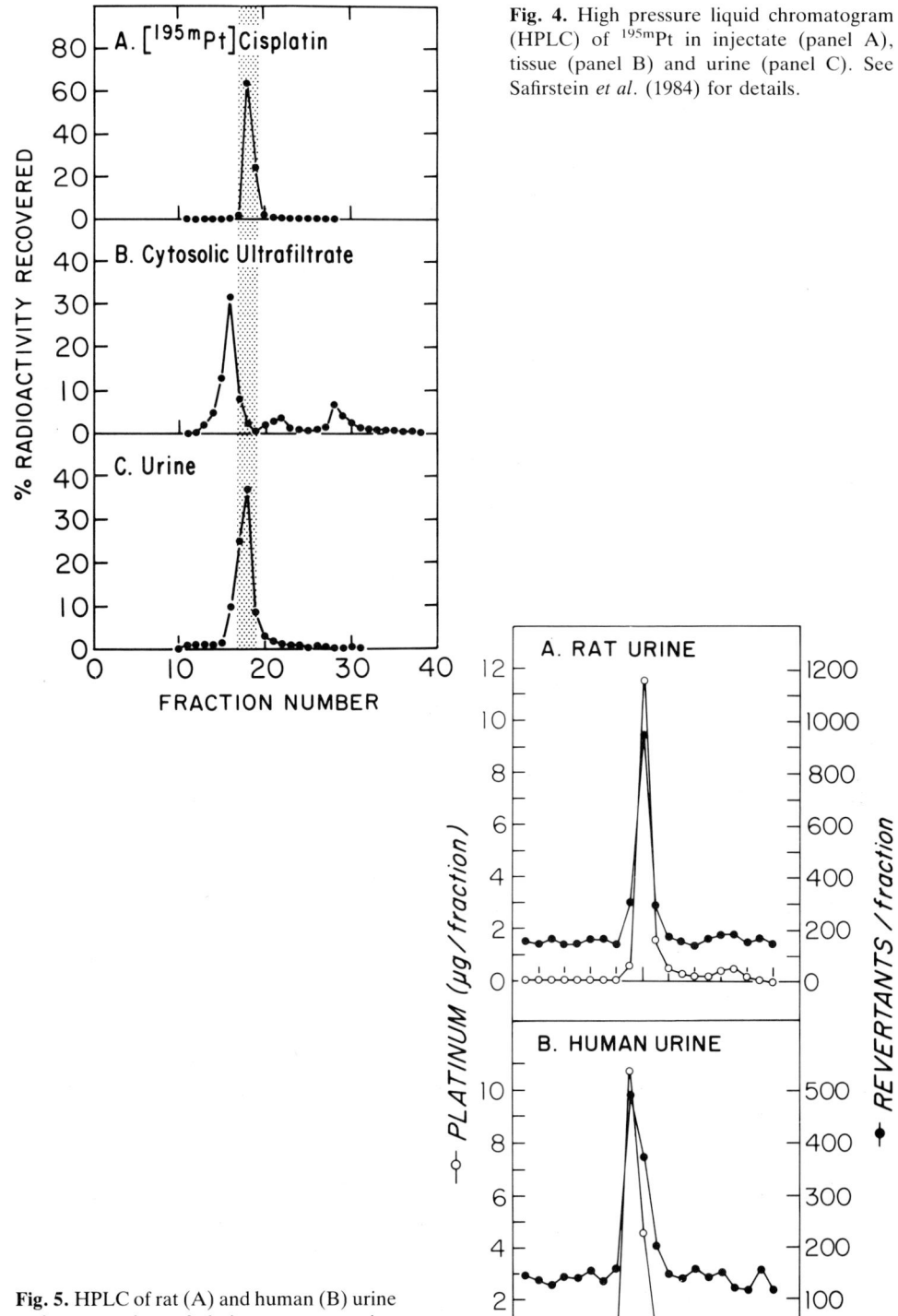

Cisplatin nephrotoxicity mechanisms 331

Fig. 4. High pressure liquid chromatogram (HPLC) of ^{195m}Pt in injectate (panel A), tissue (panel B) and urine (panel C). See Safirstein *et al.* (1984) for details.

Fig. 5. HPLC of rat (A) and human (B) urine and a comparison of platinum concentration obtained by atomic absorption with mutagenic activity in each fraction. (See Safirstein *et al.* 1983) for details.

C. Physiological aspects of cisplatin-induced nephrotoxicity

1. Cisplatin-induced polyuria

Polyuria uniformly accompanies cisplatin administration and occurs in two distinct phases (Table 4). Urine osmolality initially falls over the first 24–48 h after it is given but glomerular filtration rate (GFR) in this phase is normal. This early polyuria usually improves spontaneously. A second phase of increased volume and reduced osmolality occurs between 72 and 96 h after cisplatin. This later phase is accompanied by reduced GFR and is persistent.

The early phase of polyuria responds to large doses of vasopressin (Clifton et al., 1982). Blood values of vasopressin are low during this phase and cisplatin reduces release or synthesis of vasopressin from isolated pituitary cells (Clifton et al., 1982). Prostaglandins may also be involved in the early concentrating defect as the polyuria is corrected when aspirin, an inhibitor of prostaglandin synthesis, is given (Table 5). Aspirin has no effect on the later polyuria. High rates of prostaglandin production by renal cortical and medullary microsomes are also present for the first 72 h and this too could be partially inhibited by aspirin.

The later defect in renal concentrating ability has no such dependence on vasopressin (Fig. 6) or prostaglandins. Papillary solute content is uniformly

Table 4. Cisplatin-induced polyuria

	Control	24 h	48 h	72 h	96 h
U_{osm}	2065 ± 108	868 ± 249*	1048 ± 151*	736 ± 68*	945 ± 64*
V_u	6.6 ± 0.8	17.1 ± 3.7*	14.8 ± 0.7*	15.7 ± 2.9*	14.3 ± 2.2*
P_{Cr}	0.42 ± 0.01	0.45 ± 0.03	0.60 ± 0.15	1.2 ± 0.17*	1.6 ± 0.1*

U_{osm} urine osmolality (mOsm/kg H_2O); V_u, daily urine volume (ml/24 h); P_{Cr}, plasma creatinine (mg%). $n = 6$.
*$P < 0.05$ versus control.

Table 5. Prostaglandin production (conversion of [^{14}C]arachidonate into PGE_2) by kidney medullary microsomes of rats treated with cisplatin alone (CP) and cisplatin plus aspirin (ASA), 300 mg/kg orally, 1 h before and daily after CP, 5 mg/kg, intraperitoneally.

	CP (6)		CP plus ASA (6)	
	U_{osm} (mOsm)	PGE_2 (% conv.)	U_{osm} (mOsm)	PGE_2 (% conv.)
B	2065 ± 108	13.6 ± 0.4	1904 ± 65	4.1 ± 0.5*
Day after CP				
1	868 ± 145†	32.4 ± 2.0†	1672 ± 145*	22.3 ± 0.3†*
2	1048 ± 151†	22.6 ± 0.6†	1703 ± 251*	7.3 ± 0.3†*
3	736 ± 68†	28.8 ± 0.8†	1264 ± 129†*	10.6 ± 0.3†*
4	945 ± 64†	12.1 ± 1.0	912 ± 140†	5.3 ± 0.5*

Mean values ± SEM for daily urine osmolality (U_{osm}) and PGE_2 synthesis (% arachidonate conversion) are shown. *$P < 0.05$ CP plus ASA versus CP; †$P < 0.05$ compared to baseline (B); (n) = number of animals.

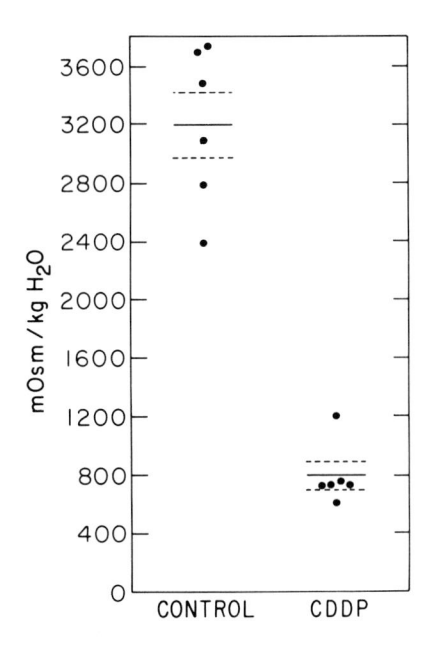

Fig. 6. Individual values for urine osmolality after 12–24 h of water deprivation and ADH administration in control and cisplatin-treated animals (CDDP).

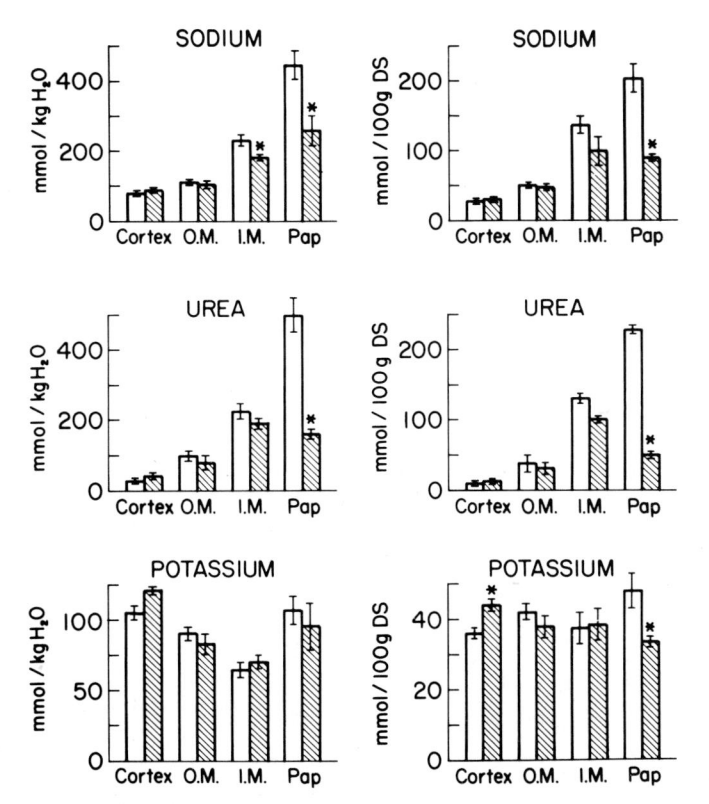

Fig. 7. Mean values ±SE for solute concentration in tissue samples from six control (open bars) and six cisplatin-treated animals (hatched bars) 5–7 days after a single dose of cisplatin, 5 mg/kg. Solute content was determined after 24 h without water and after 1000 mU arginine vasopressin. *$P < 0.05$.

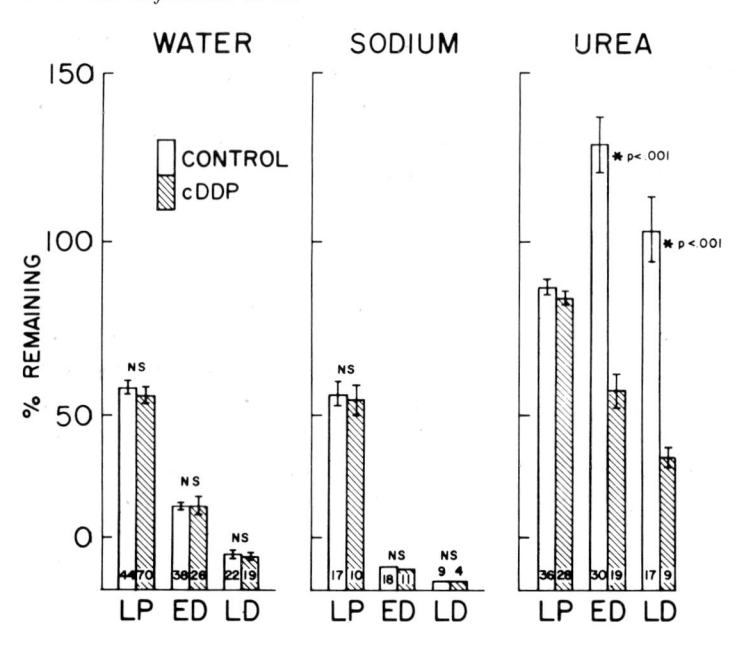

Fig. 8. Mean values ±SE for percentage of filtered water and solute remaining along late proximal (LP) and early (ED) and late distal (LD) tubule of superficial nephrons in control and cisplatin-treated animals (CDDP). Numbers of punctures at each site is shown.

reduced at this phase of the polyuria (Fig. 7) and neither elevated rates of fluid and solute flows from superficial nephrons (Fig. 8) nor an altered ability to generate a normal transepithelial solute gradient at the thick ascending limb explain the polyuria (Safirstein et al., 1982). In addition, movement of water and urea along the distal tubule is not different in control and cisplatin-treated animals, and the ability of this nephron segment to generate and maintain an increasing gradient for urea is maintained. The most prominent abnormality of solute transport during this phase of the polyuria is the lack of addition of urea to fluid in the loop of Henle. Urea is reabsorbed from, not added to, loop fluid in cisplatin-treated rats consistent with a reversal of the urea concentration gradient in the medulla. To the extent that medullary hypertonicity is dependent on urea addition in the loop such diminished recycling may account for some of the loss of medullary tonicity. Papillary blood flow is not increased during cisplatin-induced polyuria, and thus can not explain the loss of medullary hypertonicity (Safirstein et al., 1982). Taken together, these data indicate that there is diminished fluid reabsorption either in deeper nephrons not accessible to micropuncture or in collecting ducts of cisplatin-treated animals.

2. Cisplatin-induced hypomagnesaemia

Hypomagnesaemia is a particularly common complication of cisplatin administration in humans (Schilsky & Anderson, 1979; Schilsky, Barlock & Ozols, 1980) and persistent excretion of magnesium in the presence of severe hypomagnesaemia suggests that the hypomagnesaemia is due to a renal defect in magnesium reabsorption (Schilsky & Anderson, 1979). Recent studies in a rat model of this syndrome suggest that abnormal magnesium excretion may be due to a defect in magnesium transport in juxtamedullary nephrons or collecting ducts (Mavichak et al., 1986), much like the situation that exists for defective water transport described above.

3. Glomerular filtration and renal haemodynamics during cisplatin-induced renal failure

Inulin clearance initially falls 48–72 h after cisplatin administration in the rat (Fig. 9) and is unchanged from control prior to this time. The decrease in inulin clearance is persistent indicating that the recovery of renal function is partial even after a single exposure to the drug. Single nephron glomerular filtration rate (SNGFR) measured at end proximal tubule sites is also reduced and the fall in SNGFR is not due to abnormal inulin permeability across the superficial proximal convoluted tubule as early and late proximal tubule SNGFR are identical (Fig. 10).

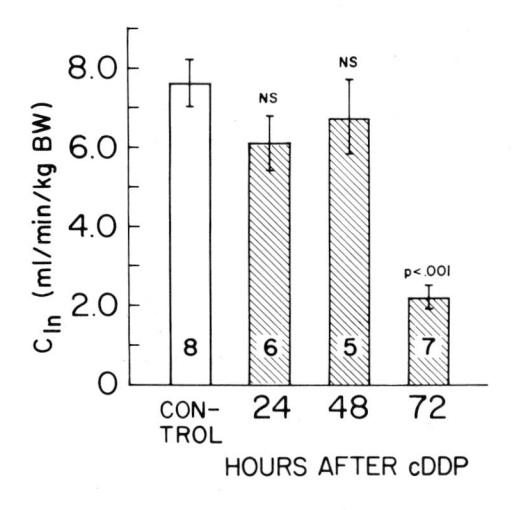

Fig. 9. Mean values ±SE for two kidney inulin clearances in control and cisplatin-treated animals. Number of animals studied are shown in bars.

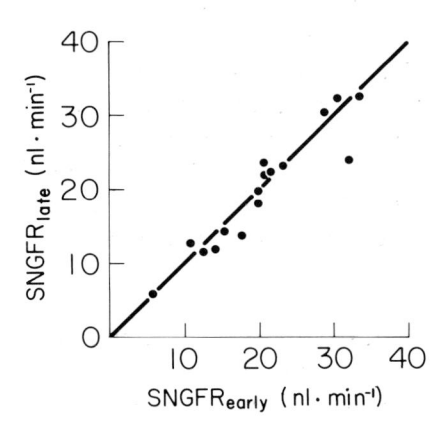

Fig. 10. Individual values for single nephron glomerular filtration rate (SNGFR) determined in early and late proximal tubule segments of the same nephron. Line of identity is indicated by solid line.

Abnormal inulin permeability beyond the proximal convoluted tubule does occur (Fig. 11) and is likely to occur at the site of the severely necrotic P3 segment of the proximal tubule. Thus the decline in inulin clearance at 3 days after cisplatin is due to both a real decline in ultrafiltration rate and abnormal inulin permeability.

The early reduction in GFR is accompanied by several changes in the determinants of GFR (Yuhas & Culo, 1980; Winston, Daye & Safirstein, 1983; Winston & Safirstein, 1985). Renal plasma flow (RPF), whole kidney GFR, single nephron (SN) GFR, and stop-flow pressure (PSF) are reduced compared to controls (Figs. 12 and 13). As arterial pressure is similar in control and cisplatin-treated animals,

Fig. 11. Urinary recovery of early proximal tubule microinjected radiolabelled inulin in control and cisplatin-treated nephrotoxic rats.

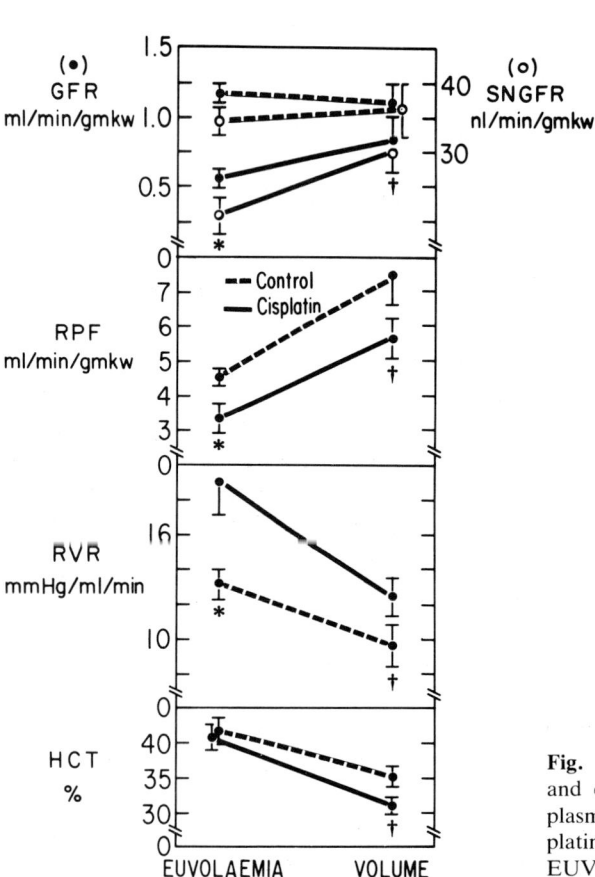

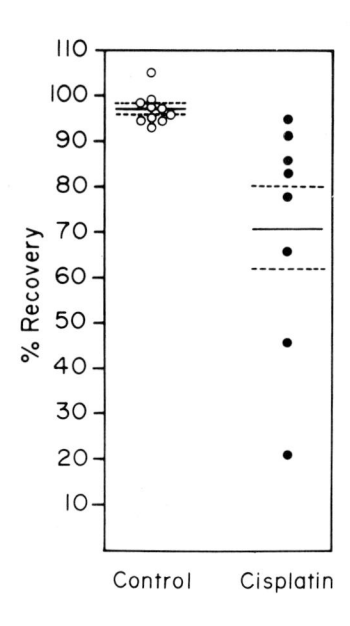

Fig. 12. Renal haemodynamics in control and cisplatin-treated rats before and after plasma volume expansion. *$P < 0.05$ cisplatin euvolaemia (EUV) versus control EUV; †$P < 0.05$ cisplatin volume expanded (VE) versus control VE.

these changes in blood flow indicate elevated renal vascular resistance. Reduced RPF is partially reversible following the rapid infusion of isoncotic plasma equivalent to 5% of the body weight. GFR and SNGFR increase but they fail to return to normal. This increase in GFR and SNGFR as RPF rises confirms the importance of reduced RPF in early cisplatin-induced acute renal failure (ARF). The failure of PSF and RPF to increase after volume expansion in cisplatin animals to levels comparable to volume expanded controls, however, suggests persistent elevation of renal resistance in cisplatin treated animals.

PT is the same as control in euvolaemic and volume expanded animals and it is unlikely that intratubular obstruction plays an important role in early cisplatin-induced ARF.

Since at least one study has demonstrated the reversibility of nephrotoxic ARF by inhibiting angiotensin II formation (Schor et al., 1981), we infused captopril, an inhibitor of angiotensin I converting enzyme, in an attempt to reverse the fall in GFR. Rats were injected with cisplatin (5 mg/kg) and 3 days later surgically prepared for clearance studies. Aged matched control animals given vehicle alone were prepared in a similar fashion. Euvolaemic rats ($n = 6$) were studied before and 60 min after a constant infusion of captopril (100–200 µg/kg/min i.v.). This dose, which effectively inhibits angiotensin II formation by the kidney (Schor et al., 1981), had no effect on inulin clearance (2.1 ml/min before and 2.0 ml/min after) or systemic blood pressure. To test whether chronic reduction in angiotensin II formation before and during the induction of renal failure might prove more effective, we gave rats housed in individual metabolic cages captopril (100 mg/kg/day) in their drinking water 3 days before and for 6 days after cisplatin. Blood urea nitrogen (BUN) was measured in these animals 4 and 6 days after cisplatin and compared to a group of cisplatin-treated rats who were not given captopril. No significant difference in BUN of captopril-treated versus control was observed at 4 (51 ± 10 versus 52 ± 7) or 6 days (53 ± 17 versus 59 ± 8) after cisplatin. Similar negative results were obtained when verapamil, a Ca^{++} channel blocker which inhibits the microvascular effects of angiotensin II in the kidney (Ichikawa, Miele & Brenner, 1979), was systematically infused (20–40 µg/kg/min i.v.) in a protocol similar to that used with captopril above. Inulin clearance in three animals before verapamil (1.5 ± 0.3 ml/min) was not different from that after verapamil (1.3 ± 0.2 ml/min). These studies suggest that the renin–angiotensin system does not play a significant role in cisplatin induced reductions in GFR.

D. Mechanism of protection of cisplatin nephrotoxicity by hypertonic solutions and frusemide

The mechanism by which mannitol, hypertonic saline and frusemide ameliorate cisplatin-induced acute renal failure is unknown. As mannitol and frusemide reduce the concentration of platinum in the urine, it has been suggested that this is the mechanism by which these agents attenuate cisplatin nephrotoxicity (Cvitkovic et al., 1977; Pera, Zook & Harder, 1979). However, neither platinum content in the plasma or kidney nor the degree of cellular necrosis it produces are modified by these diuretics. Platinum is not reabsorbed to an important degree after its intratubular microinjection and, therefore, platinum content in the cell should not be dependent on its luminal concentration. That prediction is confirmed in those studies quoted above. Therefore, it appears that other effects of mannitol or frusemide should be considered.

Prior hydration with hypertonic salt seems to reduce cisplatin-induced ARF (Litterst, 1981; Ozols *et al.*, 1984). As previous studies indicated that the degree of azotaemia produced by cisplatin was highly dependent on the sodium chloride content of the vehicle used for its administration (Litterst, 1981) it has been suggested that the increase in chloride concentration in the urine that occurs after hypertonic salt infusion may reduce the conversion of cisplatin to toxic aquated metabolites, a process known to be sensitive to Cl^- ion concentration. Yet mannitol, which is also protective, should lower Cl^- ion concentration in the urine. Furthermore, we recently confirmed an earlier report that diabetic animals given an otherwise nephrotoxic dose of cisplatin (5 mg/kg) are resistant to cisplatin nephrotoxicity (Safirstein, Brod-Miller & Dikman, 1983; Morales *et al.*, 1980). In studies on the mechanism of such protection we found chloride concentration in the urine to be reduced as expected. These findings cast doubt on the notion that urinary chloride concentration plays an important role in cisplatin nephrotoxicity.

On the other hand, mannitol and frusemide modify the abrupt changes in renal blood flow (RBF) and tubule obstruction that attend a variety of nephrotoxic insults (Wilson *et al.*, 1967; Montoreano *et al.*, 1971; Bailey *et al.*, 1973; Patak *et al.*, 1979; Hanley & Davidson, 1981). In each of these situations, acute renal failure emerges at a time when the vasodilation and diuresis produced by these agents are still present. It is thought that both of these effects are necessary to ameliorate the fall in GFR (Patak *et al.*, 1979). How mannitol and frusemide ameliorate cisplatin-induced reductions in GFR three days after these agents are given, however, is not immediately apparent. Hypertonic saline also produces vasodilation when renal perfusion is low (Johnston *et al.*, 1979), but here again the effect has been examined only acutely at the time of its administration. It may be that the response of the renal vasculature to an as yet unidentified vasoconstrictor at the time of emerging cisplatin-induced ARF is modified by each of these agents. Mannitol reduces the vasoconstrictive effects of noradrenaline and renal nerve stimulation in a number of vascular beds (Schlor, Ichikawa & Brenner, 1980) when given acutely and may have similar longer term effects on the renal vasculature. Persistent morphological (Krishnamurty *et al.*, 1977) and transport (Hanley & Davidson, 1981) effects of mannitol have been observed that do not depend on its continued administration. Detecting these effects on the renal and systemic vasculature, as well as detecting qualitative and quantitative differences in the way these agents affect the renal microvasculature at the time of cisplatin-induced ARF, may not only bring new understanding of the mechanism of the renal failure, but may lead to the design of even more effective ways of applying these hydration manoeuvres.

E. Studies on the mechanism of renal cytotoxicity

We have studied renal cell respiration and DNA replication after cisplatin exposure as they are of suspected pathogenic importance in cisplatin nephrotoxicity. Studies of the former were performed in an isolated tubule suspension enriched in the P3 segment of the proximal tubule. A distinct advantage of this system is that intracellular organelles are exposed to the toxin in a manner similar to that present *in vivo* as the toxin must pass through the plasma membrane.

Tubules were isolated from tissue taken from the outer stripe of the outer medulla, an area in which the P3 segment predominates, using collagenase digestion and Percoll gradient centrifugation as described by Vinay et al. (1981). The final tubule suspension is almost exclusively comprised of proximal straight tubules. The oxygen consumption of these tubules was measured under the following conditions: (1) basal O_2 consumption in the presence of available substrates (glucose, alanine, lactate and butyrate); (2) uncoupled rates of respiration in the presence of 10 μM carbonyl-cyanide-m-chlorophenyl hydrazone (CCCIP); and (3) respiration after the addition of the ionophore nystatin, 40 μg/mg protein. Nystatin, by increasing cell membrane permeability to sodium and potassium raises intracellular sodium concentration and stimulates Na^+/K^+ pump activity, increases ADP generation and thus stimulates mitochondrial respiration. These studies were performed in tubules from control rats exposed to cisplatin (10^{-5}–10^{-3} M) and transplatin (10^{-5}–10^{-3} M) *in vitro*, as well as in tubules from rats given 5 mg/kg cisplatin and sacrificed 12 h to 6 days later.

The results of the *in vitro* studies are summarized in Fig. 14. Incubation of the tubules with cisplatin inhibited basal and stimulated rates of oxygen consumption at very high concentrations (10^{-3} M) only. Transplatin, which is neither antineoplastic nor nephrotoxic, but also binds to DNA and protein, decreases respiration at lower concentrations (10^{-4} M) and is a more potent inhibitor of respiration than cisplatin.

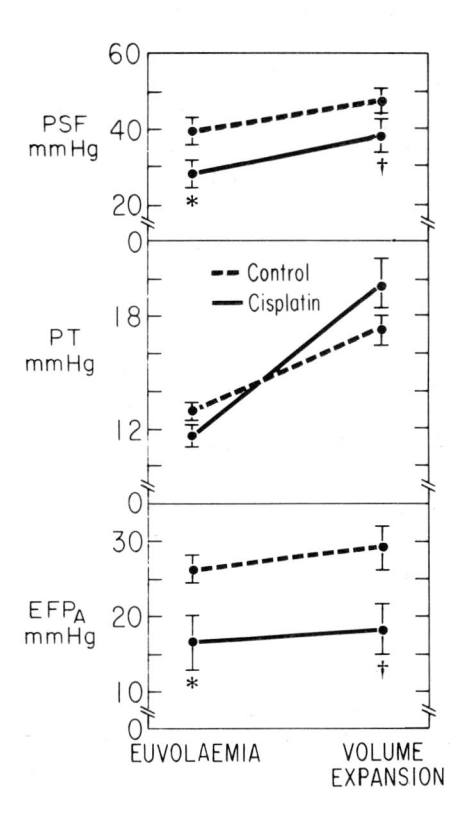

Fig. 13. Glomerular and tubular hydrostatic pressure in control and cisplatin-treated rats before and after plasma volume expansion. *$P < 0.05$ control volume expansion versus cisplatin volume expansion.

The basal rate of respiration in tubules isolated from rats given a nephrotoxic dose of cisplatin is normal up to 4 days after cisplatin, a time when plasma urea concentration is already elevated (Fig. 15). No consistent change in uncoupled or nystatin-stimulated rates of respiration was observed over a similar period of time (Fig. 16). Platinum content of tubules incubated with 10^{-3} M cisplatin *in vitro* is 64.3 ± 16.2 nM Pt/mg protein and much higher than that in tubules isolated from

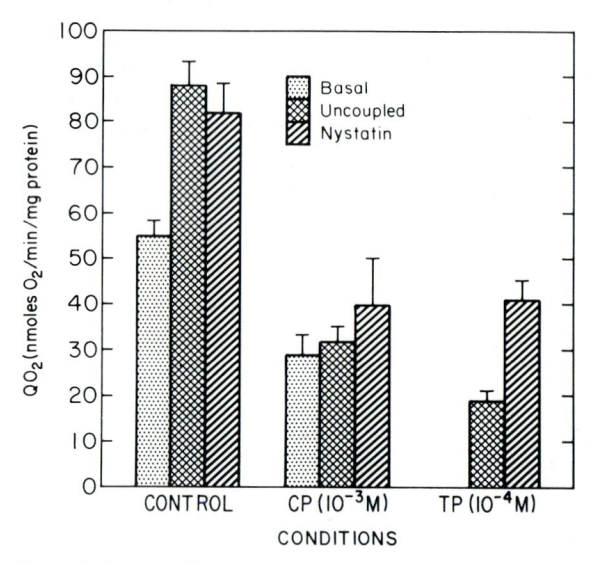

Fig. 14. *In vitro* effect of cisplatin (CP) and transplatin (TP) on tubule respiration. Rat kidney tubules were isolated from the outer stripe of the outer medulla of normal rats by collagenase digestion and Percoll gradient centrifugation. Oxygen consumption (QO_2) was measured in tubules after a 90 min period of incubation with cisplatin (CP) or transplatin (TP) at the doses indicated. Respiration was measured under basal and stimulated conditions after the addition of 10 μM carbonyl-cyanide-m-chlorophenyl hydrazone (uncoupled) or nystatin (40 μg/mg protein). Basal and stimulated rates of respiration were inhibited by CP and TP under these conditions.

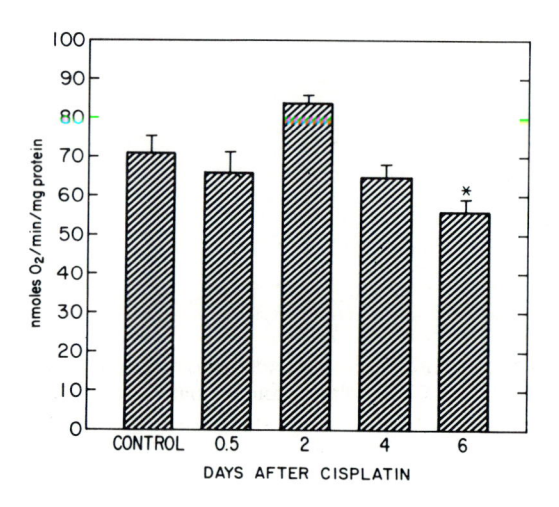

Fig. 15. *In vivo* effect of cisplatin on basal respiration 12 h, 2, 4 and 6 days after cisplatin (5 mg/kg). Basal respiration was significantly decreased in tubules isolated from animals 6 days after cisplatin but not before. *$P < 0.05$ compared to control.

Cisplatin nephrotoxicity mechanisms 341

rats given cisplatin *in vivo* (0.38 ± 0.07 nM Pt/mg protein). The results of these studies would seem to indicate that neither the renal cell mitochondria nor the membrane associated Na$^+$–K$^+$ ATPase are important early pathogenetic targets of cisplatin.

The results of studies on DNA turnover in renal tissue were more encouraging (Fig. 17). DNA turnover was examined in tissue from the outer cortex and the outer stripe of the outer medulla 1, 2, 3, 4 and 7 days after cisplatin at a dose of 5 mg/kg. DNA turnover is expressed as the specific activity of ^{3}H-thymidine in DNA 1 h after the injection of the radiolabel. DNA turnover in cisplatin treated rats initially decline significantly from the low control values on day 1. By day 3 DNA turnover had returned to control levels and by day 7 DNA turnover had nearly increased 5-fold. These findings are similar to those reported before (Taylor, Tew & Jones, 1976) except that DNA has been isolated from specific regions in these studies rather than the kidney as a whole. The fall in DNA turnover on day 1

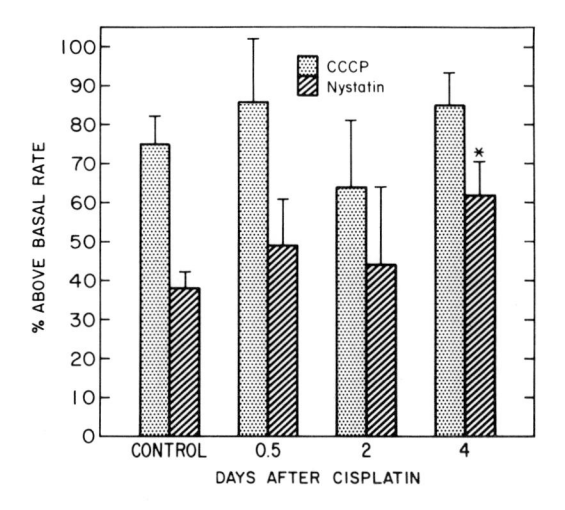

Fig. 16. *In vivo* effect of cisplatin on stimulated rates of respiration in tubules isolated from rats after cisplatin. CCCP refers to O$_2$ consumption after addition of the uncoupler carbonyl-cyanide-m-chloro-phenyl hydrazone, 10 μM. *$P < 0.05$ compared to control.

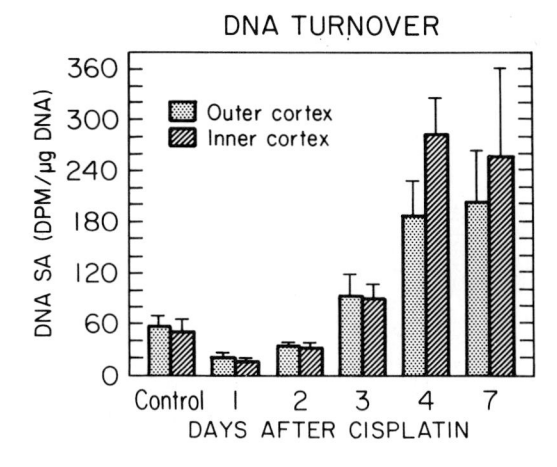

Fig. 17. Thymidine incorporation in DNA isolated from the outer cortex and the outer stripe of the outer medulla in rats at various times after a 5 mg/kg dose of cisplatin.

precedes the occurrence of cellular necrosis so characteristic of this drug and the later increase in DNA turnover coincides with the regeneration of the damaged areas of the kidney.

The inhibition of renal DNA replication is reminiscent of cisplatin's effect on tumour and normal cells in culture and suggests that renal DNA is damaged by cisplatin. It is of interest that both the outer cortex and outer stripe of the outer medulla have reduced DNA synthesis 1 day after cisplatin recalling that only the cells of the pars recta that predominate in the outer stripe undergo necrosis. At least three possibilities may be considered. First, inhibition of DNA synthesis may be irrelevant to the cytotoxicity. Its occurrence so early after exposure to cisplatin and its importance in cytotoxicity elsewhere are not consistent with that possibility. Second, cells of the outer cortex can repair their DNA lesions while those of the pars recta cannot. Studies in cells whose repair processes are deficient show that cisplatin is especially toxic in them (Fraval, Rawlings & Roberts, 1978) making such a possibility likely. Third, it may be that the levels of the DNA adducts formed in the pars recta cells are lethal while lower levels in the earlier proximal segments are not. Further studies will be necessary to determine the importance of this observation.

F. Summary

The vulnerability of the kidney to cisplatin, and the P3 segment of the proximal tubule in particular, may be related to the predominant role of the kidney in the excretion of the drug. Cisplatin is biotransformed in the kidney to a compound that may no longer be toxic. By inhibiting the renal uptake of cisplatin or increasing the production of this biotransformed product, it may be possible to reduce its nephrotoxicity. A recent report of the effective use of quinine to reduce cisplatin-induced renal failure in chickens is encouraging (Bird, Walser & Quebbemann, 1984). In cisplatin nephrotoxicity, as in other forms of nephrotoxic renal damage, reduced renal blood flow and diminished renal conservation of water are common physiological derangements. The mediator(s) of the vasoconstriction is unknown. One particularly interesting feature of its nephrotoxicity is the 48 h period that precedes overt renal failure. As changes in renal cell function almost certainly occur before the kidney fails, it may be possible to explore the early primary physiological and biochemical determinants of the renal failure it produces. It appears that cisplatin-induced renal failure is an ideal model for the study of renal failure in general.

References

Arias, I. M., Fleischmer, G., Kirsch, R., Mushkin, S. & Gatmaitan, Z. (1976) On the structure, regulation and function of ligandin. *Glutathione; Metabolism and Function* (ed. by I. M. Arias and W. B. Jakoby), pp. 175–187. Raven Press, New York.

Aull, J. L., Allen, R. L., Bapat, A. R., Daron, H. H., Friedman, M. E. & Wilson, J. F. (1979) The effects of platinum complexes on seven enzymes. *Biochimica et Biophysica Acta*, **571**, 352–358.

Bailey, R. R, Natale, R., Turnbull, D. I. & Linton, A. L. (1973) Protective effect of furosemide in acute tubular necrosis and actue renal failure. *Clinical Science and Molecular Medicine*, **45**, 1–17.

Berry, J.-P., Pauwells, C., Tlouzeau, S. & Lespinats, G. (1984) Effect of Selenium in combination with cis-diamminedichloroplatinum (II) in the treatment of murine fibrosarcoma. *Cancer Research*, **44**, 2864–2868.

Bird, J. E., Walser, M. M. & Quebbemann, A. J. (1984) Protective effect of organic cation transport inhibitors in cis-diammine dichloroplatinum-induced nephrotoxicity, *Journal of Pharmacology and Experimental Therapy*, **231**, 752–758.

Borch, R. F. & Pleasants, M. E. (1979) Inhibition of cis-platinum nephrotoxicity by diethyldithiocarbamate rescue in a rat renal model. *Proceedings of the National Academy of Science of the United States of America*, **76**, 6611–6614.

Chopra, S., Kaufman, J. S., Jones, T. W., Hong, W. K., Gehr, M. K., Hamburger, R. J., Flamenbaum, W. & Trump, B. J. (1982) Cis-diamminedichloroplatinum-induced acute renal failure in the rat. *Kidney International*, **21**, 54–64.

Clifton, G., Pearce, C., O'Neill, W., Shah, S. & Wallin, J. (1982) Early polyuria in the rat following single dose cis-dichlorodiammine platinum (II). *Journal of Laboratory and Clinical Medicine*, **100**, 659–670.

Cvitkovic, B., Spaulding, J., Bethune, V., Martin, J. & Whitemore, W. F. (1977) Improvement of cis-dichlorodiammineplatinum therapeutic index in an animal model. *Cancer*, **39**, 1357–1361.

Daley-Yates, P. T. & McBrien, D. C. H. (1982) The inhibition of renal ATPase by cisplatin and some biotransformation products. *Chemico-Biological Interactions*, **40**, 325–334.

Fraval, H. N. A., Rawlings, C. J. & Roberts, J. J. (1978) Increased sensitivity of UV repair deficient human cells to DNA bound platinum products which unlike thymine dimers are not recognized by an endonuclease extracted from Micrococcus luteus. *Mutation Research*, **51**, 121–132.

Goldstein, M. H. & Safirstein, R. (1981) Functional characteristics of chronic tubulo-interstitial disease after repeated doses of cisplatin. Abstracts, 8th International Congress of Nephrology, June 1981, p. 229.

Hanley, M. J. & Davison, K. (1981) Prior mannitol and furosemide infusion in a model of ischemic actue renal failure. *American Journal of Physiology*, **241**, F556.

Harder, H. C. & Rosenberg, B. (1970) Inhibitory effects of antitumor platinum compounds on DNA, RNA, and protein synthesis in mammalian cells in vitro. *Cancer*, **6**, 207–216.

Harder, H. C., Smith, R. G. & LeRoy, E. (1976) Template-primer inactivation by cis- and trans-dichlorodiammine platinum for human DNA polymerase a, b, and Rausher murine leukemia virus reverse transcriptase as a mechanism of cytotoxicity. *Cancer Research*, **36**, 3821–3829.

Howle, J. A. & Gale, G. R. (1970) Cis-dichlorodiammine platinum II persistent and selective inhibition of deocyribonucleic acid synthesis in vitro. *Biochemistry and Pharmacology*, **19**, 2757–2762.

Ichikawa, I., Miele, J. F. & Brenner, B. M. (1979) Reversal of renal cortical actions of angiotensin II by verapamil and manganese. *Kidney International*, **16**, 137–147.

Jacobs, C., Kalman, S. M., Tretton, M. & Weiner, M. W. (1980) Renal handling of cis-diammine dichloroplatinum (II). *Cancer Treatment Reports*, **64**, 1223–1226.

Johnston, P. A., Bernard, D. B, Donohoe, J. F., Perrin, N. S. & Levinsky, N. G. (1979) Effect of volume expansion on hemodynamics of the hypoperfused rat kidney. *Journal of Clinical Investigation*, **64**, 550–558.

Kohl, H. H., Friedman, M. E., Melius, P., Mora, E. C. & McAuliffe, C. A. (1979) Enhanced inhibition of both cellular protein synthesis and malate dehydrogenase by aged aquoplatinum (II) complexes. *Chemico-Biological Interactions*, **24**, 209–215.

Krishnamurty, V. S. R, Adams, H. R., Smitherman, T. C. et al. (1977) Influence of mannitol on contractile responses of isolated perfused arteries. *American Journal of Physiology*, **232**, H59–H66.

Lecointe, P., Macquet, J.-P. & Butour, J.-L. (1979) Correlation between the toxicity of platinum drugs to L1210 leukemia cells and their mutagenic properties. *Biochemical and Biophysical Research Communications*, **90**, 209–213.

Levi, J., Jacobs, C., Kalman, S., McTigue, M. & Weiner, M. W. (1980) Mechanism of cis-platinum nephrotoxicity I. Effects on sulfhydryl groups in rat kidneys. *Journal of Pharmacology and Experimental Therapy*, **213**, 545–550.

Litterst, C. L., Torres, I. J. & Guarino, A. M. J. (1977) Plasma levels and organ distribution of platinum in the rat, dog, and dog fish following intravenous administration of cis-DDP(II). *Clinical Hematology and Oncology*, **7**, 169–178.

Litterst, C. L. (1981) Alterations in the toxicity of cis-dichlorodiammine platinum II and in tissue localization of platinum as a function of NaCl concentration in the vehicle of administration. *Applied Pharmacology*, **61**, 99–108.

Mavichak, V., Wong, N. L. M., Quamme, G. A., Magil, A. B., Sutton, R. A. L. & Dirks, J. H. (1986) Studies on the pathogenesis of cisplatin-induced hypomagnesemia in rats. *Kidney International* (in press).

Grigor Dr Ozols told us in a previous paper that chloride protects the kidney from cisplatin. Can you explain this mechanism?

Safirstein As I indicated in my paper, there is ample evidence to suggest that aquation of cisplatin in the urinary space is not a determinant of its renal toxicity.
1 The area of damage in the kidney (the terminal portion of the proximal tubules) has a chloride concentration 30% higher than plasma and much higher than is necessary to inhibit aquation completely.
2 Mannitol, which is equally as effective as hypertonic saline in ameliorating cisplatin nephrotoxicity, lowers urinary chloride concentration.
3 Rats partially protected by mannitol from cisplatin nephrotoxicity have the same renal content and cytotoxicity of cisplatin as unprotected animals, indicating that no modification of its cytotoxicity has occurred.

As in other forms of nephrotoxic renal failure such as glycerol, ischaemia and $HgCl_2$, hydration in some way partially dissociates the cytotoxic effects of nephrotoxins and their effect on GFR. I think the data is now overwhelmingly against any role for urinary aquation of cisplatin in its nephrotoxicity.

Schmoll Does frusemide protect the kidney or does it enhance cisplatin nephrotoxicity? We hear conflicting reports.

Safirstein The literature is very confusing. I think frusemide works under well controlled circumstances. I suspect that when excess fluid loss induced by frusemide is carefully prevented then it protects. However, if extracellular fluid depletion is not corrected, then frusemide might actually potentiate nephrotoxicity.

Effect of cisplatin on renal haemodynamics and tubular function in the dog kidney

GEDSKE DAUGAARD,[1] U. ABILDGAARD,[2]
N. H. HOLSTEIN-RATHLOU,[3] O. AMTORP[2] and
P. P. LEYSSAC[3] [1]*Department of Oncology ONB, The Finsen Institute, Copenhagen,* [2]*Department of Cardiology, Gentofte Hospital, and* [3]*University Institute of Experimental Medicine, Copenhagen, Denmark*

Summary
Administration of cisplatin (5 mg/kg) to dogs results in polyuric renal failure due initially to a proximal tubular functional impairment. 48–72 h after the cisplatin administration the depressed renal function can be attributed to impairment of proximal as well as distal tubular reabsorptive capacities associated with increased renal vascular resistance. The polyuria seems to be due to the impaired reabsorption rate in the distal nephron segments.

Key words. Cisplatin, renal blood flow, glomerular filtration rate, natriuresis, tubular function, lithium clearance method, dogs.

Introduction
Cisplatin (cis-diamminedichloroplatinum (II)), a coordination complex of platinum, is widely used for cancer chemotherapy, but like other heavy metals it has an associated dose-limiting nephrotoxic effect (Chopra *et al.*, 1982; Safirstein *et al.*, 1981).

In order to elucidate and localize the nephrotoxic actions of cisplatin, we have taken advantage of the lithium clearance method. The lithium clearance (C_{Li}) method is based on evidence indicating that lithium is reabsorbed almost exclusively in the proximal tubules in parallel with sodium and water (Thomsen, 1984). It is therefore a measure of the delivery of fluid from the end of the straight segment proximal to the thin descending limb of Henle's loop. Thus, when the lithium clearance method is used in concert with measurements of glomerular filtration rate and sodium and water excretion rates it is a noninvasive method for assessing the absolute and fractional reabsorption rates of sodium and water in the proximal as well as the more distal segments of the nephron in animals and patients (Thomsen, 1984; Thomsen, Holstein-Rathlou & Leyssac, 1981).

The present study was designed to investigate the early effects of cisplatin administration to dogs by simultaneous and serial measurements of renal and

Correspondence: Dr Gedske Daugaard, Department of Oncology ONB, The Finsen Institute, Strandboulevarden 49, DK-2100 Copenhagen, Denmark.

systemic haemodynamics, glomerular filtration rate (GFR) and tubular reabsorption rates of sodium and water.

Methods

Studies were performed on twenty mongrel dogs (17–32 kg), starved overnight, but allowed free access to water.

Experimental preparation

The animals were neurolept anaesthetized with fentanyl and N_2O (5). The kidneys were exposed through a median laparotomy. Electromagnetic flow probes (Statham SN-68918) were placed around the renal arteries to measure the renal blood flow (RBF). The ureters were cannulated close to the kidneys for collection of urine. Throughout the experiment RBF, mean aortic pressure (MAP), mean pulmonary pressure (MPAP), ECG and body temperature were continuously recorded. Priming doses of 3 µCi/kg ^{51}Cr-EDTA and 88 µmol/kg of lithium carbonate were administered i.v. dissolved in 15 ml of isotonic saline followed by a sustaining infusion of 0.015 µCi/kg/min of ^{51}Cr-EDTA and 0.20 µmol/kg/min lithium in isotonic saline, sufficient to maintain the plasma concentration of ^{51}Cr-EDTA and lithium at a constant level.

Experimental procedure

The animals were allowed to stabilize for 60–90 min to recover from surgery. The animals were divided into three experimental groups:

(a) Six dogs were studied immediately after infusion of cisplatin. During reference conditions urine was collected in three successive 20 min clearance periods. At the middle of each period RBF, cardiac output (CO), MAP, MPAP and heart rate (HR) were measured and blood samples were drawn. Following measurements during reference conditions, a dose of 5 mg/kg cisplatin dissolved in sterile water (1 mg/ml) was infused i.v. over a 30 min period (0.17 ml/kg/min) with a corresponding reduction of the infusion rate of Ringer's solution. At the same time urine collection was started in 20 min periods (from 0 to 160 min) and measurements were made as described above.

(b) In six dogs the cisplatin infusion was replaced with sham infusion of Ringer's solution (0.17 ml/kg/min) (time control). Urine and blood samples and haemodynamic variables were obtained according to the time schedule mentioned above.

(c) Eight dogs were studied 48 h ($n=6$) to 72 h ($n=2$) after administration of cisplatin at a dose of 5 mg/kg. Venous blood samples for determination of haemoglobin concentration, haematocrit and plasma concentrations of protein, creatinine and urea were obtained every 24 h. On the day of the experiments reference measurements were performed as mentioned in group (a).

Calculations

The renal clearances of ^{51}Cr-EDTA, lithium (C_{Li}) and sodium (C_{Na}) were calculated from the urine excretion rates and mid-point plasma concentrations of ^{51}Cr-EDTA, lithium and sodium respectively as: $C = (U/P)*V$, where U/P denotes the urine to plasma concentration ratio of the substance and V the rate of urine flow.

The clearance of ^{51}Cr-EDTA was used as a measure of glomerular filtration rate (GFR). The fractional proximal reabsorption rates (FPR) were calculated as $1-(C_{Li}/GFR)$. The absolute proximal reabsorption rates (APR) were calculated as $GFR - C_{Li}$. The fractional distal reabsorption rates of water (FDR$_{H_2O}$) and of sodium (FDR$_{Na}$) in per cent of the delivery to the loop of Henle were calculated as $1 - (V/C_{Li})$ and $1 - (C_{Na}/C_{Li})$, respectively. Absolute distal reabsorption rates of water (ADR$_{H_2O}$) and of sodium (ADR$_{Na}$) were calculated as $C_{Li} - V$ and $(C_{Li} - C_{Na}) \times P_{Na}$, respectively.

Results

Haemodynamic variables, plasma sodium, plasma potassium and plasma osmolarity did not differ among the groups, and remained constant throughout the experiments.

The intravenous infusion of cisplatin in group (a) produced no significant changes in RBF or GFR, but an immediate and significant increase in V, C_{Na} and C_{Li} ($82\pm17\%$, $96\pm23\%$ and $59\pm15\%$) in the first 20 min period (Table 1), and thereafter V, C_{Na} and C_{Li} remained significantly higher than the pretreatment reference value.

In group (a) the fractional as well as absolute rates of proximal reabsorption decreased significantly in the first 20 min by $21\pm5\%$ and $18\pm6\%$ respectively, and both remained significantly decreased during the rest of the study period. The

Table 1. Measured and calculated renal function variables in group (a), (b) and (c)

	Group a		Group b (sham infusion)		Group c
	Reference pretreatment value	First 20 min period	Reference pretreatment value	First 20 min period	
RBF ml/min	211±11	214±17	212±13	205±22	143±14*
GFR ml/min	50.0±4.1	51.0±3.7	48.6±3.7	50.3±3.7	10.7±1.1*
V ml/min	0.38±0.07	0.73±0.12*	0.28±0.06	0.25±0.05	1.09±0.11*
C_{Na} ml/min	0.33±0.11	0.65±0.14*	0.18±0.08	0.17±0.06	0.63±0.10*
C_{Li} ml/min	15.54±2.21	23.56±3.9*	13.73±1.47	14.15±2.65	6.29±0.61*
FPR	0.68±0.03	0.56±0.04*	0.71±0.02	0.72±0.01	0.35±0.07*
APR ml/min	33.19±2.23	27.22±1.59*	34.10±3.98	34.56±1.74	4.4±0.9*
FDR$_{Na}$	0.982±0.004	0.969±0.008	0.989±0.004	0.991±0.003	0.897±0.012*
ADR$_{Na}$ mmol/min	2.16±0.30	3.28±0.53*	1.99±0.21	2.19±0.26	0.82±0.08*
C_{osm} ml/min	1.53±0.37	1.94±0.40			1.08±0.09*

RBF = renal blood flow, GFR = glomerular filtration rate, V = water excretion rate, C_{Na}, C_{Li} and C_{osm} = sodium, lithium and osmolal clearance, FPR and APR = fractional and absolute proximal reabsorption rates, FDR$_{Na}$ and ADR$_{Na}$ = fractional and absolute distal reabsorption rates of sodium. Data are expressed as means ± SEM. All values are compared with the reference value in group (a). * indicates $P < 0.05$.

calculated absolute distal rate of reabsorption of sodium (ADR$_{Na}$) increased significantly in the first 20 min period by 55±15% and then remained at this signficantly increased level during the study compared with the reference value. In contrast, the fractional distal reabsorption of sodium decreased insignificantly ($0.1 > P > 0.05$).

Haemoglobin, haematocrit and plasma electrolytes did not change significantly during the observation period of 48–72 h in group (c), while plasma creatinine and plasma urea increased significantly from 96±3 µmol/l to 178±10 µmol/l and from 3.9±0.2 mmol/l to 11.7±1.4 mmol/l, respectively.

The mean values of RBF, GFR and C_{Li} were significantly lower and V and C_{Na} significantly higher in group (c) than in group (a) animals (pretreatment values). Furthermore, 48–72 h after administration of cisplatin (group c) absolute as well as fractional reabsorption rates in proximal and distal nephron segments were significantly lower than reference values obtained in group (a) animals (pretreatment values). It seems notable that free water clearance in the cisplatin treated animals was close to zero.

Discussion

The lithium clearance method used in this study has been widely utilized in humans (Thomsen, 1984), in rats (Thomsen et al., 1981) and in dogs (Abildgaard, Holstein-Rathlou & Leyssac, 1986). Abildgaard et al. (1986) have justified the use of the method as a reliable measure of proximal tubular function in dog kidneys during different experimental conditions.

In the present study, a prompt and marked increase in sodium and water excretion and a rise of C_{Li} was observed minutes to hours (group a) after the cisplatin administration. This occurred without measurable changes in GFR and RBF and it was not associated with significant alterations in MAP, HR, CO, Hct or plasma sodium. The increase in C_{Li} and in the fractional lithium clearance (C_{Li}/GFR) indicates an increased fluid delivery out of the proximal tubules caused by a decrease in absolute as well as in fractional proximal reabsorption rates, strongly suggesting that cisplatin induced nephrotoxicity is initiated by a primary proximal tubular functional impairment.

Forty-eight to 72 h after the administration of cisplatin (group c) RBF and C_{Li} had decreased to about 50% of control values, and there was a marked decrease in the filtered load (GFR), indicating a pronounced further reduction in absolute proximal reabsorption rates, and also a further decrease in proximal fractional reabsorption. This observation suggests a progression of the initial impairment of proximal tubular function observed in group (a). The marked decrease in GFR associated with a reduction in RBF suggests that increased renal vascular resistance also develops with time and contributes to the cisplatin induced nephrotoxicity.

Furthermore, in group (c) animals the decreased rate of fluid flow from the end of the proximal straight segment into the thin descending limb of Henle's loop (C_{Li}) was associated with a marked decrease not only in absolute, but also in fractional sodium and water reabsorption rates in more distal nephron segments. As a consequence the urine flow and sodium excretion rate actually increased in accordance with the findings in the rat (Safirstein et al., 1981). This observation indicates that, in addition to its proximal effect, the delayed impairment of tubular function caused by cisplatin had also progressed to involve the more distal segments of the nephron.

In conclusion, administration of cisplatin (5 mg/kg) to dogs results in polyuric renal failure due initially to a proximal tubular functional impairment. Forty-eight to 72 h after the cisplatin administration the depressed renal function can be attributed to impairment of proximal as well as distal tubular reabsorptive capacities associated with increased renal vascular resistance. The polyuria seems to be due to the impaired reabsorption rate in the distal nephron segments.

Acknowledgement
This study was supported by grants from the Danish Cancer Society.

References
Abildgaard, U., Holstein-Rathlou, N. H. & Leyssac, P. P. (1986) Effect of renal sympathetic nerve activity on tubular sodium and water reabsorption in dog kidneys as determined by the lithium clearance method. *Acta Physiologica Scandinavica*, **126**, 251–257.
Chopra, S., Kaufman, J. S., Jones, T. W., Hong, W. K., Gehr, M. K., Hamburger, R. J., Flamenbaum, W. & Trump, B. J. (1982) Cis-diamminedichloroplatinum induced acute renal failure in the rat. *Kidney International*, **21**, 54.
Safirstein, R., Miller, P., Dikman, S., Leyman, N. & Chapiro, C. (1981) Cisplatin nephrotoxicity in rats — Defect in papillary hypertonicity. *American Journal of Physiology*, **241**, F175–F185.
Thomsen, K. (1984) Lithium clearance. A new method for determining proximal and distal tubular reabsorption of sodium and water. *Nephron*, **37**, 217–223.
Thomsen, K., Holstein-Rathlou, N. H. & Leyssac, P. P. (1981) Comparison of three measures of proximal tubular reabsorption: Lithium clearance, occlusion time and micropuncture. *American Journal of Physiology*, **241**, F348–F355.

Discussion

Vogelzang Do you have a hypothesis to account for the increased vascular resistance in the kidney following cisplatin?

Daugaard No, we do not know why this occurs. Renal blood flow decreases but we cannot explain the mechanism.

Vogelzang Do you know whether cisplatin affects gastro-intestinal transport of fluid and electrolytes, because many patients develop diarrhoea?

Daugaard I have no information on the causation of cisplatin-induced diarrhoea.

Altered renin and aldosterone excretion in patients treated for metastatic germ cell tumours

G. J. BOSL, S. P. LEITNER, S. A. ATLAS, J. E. SEALEY, J. J. PREIBISZ and E. SCHEINER *The Solid Tumor Service and the Physiology Service, Department of Medicine, Memorial Sloan-Kettering Cancer Center, and the Hypertension Laboratory, Department of Medicine, The New York Hospital, Cornell University Medical College, New York, U.S.A.*

Summary

Twenty-four patients with metastatic germ cell tumours were studied for abnormalities in the renin–aldosterone axis and for persistent abnormalities of renal function 9+ to 54+ months following completion of cisplatin based chemotherapy. Increased plasma renin activity and aldosterone were identified in fourteen of nineteen (79%) patients. The mean serum magnesium was subnormal. Statistically lower serum phosphorus levels, and higher urea and creatinine levels were also observed. No patient was hypertensive or on diuretics at the time of study. Since vascular toxicity has been reported after cisplatin based chemotherapy and hypomagnesaemia and increased plasma renin activity have been linked to cardiovascular events, these data imply that germ cell tumour patients treated with cisplatin based chemotherapy should be carefully observed for delayed cardiovascular toxicity.

Key words. Renin, aldosterone, germ cell tumour.

Introduction

The success of treatment of patients with metastatic germ cell tumours is dependent upon the use of high dose cisplatin. Nephrotoxicity is the most common acute and chronic toxicity associated with the use of this drug, and is usually manifest as a decreased creatinine clearance and hypomagnesaemia (Shilsky & Anderson, 1979). However, reports of Raynaud's phenomenon, myocardial infarction, and hypertension suggest that vascular toxicity may be a delayed consequence of cisplatin based chemotherapy (Samuels, Johnson & Holoye, 1975; Edwards, Lane & Smith, 1979; Vogelzang, Frenning & Kennedy, 1980; Vogelzang et al., 1981; Harrell, Sibly & Vogelzang, 1982; Vogelzang, 1984).

Given that cisplatin induced renal tubular damage in both rat and man, renin and aldosterone excretion might be altered. We, therefore, evaluated a group of patients treated with cisplatin based chemotherapy for metastatic germ cell

Correspondence: George J. Bosl, Memorial Hospital, 1275 York Avenue, New York, NY 10021, U.S.A.

tumours for persistent alterations in renal function and abnormalities in renin and aldosterone excretion.

Patients and Methods

Twenty-four patients were evaluated (9+ to 54+ months) after chemotherapy for metastatic germ cell tumour. Twenty-one patients had received VAB-6 (cyclophosphamide + vinblastine + bleomycin + cisplatin + actinomycin) (Vugrin et al., 1981; Bosl et al., 1986) and three received etoposide + cisplatin (Bosl et al., 1985). All patients were studied in the Clinical Research Center of The New York Hospital–Cornell University Medical College. None of the patients were hypertensive either at the time of the study or on past history.

A 24 h urine for sodium and creatinine was obtained in nineteen patients and for aldosterone in sixteen patients. Blood was collected for baseline supine plasma renin activity (PRA) and aldosterone, and after 1 h of ambulation, repeat values for PRA and aldosterone were obtained. At that time, blood was also obtained for serum magnesium, total ionized calcium, electrolytes, blood urea nitrogen, and creatinine. A 3 h oral water loading test was performed and the initial and minimum urine osmolality values were obtained.

The complete details of the methods of this study and of the assays performed have been published elsewhere (Bosl et al., in press).

Results

Of the nineteen patients who had both a 24 h urine for sodium and blood obtained for PRA and aldosterone, fourteen (79%) had elevated levels of ambulatory PRA. The mean elevated value was 15.2 ± 1.5 ng/ml/h and the mean ambulatory PRA for all nineteen patients was 10.9 ± 1.8 ng/ml/h. The PRA was normally responsive to changes in posture with the mean supine PRA of 4.7 ± 0.6 ng/ml/h. Similarly, plasma aldosterone levels were elevated with a mean ambulatory plasma aldosterone of 25.2 ± 3.2 ng/dl and supine levels of 10.7 ± 1.9 ng/dl. The ambulatory PRA was correlated with both ambulatory plasma aldosterone as well as 24 h urinary aldosterone excretion. The mean urinary aldosterone excretion was 11.7 ± 2.9 mg/day. All patients had 24 h urine sodium values above 50 meq/day.

Evidence of persistent renal injury was noted in all patients studied. Fourteen patients had asymptomatic hypomagnesaemia (< 1.5 meq/l), four patients had values above 1.1 meq/l, and one patient had a value of 0.5 meq/l. Serum phosphorus levels were higher prior to treatment (3.64 ± 0.11 mg/dl) than at the time of study (3.06 ± 0.09 mg/dl) ($P < 0.001$) and the blood urea nitrogen was significantly greater at the time of study (17.13 ± 1.17 mg/dl) than before treatment (13.96 ± 0.77 mg/dl) ($P < 0.01$). The mean peak serum creatinine during chemotherapy (1.40 ± 0.03 mg/dl) was significantly greater than that observed prior to starting chemotherapy (0.99 ± 0.03 mg/dl) ($P < 0.001$). The higher peak creatinine during treatment was significantly correlated with a lower serum magnesium at the time of study ($P < 0.0001$; $R = 0.79$). There was a suggestion that the mean serum potassium was lower at the time of study than prior to treatment (4.1 ± 0.1 meq/l vs 4.5 ± 0.1 meq/l, respectively), but a test for significance was not performed due to the fact that these values were obtained from different laboratories.

No significant relationship was found between serum magnesium, calcium and abnormal PRA.

Following the 3 h water loading tests, all patients had a normal diminution of serum osmolality. The mean value decreased from 848 ± 41 meq/l to 75 ± 4 meq/l. There was a trend toward a lower maximum urine osmolality in patients with high peak creatinine values during treatment, but this value did not reach statistical significance.

Discussion

There is no question that cisplatin combination chemotherapy has dramatically changed the prognosis of patients with metastatic germ cell tumours. However, it is to be expected that late toxicities will occur as a consequence of this therapy in cured patients. That the late toxicity after the treatment of a germ cell tumour is not related to the development of a second malignancy is probably related to the short course of therapy as opposed to the prolonged courses of therapy and radiotherapy in patients with Hodgkin's disease. However, it comes as something of a surprise that the major late toxicity in patients with germ cell tumours may be vascular. At least in part, this may be a consequence of both direct drug induced endothelial toxicity and hypomagnesaemia. Raynaud's phenomenon and hypertension have both been reported after vinblastin + bleomycin with and without cisplatin (Samuels et al., 1975; Vogelzang et al., 1981) and the degree of hypomagnesaemia seemed to be correlated with the frequency of Raynaud's phenomenon (Vogelzang, Torkelson & Kennedy, 1985).

However, other mechanisms may also be operative. Renal plasma flow decreases after cisplatin based chemotherapy (Meijer et al., 1983). This could lead to increased PRA. The combination of low magnesium and increased PRA is associated with an increased risk of cardiovascular events in patients with essential hypertension (Resnick, Laragh & Sealey, 1983). Additionally, magnesium depleted rats develop reduced terminal arteriolar lumen sizes, and significant arterial hypertension (Altura et al., 1981) and decreased cardiac muscle magnesium content has been implicated in sudden ischaemic cardiac deaths in soft water areas of Europe (Chipperfield & Chipperfield, 1978). Lastly, dog coronary arteries maintained in a hypomagnesaemic medium are hypercontractile when exposed to several agents (Turlapaty & Altura, 1980), supporting the observation of a greater frequency of Raynaud's phenomenon in cisplatin treated hypomagnesaemic patients.

The absence of hypertension in this group of treated patients, however, suggests that other mechanisms of increased PRA and aldosterone excretion might also be operative. Chronic salt wasting could be a consequence of cisplatin based chemotherapy, resulting in an elevated PRA as a compensatory mechanism. Neither hyponatraemia nor signs of volume depletion would be necessary since compensation could occur through hyperaldosteronism.

Continued long term observation of cisplatin treated patients with germ cell tumours is necessary if the early signs and symptoms of late toxicity are to be detected. Since the major end organ toxicity of cisplatin is renal in nature, the late toxicities of this therapy should also be expected to stem from this major end organ toxicity. Perhaps the use of less nephrotoxic cisplatin analogues will obviate the potential for late vascular toxicity, but only careful clinical trials designed to study both efficacy and long term toxicity will be able to answer these questions.

Acknowledgements
This work was supported in part by grants from The National Institutes of Health CA-05826, RR47, and HL-18323 SCOR, Contract CM-07337. Dr Atlas is a recipient of the Research Career Development Award (HL00570).

References
Altura, B. M., Altura, B. J., Gebrewold, A., et al. (1984) Magnesium deficiency and hypertension: correlation between magnesium-deficient diets and microcirculatory changes *in situ*. *Science*, 223, 1315–1317.

Bosl, G. J., Gluckman, R., Geller, N., Golbey, R. B., Whitmore, W. F., Herr, H., Sogani, P., Morse, M., Martini, N., Bains, M. & McCormack, P. (1986) VAB-6: An effective chemotherapy regimen for patients with germ cell tumors. *Journal of Clinical Oncology*, 4, 1493–1499.

Bosl, G. J., Leitner, S. P., Atlas, S., Scaley, J. E., Preibeisz, J. & Scheiner, E. Increased plasma renin and aldosterone in patients treated for metastatic germ cell tumors. *Journal of Clinical Oncology* (in press).

Bosl, G. J., Yagoda, A., Golbey, R. B., Whitmore, W., Herr, H., Sogani, P., Morse, M., Vogelzang, N., & MacDonald, G. (1985) The role of etoposide-based chemotherapy in the treatment of patients with refractory or relapsing germ cell tumors. *American Journal of Medicine*, 78, 423–428.

Chipperfield, B. A. & Chipperfield, J. R. (1978) Differences in metal content of the heart muscle in death from ischemic heart disease. *American Heart Journal*, 95, 732–737.

Edwards, G. S., Lane, M. & Smith, F. E. (1979) Long-term treatment with cis-dichlorodiamminoplatinum (II) – vinblastine – bleomycin: Possible association with severe coronary artery disease. *Cancer Treatment Reports*, 63, 551–552.

Harrell, R. M., Sibley, R. J. & Vogelzang, N. J. (1982) Renal vascular lesions after chemotherapy with vinblastine, bleomycin, and cisplatin. *American Journal of Medicine*, 73, 429–434.

Meijer, S., Sleijfer, D. T., Mulder, N. H., Sluiter, W. J., Marrink, J., Schraffordt Koops, H., Brouwers, T. M., Oldhoff, J., van der Hem, G. K. & Mandema, E. (1983) Some effects of combination chemotherapy with cis-platinum on renal function in patients with nonseminomatous testicular cancer. *Cancer*, 51, 2035–2040.

Resnick, L. M., Laragh, J. H. & Sealey, J. E. (1983) Divalent cations in essential hypertension: Relationships between serum ionized calcium, magnesium, and plasma renin activity. *New England Journal of Medicine*, 309, 888–891.

Samuels, M. L., Johnson, D. E. & Holoye, P. Y. (1975) Continuous intravenous bleomycin (NSC-49842) in stage III testicular neoplasia. *Cancer Chemotherapy Reports*, 59, 563–570.

Shilsky, R. L. & Anderson, T. (1979). Hypomagnesaemia and renal magnesium wasting in patients receiving cisplatin. *Annals of Internal Medicine*, 90, 929–931.

Turlapaty, P. D. M. V. & Altura, B. M. (1980) Magnesium deficiency produces spasms of coronary arteries: relationship to etiology of sudden ischemic heart disease. *Science*, 208, 198–200.

Vogelzang, N. J. (1984) Vascular and other complications of chemotherapy for testicular cancer. *World Journal of Urology*, 2, 32–37.

Vogelzang, N. J., Bosl, G. J., Johnson, K. & Kennedy, B. J. (1981) Raynaud's phenomenon: A common toxicity after combination chemotherapy for testicular cancer. *Annals of Internal Medicine*, 95, 288–292.

Vogelzang, N. J., Frenning, D. H. & Kennedy, B. J. (1980) Coronary artery disease after treatment with bleomycin and vinblastine. *Cancer Treatment Reports*, 64, 1190–1160.

Vogelzang, N. J., Torkelson, J. L. & Kennedy, B. J. (1985) Hypomagnesaemia, renal dysfunction, and Raynaud's phenomenon in patients treated with cisplatin, vinblastine, and bleomycin. *Cancer*, 56, 2765–2770.

Vugrin, D., Herr, H. W., Whitmore, W. F., Sogani, P. C. & Golbey, R. B. (1981) VAB-6 combination chemotherapy in disseminated cancer of the testis. *Annals of Internal Medicine*, 95, 59–61.

Discussion

Rustin Do you think that elevated plasma renin levels with normal blood pressure could be due to compensation against platinum-induced autonomic nephrotoxicity? I have definitely seen this in association with postural hypotension.

Bosl I have no direct data in this matter. No patient had orthostatic hypotension or overt peripheral neuropathy. It is certainly possible, however, that increased plasma renin activity is compensatory to some other event and not related to intrarenal vascular toxicity. We have not detected any evidence of peripheral neuropathy which may indicate that the autonomic nervous system was similarly unaffected.

Rankin Is there any correlation between the development of Raynaud's phenomenon and the presence of high plasma renin levels?

Bosl I cannot comment on such a correlation. The VAB-6 regimen at Memorial Hospital has not been associated with a single case of Raynaud's phenomenon among 166 patients. I am very aware of the existence of this complication and I look for it. The absence of this disease in our patients may be related to the lower doses of velban and bleomycin which we use.

Einhorn This is a very elegant study but I am not sure of its clinical significance. We have followed 175 patients for a minimum of 5 years after PVB treatment, and we have not seen any evidence of treatment-related hypertension. Blood pressure is not significantly elevated over baseline levels. We have had a few patients with mild hypertension or a strong family history of hypertension, who had a sudden acceleration in their diastolic blood pressure when they started cisplatin therapy. This went back to baseline levels after cessation of therapy. In patients with no family history of hypertension we have seen no clinical problems related to their blood pressure.

Bosl We also have not had any clinical problems with hypertension and I do not know the long-term clinical significance of our findings.

Several investigators have suggested that small vessel disease does exist and it is possible that this will lead to hypertension in the long term. We should be observing these patients over a prolonged period for cardiovascular effects. I do not think we will be seeing metastatic tumours in the long term but long-term follow-up is indicated in case second tumours or cardiovascular complications arise.

Safirstein We may be concentrating unnecessarily on the occurrence of hypertension. The real significance of Dr Bosl's work is that high renin levels may be a marker for end organ damage, not only in the kidney, but also in the heart, nervous system and liver. Other vasoactive substances may also be elevated such as AVP (vasopressin), prostaglandins and others indicative of organ damage. The organ defects may be subclinical now but will become manifest later. Organ function tests should be performed under stress in order to detect minor alterations.

Bosl We looked at serum vasopressin levels both before and after water loading and found normal levels and normal suppression.

ototoxicity. The incidence of hearing loss is highest in patients receiving single high dose injections (Reddel et al., 1982). This finding may suggest a correlation between ototoxicity and the peak level of cisplatin in plasma. The complex pharmacology of cisplatin with a second slow phase of elimination (Frick et al., 1979) indicates that the interval between the times of administration is also of importance for development of ototoxic changes.

The total platinum concentration can be determined by atomic absorption spectrometry (Le Roy et al., 1977) which is a complex procedure and not performed routinely. Cisplatin binds extensively to albumin and other serum proteins and the active cytotoxic component of cisplatin is in the unbound fraction. The total level of platinum in serum therefore does not reflect the level of active drug present.

Several risk factors for ototoxicity have been suggested but there is so far no known indicator that predicts the level of susceptibility. A pre-existing hearing loss does not seem to potentiate the ototoxic effect of cisplatin (Piel et al., 1974).

The incidence and severity of hearing loss reported in different clinical studies varies. Many studies are not directly comparable because of different dose schedules, variations in hearing test conditions, lack of a standardized definition of significant change in hearing thresholds, and loss of patients since they are too ill to perform serial audiograms. Even if the effect on hearing were to be found to be more severe with increasing doses of single injections, ototoxicity also occurs in a cumulative manner after several low dose injections (Aguilar-Markulis et al., 1981).

Nephrotoxicity has been ameliorated by using prehydration of the patients and thereafter mannitol or frusemide induced diuresis (Hayes et al., 1977). The incidence and severity of ototoxicity has, however, not significantly been altered by this method of protective administration. In addition, ototoxicity is a rare side effect of frusemide and other loop diuretics. In animal experimental studies loop diuretics have been found to potentiate the ototoxic effect of cisplatin (Brummett, 1981). No clinical studies have shown this type of interaction.

Morphological studies of inner ear damage after cisplatin administration have been performed most often on guinea-pigs (Fleischman et al., 1975; Estrem et al., 1981), although rhesus monkeys and humans have also been studied (Wright & Schaefer, 1982). The primary mechanism of cisplatin responsible for the damage to the cochlea is not known. The most notable morphological alteration in the inner ear caused by cisplatin administration is a destruction of the outer hair cells (OHC) of the organ of Corti. This degeneration of the OHC is most pronounced in the basal turn of the cochlea which is correlated with a high frequency hearing loss. The first row of the OHC is most severely affected. This degenerative pattern is similar to several other ototoxic agents, including the aminoglycosides. The inner hair cells (IHC) may also be destroyed but only after higher doses of cisplatin. There is some contradiction reported in the literature about the morphological alterations of the stria vascularis which may affect the blood–cochlear barrier, ranging from no damage to severe degenerative changes (Tange & Vuzevski, 1984). There is a two- to three-fold increase in platinum concentration in the stria vascularis in comparison to the organ of Corti 2 h after administration of radioactive platinum (Schweitzer et al., 1984).

In order to elucidate some of the questions about the relationship between cisplatin dosage and change in pure tone hearing thresholds, a study was undertaken on patients receiving different doses of cisplatin.

Material and Methods

This preliminary report comprises 186 women with gynaecological cancer. The patients ranged from 26 to 75 years of age (median age 57). A dose of 50 mg of cisplatin/m^2 body surface was given every 4 weeks. Cisplatin was combined with other cytostatic drugs such as adriamycin and melphalan. The cumulative doses of cisplatin varied from 35 to 1120 mg. The audiological evaluations were performed at the Department of Audiology, Karolinska Hospital. Pure-tone audiometry was performed prior to the initiation of cisplatin treatment and repeated after each subsequent treatment course. All tests were performed under optimal conditions in a sound-proof test box using a Madsen OB 822 audiometer and TDH 39 earphones (with MX 41/AR cushion) calibrated according to ISO 389.

Results

The thresholds of the audiograms were compared before and after treatment. Patients were considered to have developed significant hearing loss if they had at least a 15 dB decrease in pure-tone threshold at any frequency, or at least a 10 dB decrease at three adjacent frequencies in one ear. Forty patients showed significant auditory changes. The greatest incidence of hearing loss occurred at 6 kHz and 8 kHz. The highest value of hearing loss at 6 kHz was 30 dB, and at 8 kHz, 40 dB. No significant loss of hearing was detected in the speech frequency range 0.5–2 kHz. Furthermore, there was no relationship between prior hearing acuity and the probability of having further hearing loss.

Conclusion

A moderate dose of cisplatin (50 mg/m^2 every 4 weeks) was not found to affect significantly the cochlear function in the speech frequency range. Regular audiometric monitoring has a low cost efficiency and does not have a place in the basic follow-up studies of patients undergoing low and moderate dose cisplatin treatment. However, it is highly recommendable to follow the hearing function with repeated audiograms during treatment with higher individual doses.

References

Aguilar-Markulis, N. V., Beckley, S., Priore, R. & Mettlin, C. (1981) Auditory toxicity effects of long-term cisdichlorodiammineplatinum II therapy in genitourinary cancer patients. *Journal of Surgical Oncology*, **16**, 111–123.
Brummett, R. E. (1981) Ototoxicity resulting from the combined administration of potent diuretics and other agents. *Scandinavian Journal of Audiology*, Suppl. 14.
Estrem, S. A., Babin, R. W., Ryu, J. H. & Moore, K. C. (1981) Cisdiamminedichloroplatinum II ototoxicity in the guinea pig. *Otolaryngology: Head and Neck Surgery*, **89**, 638–645.
Fleischman, R. W., Stadnicki, S. W., Ethier, M. F. & Schaeppi, U. (1975) Ototoxicity of cis-dichlorodiammine platinum (II) in the guinea pig. *Toxicology and Applied Pharmacology*, **33**, 320–332.
Frick, G. A., Ballentine, R., Driever, C. W. & Kramer, W. G. (1979) Renal excretion kinetics of high-dose cis-dichlorodiammineplatinum (II). Administration with hydration and mannitol diuresis. *Cancer Treatment Reports*, **63**, 13–16.

Table 1. Patient characteristics

Age (yr)	Histology	Therapy	Outcome of therapy	Vascular event	Outcome
24	Teratocarcinoma, embryonal ca.	VBP	CR	Acute myocardial infarction	Died
23	Endodermal sinus	VBP	CR	Rectal infarction	Died
42	Seminoma	VBP	CR	Acute myocardial infarction	Died
58	Choriocarcinoma + embryonal ca.	VBP	NR	Cerebrovascular accident	Died
33	Embryonal ca.	VBP	NR	Acute myocardial infarction	Died

VBP = vinblastine, bleomycin and cisplatin; CR = complete response; NR = no response.

Case reports

The clinical data in the five cases are summarized in Table 1. The VBP chemotherapy regimen consisted of vinblastine 0.15 mg/kg days 1 and 2, bleomycin 30 U days 2, 9 and 16, cisplatin 20 mg/m^2 days 1–5, repeated every 3 weeks.

Patient 1

This 24-year-old white male presented with scrotal swelling. Orchidectomy showed teratocarcinoma. A retroperitoneal lymph node dissection revealed embryonal carcinoma involvement. Pulmonary nodules were noted, and chemotherapy with VBP was started. Complete remission was achieved after six cycles. He remained well for 18 months, but was then found dead. He had no history of coronary artery disease, was a nonsmoker, but was grossly obese. Pre-treatment ECG was normal. He did not receive mediastinal radiation. At autopsy, there was no evidence of tumour. There was 75% focal occlusion of the left anterior descending coronary artery, with a septal acute myocardial infarction, and 50% narrowing of the right coronary artery. The major arteries showed minimal atherosclerosis.

Patient 2

This 23-year-old white male presented with a mediastinal mass in September 1978. Thoracotomy and biopsy showed an endodermal sinus tumour. He had no testicular masses. He received four cycles of VBP, with some response. On day 16 of the fourth cycle he developed sudden rectal pain and bleeding. He died after a rapidly downhill course notable for clostridial sepsis. At autopsy the mediastinal mass was necrotic, with no evidence of viable tumour. Rectal infarction was noted, and was presumed to be the source of clostridial sepsis.

Patient 3

This 42-year-old white male presented with a large abdominal mass. Exploratory laparotomy revealed an anaplastic seminoma. Subsequent right orchidectomy showed seminoma. He received radiation therapy (35 gy) to the abdomen (but not to the mediastinum), and low dose cyclophosphamide, bleomycin and doxorubicin, followed by VBP therapy. The abdominal mass was not detectable after three cycles of VBP chemotherapy. He had no history of coronary artery disease, but had a 25 pack-year smoking history. After a 46-month interval he presented in cardiogenic shock with renal failure and died shortly thereafter. At autopsy, an extensive acute myocardial infarct, involving the entire right ventricle, posterior interventricular septum, posterior and postero-lateral left ventricle, and right atrial appendage was found. There was intimal thickening, fibrosis, and recent thrombosis of the right coronary artery. There was minimal atherosclerosis in the left anterior descending and circumflex coronary arteries. No viable tumour was found.

Patient 4
This 58-year-old white male presented with multiple pulmonary nodules, a mediastinal mass, and an enlarged submental lymph node. There were no testicular masses. Biopsy of the node showed choriocarcinoma with embryonal elements. Chemotherapy with VBP was initiated. On day 6 of cycle 1 he developed acute left hemiparesis. Brain computerized tomography was negative. The hemiparesis resolved. The patient received a further five cycles of VBP, after which he still had extensive pulmonary disease, and received cyclophosphamide, actinomycin D and methotrexate. One month later he developed worsening left hemiparesis and altered mentation. Computerized tomography was again normal. Cerebral angiography was consistent with occlusive arteritis in the right frontal and left temporoparietal regions. He died a few days later. No autopsy was performed.

Patient 5
This 33-year-old white male presented with a left scrotal mass and multiple pulmonary nodules, as well as cervical and supraclavicular lymphadenopathy. Further evaluation showed retroperitoneal adenopathy and hepatic metastases. Orchidectomy revealed embryonal carcinoma. Chemotherapy with VBP was started. He did not receive mediastinal irradiation. After four cycles he had persistent pulmonary and hepatic disease, and received VP-16 and cisplatin, without response. He was then given high dose cytosine arabinoside. On day 15 of cycle 1 he was admitted with neutropenia, sepsis and hypotension. Echocardiography showed marked right ventricular dilatation and dysfunction with minor left ventricular dysfunction. His ECG, initially normal, showed an evolving inferior infarct. A clinical diagnosis of right ventricular infarction was made. The patient died 3 days after admission. No autopsy was performed.

Discussion
The increasing number of reports of life-threatening and fatal vascular episodes following VBP therapy are of great concern. We have described five such cases in which the deaths of the patients were solely or partially due to an acute vascular event. Several case reports documenting major vascular disease following this therapy are summarized in Table 2.

There may be both acute and long-term vascular toxicity. In Kukla's four cases of cerebrovascular accident (Kukla *et al.*, 1982), and in our patient 4, symptoms developed within 48 h of the first treatment. Severe angina and acute myocardial infarction have been noted soon after vincristine (Somers *et al.*, 1976) or vinblastine (Lejonc *et al.*, 1980) therapy. Bodensteiner's patient suffered a clinically documented acute myocardial infarct after the first cycle of therapy, and a fatal myocardial infarct 7 months later, without further chemotherapy. At autopsy, coronary artery

Table 2. Vascular events reported in the literature

Authors (ref.)	No. of patients	Chemotherapy regimen(s)	Vascular events	Outcome of events
Vogelzang et al. (1980)	2	(i) VB+Act D (ii) VB+Act D,MTX, CTX, mithramycin	Coronary artery disease	2 alive
Edwards et al. (1979)	2	VBP	Coronary artery disease	2 dead
Bodensteiner (1981)	1	VBP	Myocardial infarction	1 dead
Greist et al. (1985)	6	VBP VBP+doxorubicin	Coronary artery disease	3 alive, 3 dead
Kukla et al. (1982)	4	Vincristine + BP	Cerebrovascular accident	4 dead
Cohen et al. (1983)	1	VBP	Transient hemianopsia (? neurotoxicity)	1 alive

V = vinblastine; B = bleomycin; Act D = actinomycin D; MTX = methotrexate; CTX = cyclophosphamide; P = cisplatin.

fibrosis was found (Bodensteiner, 1981). In initial toxicity studies, bleomycin was found to cause an acute necrotizing coronary arteritis in rhesus monkeys (Schaeppi et al., 1973), but the long-term potential of this lesion to result in arterial fibrosis was not assessed. Severe hypomagnesaemia causes ventricular fibrillation (Iseri, Freed & Bures, 1975), and therefore cisplatin-induced hypomagnesaemia could contribute to early cardiovascular morbidity.

Raynaud's phenomenon becomes clinically evident a mean of 10 months after starting therapy (Vogelzang et al., 1981). Coronary artery disease may occur months to years after therapy. The cause of this chronic vascular toxicity is obscure, and the relative contribution of various drugs is unknown. Autonomic neuropathy induced by vinblastine, and microvascular changes seen after bleomycin, are clearly long term in nature. Hypomagnesaemia occurs in 87% of testicular cancer patients treated with cisplatin (Vogelzang et al., 1985), and may persist for up to 3 years (Schilsky, Barlock & Ozols, 1982). Since, under hypomagnesaemic conditions, arterial smooth muscle shows increased sensitivity to agents which induce contraction (Turlapaty & Altura, 1980), cisplatin may also contribute to long-term vascular toxicity.

Based on our experience with these five patients and two previously reported (Vogelzang et al., 1980), and a careful review of the literature, we suggest that the combination of vinblastine, bleomycin and cisplatin as used in the therapy of germ cell tumours is associated with life-threatening vascular toxicities. Although there is as yet no direct evidence linking VBP chemotherapy to these vascular events, we believe that the circumstantial evidence is strong. The potential toxicity is serious, and might not ordinarily be watched for, since the age group at risk for germ cell tumours normally has a low prevalence of major vascular disease. This is particularly significant because these young patients have an excellent outlook for cure of their malignancies. We believe that it is therefore important that the possibility of an acute vascular event, either at the time of therapy or months to years later, be brought to the attention of physicians treating such patients.

References

Bodensteiner, D. C. (1981) Fatal coronary artery fibrosis after treatment with bleomycin, vinblastine, and cis-platinum. *Southern Medical Journal*, **74**, 898–899.

Cohen, R. J., Cuneo, R. A., Cruciger, M. P. & Jackman, A. E. (1983) Transient left homonymous hemianopsia and encephalopathy following treatment of testicular carcinoma with cisplatinum, vinblastine, and bleomycin. *Journal of Clinical Oncology*, **1**, 392–393.

Comis, R. L., Kuppinger, M. S., Ginsberg, S. J., Crooke, S. T., Gilbert, R., Auchincloss, J. H. & Prestayko, A. W. (1979) Role of single breath carbon monoxide-diffusing capacity in monitoring the pulmonary effects of bleomycin in germ cell tumor patients. *Cancer Research*, **39**, 5076–5080.

Dunagin, W. G. (1983) Clinical toxicity of chemotherapeutic agents: dermatologic toxicity. *Seminars in Oncology*, **9**, 14–22.

Edwards, G. S., Lane, M. & Smith, F. E. (1979) Long-term treatment with cis-dichlorodiammineplatinum (II)-vinblastine-bleomycin: possible association with severe coronary artery disease. *Cancer Treatment Reports*, **63**, 551–552.

Einhorn, L. H. (1981) Testicular cancer as a model for a curable neoplasm. *Cancer Research*, **41**, 3275–3280.

Griest, A., Roth, B., Einhorn, L. & Williams, S. (1985) Cisplatin combination chemotherapy for disseminated germ cell tumors: long term followup. (Abstract). *Proceedings of the American Society of Clinical Oncology*, **4**, C-388.

Harrell, R. M., Sibley, R. & Vogelzang, N. J. (1982) Renal vascular lesions after chemotherapy with vinblastine, bleomycin, and cisplatin. *American Journal of Medicine*, **73**, 429–433.

Iseri, L. T., Freed, J. & Bures, A. R. (1975) Magnesium deficiency and cardiac disorders. *American Journal of Medicine*, **58**, 837–846.

Kukla, L. J., McGuire, W. P., Lad, T. & Saltiel, M. (1982) Acute vascular episodes associated with therapy for carcinomas of the upper aerodigestive tract with bleomycin, vincristine and cisplatin. *Cancer Treatment Reports*, **66**, 369–370.

Lejonc, J. L., Vernant, J. P., Macquin, I. & Castagne, A. (1980) Myocardial infarction following vinblastine treatment. *Lancet*, **ii**, 692.

Schaeppi, U., Thompson, G. R., Fleishman, R. W., Baker, J. R., Rosenkrantz, H., Ilievski, V., Cooney, D. A. & Davis, R. D. (1973) Preclinical toxicologic evaluation of bleomycin in rhesus monkeys. *Cancer Chemotherapy Reports*, Part 3, **4**, 31–39.

Schilsky, R. L., Barlock, A. & Ozols, R. F. (1982) Persistent hypomagnesemia following cisplatin chemotherapy for testicular cancer. *Cancer Treatment Reports*, **66**, 1767–1769.

Somers, G., Abramow, M., Wittek, M. & Naets, J. P. (1976) Myocardial infarction: a complication of vincristine treatment. *Lancet*, **ii**, 690.

Turlapaty, P. D. M. V. & Altura, B. M. (1980) Magnesium deficiency produces spasms of coronary arteries: relationship to etiology of sudden death ischemic heart disease. *Science*, **208**, 198–200.

Vogelzang, N. J., Bosl, G. J., Johnson, K. & Kennedy, B. J. (1981) Raynaud's phenomenon: a common toxicity after combination chemotherapy for testicular cancer. *Annals of Internal Medicine*, **95**, 288–292.

Vogelzang, N. J., Frenning, D. H. & Kennedy, B. J. (1980) Coronary artery disease after treatment with bleomycin and vinblastine. *Cancer Treatment Reports*, **64**, 1159–1160.

Vogelzang, N. J., Torkelson, J. L. & Kennedy, B. J. (1985) Hypomagnesemia, renal dysfunction and Raynaud's phenomenon in patients treated with cisplatin, vinblastine, and bleomycin. *Cancer*, **56**, 2765–2771.

Discussion

Schmoll I would like to describe a new case from our Hannover series. A 21-year-old man was treated with platinum, high dose VP-16 and bleomycin, and later died of myocardial infarction. At autopsy he was found to have extensive coronary atherosclerosis. My question is, what is the mechanism of action contributing to his atherosclerosis since bleomycin is said to act more at the microvasculature level and supposedly only causes sclerosis (fibrosis) without the atheromatous component of atherosclerosis?

Vogelzang The lesion *may* be related to initial endothelial cell injury as evidenced by increased level of von Willebrand factor, followed by endothelial hyperplasia and luminal obliteration. Alternatively there may have been platelet activation and thrombosis.

Other side effects we have seen include oesophageal sclerosis which occasionally occurs and may be severe with complete or almost complete obliteration. The reason for this is unclear but is perhaps due to some kind of vascular insult to the oesophagus.

Oliver The difference in incidence of Raynaud's phenomenon between the Minnesota and the MSKCC patients could be related to the administration of bleomycin by pulse in Minnesota and by continuous infusion at MSKCC, or is it an innate difference between PVB as opposed to VAB?

Vogelzang All our patients received bleomycin injected as an i.v. bolus.

Oliver Our own experience of Raynaud's phenomenon would support this as over the last 2 years we have treated 40 patients all with continuous i.v. infusions of bleomycin having previously used pulse therapy, and Raynaud's phenomenon is no longer seen. However, this new regimen has not eliminated the other arterial complications as we have recently seen a CVA in a 30-year-old female patient with an ovarian germ cell tumour.

Vogelzang Vascular events are giving cause for concern in patients in the USA and I have heard of a patient losing several digits because of necrosis after intramuscular bleomycin and another having inferior mesenteric infarction several days after initiation of chemotherapy. Also, obliterative arteritis of the lower extremities has been seen. Vascular disease is very complex and difficult to piece together.

Levi The precise cause-and-effect relationship of these heterogeneous vascular events is difficult to explain. Could you indicate the denominator from which the illustrative cases have been drawn so that we may have some indication of the possible mechanisms? In the first Australasian germ cell tumour study, a total number of 260 patients received PVB, bleomycin being given as a bolus, and no such vascular events have been reported.

Vogelzang The denominator is difficult to define precisely because of selective patient referral. Perhaps our five PVB cases come from 150–250 patients in the Minnesota and Chicago areas so that the incidence is low.

A report from Einhorn's group indicates six vascular events from 200 patients; three of the patients are living and three are dead.

Einhorn That is correct. Let me say that trying to work out the cause-and-effect in such events is very complicated because different drug protocols have been used in different cases. We do not know if cisplatin, bleomycin or actinomycin D affects the vessels and indeed two of your patients never received platinum, but were treated with bleomycin and VP-16. In our six cases with vascular events, five had mediastinal radiotherapy so that the vessels may have been affected by chemotherapy alone or a combination of chemotherapy and radiotherapy.

In the patients we are treating there is a denominator of vascular events, but this is small, probably in the region of 1–2%. Some events may be due to chemotherapy and others are probably not. There are cases of vascular events following one course of chemotherapy but no further event after re-introduction to the same drugs. For example, CVA was seen after initial but not after subsequent drug therapy, and myocardial infarction has occurred initially but not repeated after resumption of chemotherapy. Can we ascribe these complications purely to the effect of drugs, or should we also consider factors such as the level of hydration, or the anti-emetics used along with the chemotherapeutic agents?

Vogelzang In young patients with atypical and unexpected vascular complications I think we must consider the drugs as the most likely aetiological factor. Careful autopsies must be performed if death occurs following vascular events. I have even shocked pathologists by personally dissecting out all the digital arteries and surprised them by demonstrating a substantial degree of endothelial hyperplasia. Information from clinical data will be slow to collect, but we have material available and we must be prepared to look for it.

Schmoll Yes, we must follow these patients carefully and if they are killed accidentally we must try to perform an autopsy.

Einhorn I believe that in animal models, vascular abnormalities have not been detected following single agent platinum therapy, although this has been looked for very carefully.

Vogelzang It is my hypothesis that bleomycin and vinblastine are more important than cisplatin in the causation of vascular events.

Testicular cancer and fertility

J. G. BERTHELSEN *Laboratory of Reproductive Biology, University Department of Obstetrics and Gynaecology Y, Rigshospitalet, Copenhagen, and University Department of Gynaecology and Obstetrics, Herlev Hospital, Copenhagen*

Summary

Before treatment, a little over one-half of patients with testicular cancer have fathered children, while one-fifth have a history of sterility. Radiotherapy with a gonadal dose of less than 1.5 Gy seems to do little permanent damage to fertility. Following cisplatin-based combination chemotherapy, a number of conceptions have been reported. The newer regimens affect spermatogenesis less than earlier ones due to a lower toxicity of the drugs and shorter duration of the treatment. New modifications of retroperitoneal lymphadenectomy may save ejaculatory ability in over one-half of the patients. It is uncertain whether this procedure is less detrimental to fertility than the cisplatin-based combination chemotherapy. Even though semen quality is often poor before treatment, cryopreservation of semen should be considered since *in vitro* fertilization may be successful even with very poor semen quality. There are no indications in the literature of permanent adverse genetic effects of the treatment.

Key words.   Testicular cancer, fertility, radiotherapy, chemotherapy.

Introduction

Due to the increasingly successful treatment of testicular germ cell cancer, fertility and genetic implications of the disease and the treatment have gained major importance.

The effect on spermatogenesis of the disease itself and the treatment has been studied on semen samples and testicular biopsy specimens over the past decade (Thachil, Jewett & Rider, 1981; Berthelsen & Skakkebæk, 1983; Berthelsen, 1984a). However, when assessing the actual effect on fertility, laboratory tests are of no avail, and nothing short of computing conception rates will reveal the true picture. This type of work is only in its infancy at the moment.

The present report reviews data on conceptions before and after the various treatments for testicular cancer and deals briefly with the genetic implications of the treatment.

Methods

Reports on fertility in patients with testicular cancer should include details of age, type and stage of the tumour, and the treatment. It should be clearly stated whether

Correspondence: Jørgen G. Berthelsen, Laboratory of Reproductive Biology, Afsnit 4052, Rigshospitalet, DK-2100 Copenhagen Ø, Denmark

the sample of patients is biased with respect to the entire population of patients with testicular cancer in that particular area. Fertility data include: age and sex of children, length of period of infertility, or whether conception is desired. Data on early spontaneous abortions are usually not well remembered/recorded and should be left out in retrospective surveys.

The mere number of children conceived is a rather crude measure of fertility, since it does not take into account the time needed for the conceptions to occur. Therefore, conception rates should be computed. For this purpose, 'life table' analysis of the cumulative probability of conception is very well suited (Scammell et al., 1985) and easily amenable to statistical comparison between groups of treated patients and/or suitable reference groups.

As will be seen in the following, these techniques have not yet been implemented and usually few details are given in the reports on fertility in patients with testicular cancer.

Fertility before treatment
Many patients have not yet completed their family prior to treatment for testicular cancer. A little over one-half of the patients have fathered children while one-fifth have not been able to conceive in spite of a wish to do so (Table 1).

The proportion of infertile couples in these studies is probably higher than in the general population of the same age. This would not be surprising since histological analysis has shown that one-fourth of these patients have totally or partially disrupted spermatogenesis in the contralateral testis at the time of diagnosis of the tumour (Berthelsen & Skakkebæk, 1983).

Few details are given on the actual number and sex of the children. However, in our own survey of 179 patients with testicular cancer (Berthelsen & Rørth, unpublished, Table 1) 34% had no children, 26% had one child, 27% had two children and 13% had three or more children. The ratio of boys to girls was 0.86, which is not significantly different from the expected 1.05.

Fertility after treatment
Conceptions during the first 2 post-treatment years have been rare. Not only are patients advised not to have children during or immediately after treatment, but, in addition, radiotherapy and chemotherapy have usually rendered the men azoospermic for at least 1–2 years (Thachil et al., 1981; Drasga et al., 1983; Berthelsen, 1984a).

Besides removal of the diseased testis, three main treatment modalities have been used during the past two decades: irradiation of the regional lymph nodes +/− adjuvant chemotherapy, combination chemotherapy, and retroperitoneal lymphadenectomy (DATECA Working Group, 1983; Lange et al., 1983).

Radiotherapy +/− adjuvant chemotherapy. Radiation to the para-aortic and ipsilateral common and superficial iliac lymph nodes of 40 Gy gives scattered irradiation to the remaining testis of 0.2–1.3 Gy (Berthelsen, 1984a). In the past, adjuvant chemotherapy such as vincristine and bleomycin often was given to nonseminoma cases. In spite of the vast number of patients treated with radiotherapy +/− adjuvant chemotherapy, little data on fertility is available (Table 2).

Table 1. Fertility in patients with testicular cancer before treatment

Authors	Age in years (mean (range))	Men with children (No. (%))	Men without children Infertile	Men without children Not wished conception	No. and sex of children
Haubrich & Harms, 1973	(20–64)	43 (69)	12	7	?
Orecklin et al., 1973	33 (16–60)	42 (63)	10	25	?
Bracken & Johnson, 1976	?	47 (59)	33		116
Kuber et al., 1980	35 (20–85)	112 (48)	122		?
Drasga et al., 1983	28 (17–50)	36 (52)	33		?
Johnson et al., 1984	29 (19–51)	9 (50)	9		?
Fritz & Weissbach, 1985	29 (18–44)	72 (58)	52		?
Furuhata & Ogawa, 1985	?	18 (78)	5		?
Nijman et al., 1985	28 (?)	11 (20)	33	10	?
Berthelsen & Rørth, unpub.	36 (19–81)	119 (63)	25	35	219
Total		509 (55)	411		M:F = 0.856*

*F = girls, M = boys.

Table 2. Fertility in patients with testicular cancer after radiotherapy

Authors	Radiation dose	Age in years (mean (range))	No. of patients	No. of patients with children (%)	No. and sex of children	Time after therapy in months (mean (range))
Amelar et al., 1971	30–55 Gy	31 (19–35)	7	3 (43)	1 M, 3 F*	48 (26–72)
Orecklin et al., 1973	30–45 Gy	33 (16–60)	37	16 (43)	?	? (12–240)
Smithers et al., 1973	40 Gy	?	446	36 (8)	52 children	?
Kuber et al., 1980	30–45 Gy	35 (20–85)	234	4 (2)	?	? (36–60)
Panduro (cited by Berthelsen 1984b)	30–40 Gy	?	124	49 (40)	?	?
Furuhata & Ogawa, 1985	?	?	23	9 (39)	?	?
Senturia et al., 1985	30 Gy	?	?	27	40 children	? (1–120)
Total				117/871 (13%)		

*F = girls, M = boys.

The survey of Panduro (cited in Berthelsen, 1984b) indicated that approximately two-thirds of those wishing to have children were able to do so. This suggests that little permanent damage to fertility is done by such radiotherapy and adjuvant chemotherapy.

Combination chemotherapy. Early reports on semen quality and fertility after combination chemotherapy for advanced testicular cancer showed azoospermia or extremely poor semen quality (Fosså et al., 1980) and very few conceptions. However, with the advent of cisplatin-based combination chemotherapy, the outlook for fertility appears much better.

The combination of cisplatin, vinblastine and bleomycin (VBP) has been widely used during the last decade as treatment for advanced stages or recurrence of testicular cancer (Einhorn & Donohue, 1977). There exists no assessment of the effect on fertility of the individual drugs; however, after treatment with three or four cycles of the drugs in combination, a temporary azoospermia develops and usually lasts for more than 12 months (Drasga et al., 1983; Lange et al., 1983). However, spermatogenesis recovers in many patients and an increasing number of reports (Table 3) documents that fertility may be preserved after treatment with VBP as well as with other modern combination chemotherapy regimens for advanced testicular cancer.

Observation times are still rather short and the reports lack sufficient details for reliable conception rates to be calculated. However, there seems to be no doubt that these regimens are less toxic to spermatogenesis than those used for instance in Hodgkin's disease (Waxman et al., 1982). This is probably caused by a lower toxicity of the drugs and a shorter duration of treatment.

Retroperitoneal lymphadenectomy. This extensive surgical procedure has lost importance with the advent of effective combination chemotherapy. However, it is still favoured by some as a diagnostic and therapeutic procedure (Lange et al., 1983). In most surveys, retroperitoneal lymphadenectomy frequently causes anejaculation by nonemission or retrograde ejaculation of semen due to surgical destruction of sympathetic paravertebral nerves and the superior hypogastric nerve plexus (Nijman et al., 1982; Chiou, Fraley & Lange, 1984). However, it is becoming apparent that graded extent of the procedure and careful delineation of the dissection may save ejaculatory ability in at least half of the patients (Chiou et al., 1984; Fosså et al., 1985a; Fritz & Weissbach, 1985; Table 4). Furthermore, sympathomimetic treatment may restore ejaculation in additional patients (Nijman et al., 1982; Lange et al., 1983; Table 4).

Clearly, the modified lymphadenectomy allows preservation of fertility in at least some patients (Table 4); however, it is still uncertain whether this procedure is less detrimental to fertility than combination chemotherapy.

Cryopreservation and in vitro *fertilization*
It is possible to store semen in the frozen state in liquid nitrogen for many years and subsequently use it for artificial insemination. The conception rate is dependent not only on the freezing and thawing techniques, but also on the prestorage semen quality bearing in mind that some deterioration always occurs during this process.

Cryopreservation of pretreatment semen samples from men with testicular

Table 3. Fertility in patients with testicular cancer after treatment with cisplatin-based combination chemotherapy

Authors	Treatment	Age in years (mean (range))	No. of patients*	No. of patients with children (%)	No. and sex of children	Time after therapy in months (mean (range))
Brenner et al., 1983	VAB-6 +/− RPLD	? (17–46)	61	1 (2)	1	?
Drasga et al., 1983	VBP 3–4 × VBP	26 (17–40) 30 (20–50)	34 25	3 (9) 8 (32)	1 M, 2 pregn.† 2 M, 3 F, 3 pregn.	? (1–36) ? (13–57)
Chiou et al., 1984	VB/VBP +/− RPLD	?	34	3 (9)	?	? (?−>18)
Fosså et al., 1985b	3–4 × VBP +/− RPLD +/− X-ray +/− other chemoth.	?	90	5 (6)	?	? (1–36)
Senturia et al., 1985	9 VBP 6 VP + etoposide 6 VB 4 other	?	?	25	30 children	? (12–132)
Total				21/244 (9%)		

VAB-6: vinblastine, dactinomycine, bleomycin, cyclophosphamide, cisplatin. VBP: cisplatin, vinblastine, bleomycin. RPLD: retroperitoneal lymphadenectomy. *Patients with vasectomy not included. †F = girl, M = boy, pregn. = pregnancy ongoing.

Table 4. Fertility in patients with testicular cancer after retroperitoneal lymphadenectomy

Authors	Additional treatment	Age in years (mean (range))	No. of patients	No. of patients with ejaculation (No. with ejaculation only after medication)	No. of patients with children (%)	Time after therapy in months (mean (range))
Bracken & Johnson, 1976	+/− radiotherapy	?	50	30 (?)	7 (14)	?
Nijman et al., 1982	6 patients: chemoth.	27 (18–42)	14	2 (10)	5 (36)*	31 (6–78)
Chiou et al., 1984	?	?	86	39 (12)	16 (19)	? (1–36)
Fosså et al., 1985a	36 patients: unilat. RPLD 61 patients: bilateral. RPLD +/− chemoth.	30 (15–60)	97	39 (3)	14 (14)	22 (?)
Fritz & Weissbach, 1985		29 (18–44)				
Radical RPLD			87	20 (?)	?	?
Modified RPLD			37	29 (?)	?	?
Total			371	159 (25)	42/247 (17%)	

RPLD: retroperitoneal lymphadenectomy. *3 boys, 1 girl, 1 spontaneous abortion.

cancer has not been extensively used since the pretreatment semen quality is often rather poor. However, recent reports demonstrate the feasibility of this procedure (Scammell et al., 1985; Schoysman, 1985).

Three conceptions occurred in eleven couples (Scammell et al., 1985). All conceptions occurred within seven cycles of treatment and in successful cases, prestorage sperm counts were 20×10^6/ml or higher with 40% or more motile sperms.

A limited amount of frozen semen will be available from each man. In order to avoid unnecessary wastage of semen, the wife should undergo a thorough fertility investigation prior to insemination. Furthermore, the timing of insemination should be based upon an accurate method of predicting ovulation, such as ultrasonic measurement of the developing follicle, LH surge detection (Scammell et al., 1985), or hCG injection.

While artificial insemination demands a large number of motile spermatozoa, it is possible to induce pregnancy by *in vitro* fertilization and embryo replacement using cryopreserved semen of much lesser quality (Mahadevan, Trounson & Leeton, 1983; Rowland et al., 1985). Since this technique is becoming increasingly available, cryopreservation should now be considered even for semen of low quality.

Genetic implications of cancer treatment

The increasing number of post-treatment pregnancies makes it pertinent to consider the risk of introducing permanent chromosome aberrations or gene mutations in the spermatogonia during treatment for testicular cancer. Such changes could be passed on to the progeny. However, it has never been possible to demonstrate an irradiation induced increase of heritable diseases in human populations. Neither does the literature carry any indication of permanent adverse genetic effects of the chemotherapeutic agents used in treatment of testicular cancer (Smithers, Wallace & Austin, 1973; Senturia, Peckham & Peckham, 1985). In spite of this, amniocentesis is often performed in post-treatment pregnancies as a safeguard against chromosome aberrations.

Concluding remarks

Testicular cancer treatment is very successful and we are now in a position where we can choose among several equally effective regimens.

Consequently, fertility is one of the factors which have to be taken into account when choosing a treatment for testicular cancer. However, knowledge of the effect on fertility of the various treatment modalities is extremely limited as demonstrated in the present paper.

This review serves as a plea for new reports on pretreatment and post-treatment fertility after the various treatment regimens giving sufficient details not only for the fortunate patients who become fathers, but also for the remaining patients.

References

Amelar, R. D., Dubin, L. & Hotchkiss, R. S. (1971) Restoration of fertility following unilateral orchiectomy and radiation therapy for testicular tumors. *Journal of Urology*, **106**, 714–718.

Berthelsen, J. G. (1984a) Sperm counts and serum follicle-stimulating hormone levels before and after radiotherapy and chemotherapy in men with testicular germ cell cancer. *Fertility and Sterility*, **41**, 281–286.
Berthelsen, J. G. (1984b) *Andrological Aspects of Testicular Cancer*. Scriptor, Copenhagen.
Berthelsen, J. G. & Skakkebæk, N. E. (1983) Gonadal function in men with testis cancer. *Fertility and Sterility*, **39**, 68–75.
Bracken, R. B. & Johnson, D. E. (1976) Sexual function and fecundity after treatment for testicular tumors. *Urology*, **7**, 35–38.
Brenner, J., Vugrin, D. & Whitmore, W. F. Jr (1983) Effect of treatment on fertility and sexual function in males with non seminomatous germ cell tumors of the testis. (Abstract C-565). *Proceedings of the American Society of Clinical Oncology*, **2**, 44.
Chiou, R-K., Fraley, E. E. & Lange, P. H. (1984) Newer ideas about fertility in patients with testicular cancer. *World Journal of Urology*, **2**, 26–31.
DATECA Working Group (1983) The Danish testicular carcinoma study. *Danish Medical Bulletin*, **30**, 1–3.
Drasga, R. E., Einhorn, L. H., Williams, S. D., Patel, D. N. & Stevens, E. E. (1983) Fertility after chemotherapy for testicular cancer. *Journal of Clinical Oncology*, **1**, 179–183.
Einhorn, L. H. & Donohue, J. P. (1977) Cis-Diamminedichloroplatinum, Vinblastine, and Bleomycin combination chemotherapy in disseminated testicular cancer. *Annals of Internal Medicine*, **87**, 293–298.
Fosså, S. D., Klepp, O., Aakvaag, A. & Molne, K. (1980) Testicular function after combined chemotherapy for metastatic testicular cancer. *International Journal of Andrology*. **3**, 59–65.
Fosså, S. D., Ous, S., Åbyholm, T. & Loeb, M. (1985a) Post-treatment fertility in patients with testicular cancer, I. Influence of retroperitoneal lymph node dissection on ejaculatory potency. *British Journal of Urology*, **57**, 204–209.
Fosså, S. D., Ous, S., Åbyholm, T., Norman, N. & Loeb, M. (1985b) Post-treatment fertility in patients with testicular cancer. II. Influence of cis-platin-based combination chemotherapy and of retroperitoneal surgery on hormone and sperm cell production. *British Journal of Urology*, **57**, 210–214.
Fritz, K. & Weissbach, L. (1985) Sperm parameters and ejaculation before and after operative treatment of patients with germ-cell testicular cancer. *Fertility and Sterility*, **43**, 451–454.
Furuhata, A. & Ogawa, K. (1985) Studies of testicular function after treatment for testicular tumor. I. Fertilization of patients with testicular tumor before and after treatment. *Japanese Journal of Urology*, **76**, 1022–1028.
Haubrich, R. & Harms, I. (1973) Unfruchtbarkeit beim einseitigen Hodenkrebs. *Strahlentherapie*, **146**, 94–103.
Johnson, D. H., Hainsworth, J. D., Linde, R. B. & Greco, F. A. (1984) Testicular function following combination chemotherapy with cis-platin, vinblastine, and bleomycin. *Medical and Pediatric Oncology*, **12**, 233–238.
Kuber, W., Lunglmayr, G., Seitz, W., Grauthoff, H. & Weissbach, L. (1980) Fertilität bei Patienten mit Seminom des Hodens. *Urologe A*, **19**, 272–275.
Lange, P. H., Narayan, P., Vogelzang, N. J., Shafer, R. B., Kennedy, B. J. & Fraley, E. E. (1983) Return of fertility after treatment for nonseminomatous testicular cancer: changing concepts. *Journal of Urology*, **129**, 1131–1135.
Mahadevan, M. M., Trounson, A. O. & Leeton, J. F. (1983) Successful use of human semen cryobanking for in vitro fertilization. *Fertility and Sterility*, **40**, 340–343.
Nijman, J. M., Jager, S., Boer, P. W., Kremer, J., Oldhoff, J. & Koops, H. S. (1982) The treatment of ejaculation disorders after retroperitoneal lymph node dissection. *Cancer*, **50**, 2967–2971.
Nijman, J. M., Koops, H. S., Kremer, J., Willemse, P. H. B., Sleijfer, D. Th. & Oldhoff, J. (1985) Fertility and hormonal function in patients with a nonseminomatous tumor of the testis. *Archives of Andrology*, **14**, 239–246.
Orecklin, J. R., Kaufman, J. J. & Thompson, R. W. (1973) Fertility in patients treated for malignant testicular tumors. *Journal of Urology*, **109**, 293–295.
Rowland, G. F., Cohen, J., Steptoe, P. C. & Hewitt, J. (1985) Pregnancy following in vitro fertilization using cryopreserved semen from a man with testicular teratoma. *Urology*, **26**, 33–36.
Scammell, G. E., White, N., Stedronska, J., Hendry, W. F., Edmonds, D. K. & Jeffcoate, S. L. (1985) Cryopreservation of semen in men with testicular tumour or Hodgkin's disease: Results of artificial insemination of their partners. *Lancet*, July 6, 31–32.

Schoysman, R. (1985) Problèmes d'infertilité après radiothérapie et chimiothérapie pour tumeurs testiculaires. *Acta Urologica Belgica*, **53**, 451–456.

Senturia, Y. D., Peckham, C. S. & Peckham, M. J. (1985) Children fathered by men treated for testicular cancer. *Lancet*, October 5, 766–769.

Smithers, D. W., Wallace, D. M. & Austin, D. E. (1973) Fertility after unilateral orchidectomy and radiotherapy for patients with malignant tumours of the testis. *British Medical Journal*, **iv**, 77–79.

Thachil, J. V., Jewett, M. A. S. & Rider, W. D. (1981) The effects of cancer and cancer therapy on male fertility. *Journal of Urology*, **126**, 141–145.

Waxman, J. H. X., Terry, Y. A., Wrigley, P. F. M., Malpas, J. S., Rees, L. H., Besser, G. M. & Lister, T. A. (1982) Gonadal function in Hodgkin's disease: long-term follow-up of chemotherapy. *British Medical Journal*, **285**, 1612–1613.

Pituitary and testicular hormonal function after treatment for germ cell tumours

G. J. BOSL and D. BAJORUNAS *The Solid Tumor Service and the Endocrine Service, Department of Medicine, Memorial Sloan-Kettering Cancer Center, and Department of Medicine, Cornell University Medical College*

Summary

The endocrine effects of cisplatin based chemotherapy in patients with germ cell tumours were studied in twenty-two patients 9+ to 24+ months after completing treatment. The mean basal FSH and stimulated LH and FSH levels were found to be elevated in treated patients when compared to untreated controls. Serum testosterone levels in treated patients were similar to those in untreated controls. Mean basal LH and FSH levels tended to return toward normal in those patients treated more than 18 months prior to study, and were lower in patients less than 25 years of age at the time of treatment when compared to those aged over 25. These data demonstrate that compensated hypogonadism is common after treatment for metastatic germ cell tumours, that young patients appear to be more resistant to the effects of cisplatin based chemotherapy, and that these effects tend to recover with time.

Key words. Pituitary, testicular, germ cell tumours.

Introduction

Most patients with metastatic germ cell tumours in the 1980s will be cured of their disease with the use of cisplatin based chemotherapy. Therapy related complications have been described after treatment in all other curable malignancies and have generally included gonadal dysfunction. The best example in the adult is Hodgkin's disease, wherein most patients who receive MOPP (nitrogen mustard, vincristine, procarbazine, prednisone) suffer gonadal dysfunction which may be persistent for long periods of time (Sherins & De Vita, 1973; Roeser, Stochs & Smith, 1978). The situation in patients with germ cell tumours is complicated by the fact that many patients have gonadal dysfunction prior to treatment (Thachil, Jewett & Rider, 1981). Therefore, we conducted a study of the pituitary–testicular axis in patients with germ cell tumours, both in those who had previously received chemotherapy and in a group who had not.

Patients and Methods

Twenty-two men who had achieved complete remission (CR) after cisplatin based chemotherapy at Memorial Sloan-Kettering Cancer Center (MSKCC) and six men

Correspondence: George J. Bosl, Memorial Hospital, 1275 York Avenue, New York, NY 10021, U.S.A.

who had not received chemotherapy were studied. Twenty-one had had a unilateral orchidectomy for diagnosis and the remaining patient had a mediastinal seminoma. Three treated patients had a history of cryptorchidism. One control patient had metastatic disease at the time of the study. The twenty-two patients who had achieved CR had been free of disease for a median of 24+ (9+ to 54+) months. Nineteen of twenty-two treated patients had received VAB-6 (cyclophosphamide + vinblastine + bleomycin + cisplatin + actinomycin) and three had received etoposide + cisplatin.

Tests of endocrine function were done in the Clinical Research Center unit at the New York Hospital–Cornell Medical Center. Blood samples were obtained for baseline levels of human chorionic gonadotrophin (hCG), luteinizing hormone (LH), follicle stimulating hormone (FSH), thyroid stimulating hormone (TSH), and prolactin. Gonadotrophin releasing hormone (GnRH) 200 µg and thyroid releasing hormone (TRH) 200 µg were administered as an intravenous bolus. Blood samples were then obtained at 30, 60 and 120 min for hCG, LH, FSH, TSH, and prolactin. Samples for T4 and T3 resin uptake were also obtained at $T = 120$ min. In thirteen treated patients, hCG stimulation was also performed. HCG 10,000 units was administered by intramuscular injection and samples for testosterone were obtained at 0, 24 and 48 h: on one patient, only a 48 h sample was obtained. An increase in the serum testosterone level of greater than 50% over the baseline value was considered a normal response (Mortimer *et al.*, 1973). Hormone assays were performed by techniques previously described (Korth-Schultz, Levine & New, 1976; Kulin & Hamwood, 1974; Odell, Rayford & Ross, 1967). All the results are stated as mean values ± SEM. However, because of the small number of untreated patients and the heteroscedasticity of treated and untreated data sets, a Wilcoxon test was performed to compare these two data sets.

Results

The results of baseline and peak LH and FSH levels are summarized in Table 1. Basal LH levels were elevated in both treated and untreated patients. However, peak LH levels were markedly higher in previously treated patients. In contrast, basal FSH levels were significantly higher in previously treated patients, as were peak levels after GnRH. Interestingly, all patients who had been treated with

Table 1. Comparison of hormone values in treated and untreated patients

	Treated	Untreated	P value*
Luteinizing hormone (mIU/ml)			
Baseline	15.9 ± 6.6	16.0 ± 5.3	NS
Peak	105 ± 8	66 ± 16	0.051
Follicle stimulating hormone (mIU/ml)			
Baseline	17.3 ± 2.8	3.8 ± 0.6	0.001
Peak	46.6 ± 6	14 ± 6	0.003

*Wilcoxon test.

etoposide + cisplatin had elevated baseline and peak LH and FSH values which were at or above the mean values in two of the three patients studied.

Testosterone levels in treated (581 ± 77 ng/dl) and untreated patients (555 ± 81 ng/dl) were not statistically different. However, one treated patient had a subnormal (157 ng/dl) testosterone level and eight of thirteen patients had a peak rise in serum testosterone less than 50% above baseline.

Within the group of treated patients, those 25 years or younger at the time of treatment had lower FSH values (8.3 ± 1.7 mIU/ml) than those older than 25 years (22.4 ± 3.6 mIU/ml) ($P = 0.01$). A trend toward a difference in LH values was observed in patients less than 25 years of age compared to those over 25 years of age at treatment, but this did not reach statistical significance ($P = 0.65$). Similarly, patients who had been studied within 18 months of completing chemotherapy had higher LH levels (20.5 ± 2.8 mIU/ml) than those who were studied more than 18 months after completing treatment (13.2 ± 1.1 mIU/ml) ($P = 0.01$). However, no statistically significant differences were found in FSH levels.

Basal thyroid and peak thyroid function tests and prolactin levels were normal in both treated and untreated patients and were not statistically significantly different.

Discussion

These data indicate that patients treated for metastatic germ cell tumours with VAB-6 and etoposide + cisplatin have nearly universal defects in gonadal hormonal function. The pattern of these abnormalities (elevated gonadotrophin levels and normal testosterone levels) indicates a compensated state of hypogonadism. The evidence indicates that younger patients are more resistant to the effects of this therapy, and that there is recovery with time. We cannot comment about fertility and sperm production since these studies were not performed. Greater than two-thirds of the patients had had a prior retroperitoneal lymph node dissection which precluded semen analysis. It is interesting to note that the control patients also had elevated LH levels indicating antecedent Leydig cell dysfunction. However, the markedly abnormal response to GnRH in treated patients when compared to control patients indicates that additional damage to the Leydig cell population is induced by chemotherapy. The consequences of the hypersecretion of gonadotrophins is unknown, but in hypothyroid patients with prolonged hypersecretion of TSH, pituitary enlargement with visual field defects has been reported (Vagenakis, Dole & Braverman, 1976).

Because of the presence of cyclophosphamide in the VAB-6 regimen, it is easy to speculate that this alkylating agent is responsible for the observed hypogonadism. However, this is extremely unlikely. Firstly, two of the three patients treated with etoposide + cisplatin had similar defects which were at or above the mean values of LH and FSH. Secondly, the LH and FSH values reported herein are similar to those reported after PVB (cisplatin + vinblastine + bleomycin) (Drasga et al., 1983). Moreover, seven of twenty-eight patients (25%) had low levels of testosterone after PVB compared to only one of twenty-two reported in this series. The two studies are not completely comparable since the study by Drasga et al. (1983) was primarily directed at fertility and did not report mean LH and FSH values. However, the frequency of low testosterone production indicates that the frequency of gonadal defects is probably similar regardless of whether cyclophosphamide is included or not.

It is encouraging to note that the younger patients seem to be resistant to the consequences of this treatment and that improvement does occur over time. This is in contrast to male patients with Hodgkin's disease who received MOPP in whom little recovery can be expected (Roesor et al., 1978; De Vita, 1981).

Conclusion

Most patients with metastatic germ cell tumours do experience gonadal damage. A state of compensated hypogonadism is essentially universal immediately after treatment and may recover to some extent over time. Fertility also probably increases over time after treatment provided that a retroperitoneal lymph node dissection had not been necessary to resect residual disease. The consequences of prolonged pituitary hypersecretion are unknown and these patients should be observed over many years in order to detect late developing pituitary enlargement.

Acknowledgements

This work was supported in part by grants #CA-5826 and RR47 and Contract CM-07337 from the National Institutes of Health.

References

DeVita, V. T. (1981) The consequences of the chemotherapy of Hodgkin's disease: The 10th David A. Karnofsky Memorial Lecture. *Cancer*, **47**, 1–13.
Drasga, R. E., Einhorn, L. H., Williams, S. D., Patel, D. N. & Stevens, E. E. (1983) Fertility after chemotherapy for testicular cancer. *Journal of Clinical Oncology*, **1**, 179–183.
Korth-Schutz, S., Levine, L. S. & New, M. I. (1976) Serum androgens in normal prepubertal and pubertal children and in children with precocious adrenarche. *Journal of Clinical Endocrinology and Metabolism*, **42**, 117–124.
Mortimer, C. H., Besser, G. M., McNeilly, A. S., Tunbridge, W. M. G., Gomez-Pan, A. & Hall, R. (1973) Interaction between secretion of the gonadtrophins, prolactin, growth hormone, thyrotrophin and corticosteroids in man: the effects of LH/FSH-RH, TRH and hypoglycemia alone and in combination. *Clinical Endocrinology*, **2**, 317–326.
Odell, W. D., Rayford, P. L. & Ross, G. T. (1967) Simplified, partially automated method for radioimmunoassay of human thyroid-stimulating, growth, luteinizing, and follicle stimulating hormones. *Journal of Laboratory and Clinical Medicine*, **70**, 973–980.
Reiter, E. O., Kulin, H. E. & Hamwood, S. M. (1974) The absence of positive feedback between estrogen and luteinizing hormone in sexually immature girls. *Pediatric Research*, **8**, 740–745.
Roeser, H. P., Stochs, A. E. & Smith, A. J. (1978) Testicular damage due to cytotoxic drugs and recovery after cessation of therapy. *Australian and New Zealand Journal of Medicine*, **8**, 250–254.
Sherins, R. J. & DeVita, V. T. (1973) Effect of drug treatment for lymphoma on male reproductive capacity; studies of men in remission after therapy. *Annals of Internal Medicine*, **79**, 216–220.
Thachil, J. V., Jewett, M. A. S. & Rider, W. D. (1981) The effects of cancer and cancer therapy on male fertility. *Journal of Urology*, **126**, 141–145.
Vagenakis, A. G., Dole, K. & Braverman, L. E. (1976) Pituitary enlargement, pituitary failure, and primary hypothyroidism. *Annals of Internal Medicine*, **85**, 195–198.

Incidence of developmental handicaps among the offspring of men treated for testicular seminoma

P. FRIED†, R. STEINFELD†, B. CASILETH* and A. STEINFELD† *New York University Medical Center, Division of Radiation Oncology, 560 First Avenue, New York NY 10016, *University of Pennsylvania School of Medicine, and †New York University Medical Center, Division of Radiation Oncology*

Summary

Although the issue of fertility in patients successfully treated for testicular seminoma seems to be resolved, it remains to be determined whether these patients can father normal, healthy children. At NYU Medical Center we have surveyed the patients treated between 1969 and 1984 who were treated with radiotherapy for testicular seminomas. The survey requested information regarding the qualitative development in offspring produced before and after radiation treatments. In the 33 patients responding we were unable to find any detrimental effect, either emotionally, physically, or developmentally in offspring sired by fathers following radiation therapy for testicular seminoma.

Key words. Developmental handicaps, seminoma, radiation therapy.

Introduction

The issue of fertility in cured seminoma patients has been well studied. Several authors have shown that, following therapy, patients are able to maintain sperm levels compatible with fertility or, at the very least, are able to maintain pretreatment sperm levels (Fossa et al., 1982; Lange, Narayan & Fralog, 1984; Tseng et al., 1984). The question that has not been qualitatively investigated; however, is whether laboratory semen values translate into the production of normal healthy children. In an attempt to answer this question, we have looked at the offspring of patients treated with radiation therapy for testicular seminoma.

Materials and Methods

From 1965 to 1984, seventy-nine patients with primary testicular seminoma were treated by the Division of Radiation Oncology at New York University Medical Center. Fifty-one patients presented with Stage I disease, twenty-eight patients with Stage II disease, and no patients with Stage III disease. Bilateral seminomas occurred in only one patient and that was a metachronous event. Stage I patients were generally treated by inguinal orchidectomy followed by unilateral pelvic para-aortic radiation to a dose of 2400 cGy. In patients with Stage II disease, upon completion of the pelvic and para-aortic treatment, a separate mediastinal port was

Correspondence: Dr Peter Fried, Division of Radiation Oncology, NYU Medical Center, 566 First Avenue, New York, NY 10016, U.S.A.

added. The results of treatment are as follows: four patients have died of disease; four patients have died of intercurrent disease; and three patients have been lost to follow-up. The sixty-eight remaining patients are all free of disease with a median follow-up time of 8 years. These sixty-eight patients were sent a questionnaire pertaining to the psychological aspects of their adjustment to the disease and its therapy (Cassileth & Steinfeld, 1986). The forty patients who responded were sent a second questionnaire dealing with the incidence of developmental handicaps in their children. This study results from thirty-three patients who responded. No consistent semen analyses were performed on these patients either prior to or following therapy. The questionnaire asked patients to identify any birth defects, physical handicaps, emotional problems or learning disabilities their offspring may suffer. The temporal relationship between the conception of each child and the delivery of radiation, as well as the possibility of children born to different mothers with the same father, was evaluated.

Results

Fifteen patients (median age at treatment 29 years old) never fathered children. (Only two of these fifteen patients have actually tried to father children.) There are fourteen patients (median age at treatment 43 years old) who fathered children before treatment, but no children following treatment. (Each of these patients stated that they did not attempt to father children following treatment.) These fourteen patients were responsible for thirty-nine pregnancies and twenty-eight children (eleven pregnancies were electively terminated). As assessed by their parents, there are twenty-two normal children and six children with problems, ranging from major birth defects incompatible with life to learning disabilities. There are four patients (median age at treatment 29) who fathered children following treatment. These patients fathered six children and, with the exception of one child who is being treated for juvenile rheumatoid arthritis, all children are described as being completely normal by their parents.

Discussion

Patients with testicular neoplasms may have decreased fertility even before the start of therapy. Semen analysis by Berthelsen & Skakkebæk (1983) showed that pretherapy sperm levels are lower in number as well as motility when compared to normal controls. This observation has been confirmed in a number of studies. The aetiology of this deficiency has not been established. Whether it is the result of a lack of a testicle, carcinoma-in-situ, cryptorchidism or some genetic defect that predisposes these patients to testicular cancer as well as low sperm levels has yet to be determined. Insufficient sperm has been further documented via biopsy of the remaining testicle. Histological abnormalities of impaired spermatogenesis, including Sertoli-cell-only pattern, hyalinized tubules, spermatogenic arrest, and carcinoma-in-situ were found (Berthelsen, 1984).

Already low sperm counts are potentially diminished by antineoplastic therapy. The effect of gamma radiation on sperm production has been well studied, especially in animals. Spermatogonia are among the most radiosensitive cells. Even modest doses of radiation will result in their death or in inhibition of division. Following radiation, there will be reduction in the number of these cells and, therefore, after a time the number of mature sperm will be reduced. If the radiation dose is so high as to kill or damage large numbers of spermatogonia, permanent sterility will result (Pizzarello & Witcofski, 1982).

Directly following radiation, there is no change in the number of mature sperm as their viability is not affected. Since they generally are unable to repair radiation damage, the potential of passing on genetic mutation exists. Of equal concern are the long-term effects which therapy may have on sperm production. A recent study in patients with Hodgkin's disease has shown that if total radiation dose to the testes is kept below 250 rads, sperm counts should return to a level compatible with fertility (Hahn et al., 1982). With modern therapy techniques, shielding of the remaining testicle, and the low doses necessary to eradicate seminoma, radiation to the remaining testicle can be kept to a minimum. Thus, following the initial decrease during and shortly after treatment, sperm levels return to pretherapy values.

The literature is replete with anecdotal reports of successful pregnancies initiated by patients following therapy for testicular cancer. The most definitive study in that regard is that of Smithers, Wallace & Austin (1973). In a mixed group of seminoma and teratoma patients, they reported on fifty-two children fathered following radiation therapy. From these numbers it is apparent that, following effective treatment sperm numbers return to a level that is compatible with reproduction. What is not dealt with in depth in his study is the quality of life of these children. Our data shows that patients, once successfully treated, can be advised that after an appropriate delay they can go on to have normal children. Though our numbers are small, the likelihood of birth defects, emotional deficits or learning disabilities is higher in the pretherapy group compared to the post-therapy group.

Survey studies with subjective questions are susceptible to bias. This is especially true when a patient is asked to rate his own children, the fear being that parents will underevaluate children's handicaps. If this is indeed true then one would assume that the pretherapy group would suffer the same bias as the post-therapy group. Therefore, comparisons can be made. From our study it is possible to conclude that patients with testicular seminoma can not only be assured (in the vast majority of cases) that they will be cured of their disease but also that they can go on to have a normal productive, as well as reproductive, life.

References

Berthelsen, J. G. & Skakkebæk, N. E. (1983) Gonadal function in men with testis cancer. *Fertility and Sterility*, **39**, 68–75.
Berthelsen, J. G. (1984) *Andrological Aspects of Testicular Cancer*. Scriptor, Copenhagen.
Cassileth, B. R. & Steinfeld, A. D. (1986) Psychological preparation of the patient and family. *Cancer* (in press).
Fosså, S. D., Klepp, O., Molno, L. et al. (1982) Testicular function after unilateral orchidectomy for cancer and before further treatment. *International Journal of Andrology*, **5**, 179–184.
Hahn, E. W., Feingold, S. M., Simpson, L. & Batata, M. (1982) Recovery from aspermia induced by low dose radiation in seminoma patients. *Cancer*, **50**, 337.
Lange, P. H., Narayan, P. & Fralog, E. E. (1984) Fertility issues following therapy for testicular cancer. *Seminars in Urology*, **11**, 264–274.
Pizzarello, D. J. & Witcofski, R. L. (1982) *Medical Radiation Biology*, Chapter 3. Lea & Febiger, Philadelphia.
Smithers, D. W., Wallace, D. M. & Austin, D. E. (1973) Fertility after unilateral orchidectomy and radiotherapy for patients with malignant tumours of the testes. *British Medical Journal*, **iv**, 77–79.
Tseng, A. J., Kessler, F. F., Broder, S. & Rothman Torti, F. M. (1984) Male fertility before and after treatment of testicular cancer. *Journal of Clinical Oncology*, March, 161.

Fertility after chemotherapy for male and female germ cell tumours

G. J. S. RUSTIN,*† D. PEKTASIDES,*
K. D. BAGSHAWE,* E. S. NEWLANDS* and
R. H. J. BEGENT*   *Cancer Research Campaign Laboratories, Department of Medical Oncology, Charing Cross Hospital, London, and †Mount Vernon Hospital, Northwood, Middx.

Summary

Gonadal function was assessed in fifty-nine men and thirty-one women who had successfully completed chemotherapy with the POMB/ACE regimen for germ cell tumours. Seventeen (81%) of the twenty-one men who had not received para-aortic radiotherapy, whose original tumour bulk was < 5 cm and whose duration of chemotherapy was < 6 months, recovered spermatogenesis compared with twelve (32%) of thirty-eight patients who had either larger tumour masses or longer courses of chemotherapy, or both. All but one of the seventeen women in whom menstruation could have been expected to recur are now menstruating. This study suggests that the great majority of patients treated with POMB/ACE chemotherapy for germ cell tumours will recover fertility.

Key words.   Germ cell tumours, fertility, toxicity.

Introduction

Men and women treated with chemotherapy for germ cell tumours are typically at the peak of their reproductive years and now that there are good prospects for cure it is important to assess the effect that therapy has on their fertility. Although it has been shown that combination chemotherapy used for treating men or women with Hodgkin's disease causes permanent gonadal dysfunction in the majority (Waxman, 1985) there have been several studies suggesting that fertility may be preserved after chemotherapy in patients with germ cell tumours and gestational trophoblastic tumours (Drasga et al., 1983; Rustin, 1983; Rustin et al., 1984). This study investigates those patients treated with POMB/ACE chemotherapy (Newlands et al., 1986) at the Charing Cross Hospital between 1977 and 1985. In particular it looks at which factors are particularly associated with the failure of recovery of fertility which might lead to some of these factors being avoided.

Male fertility

Between January 1977 and March 1984, 142 patients were treated with POMB/ACE for male germ cell tumours. Fifty-nine patients had sperm counts more than

Correspondence: Dr G. J. S. Rustin, Department of Medical Oncology, Charing Cross Hospital, London W6 8RF.

12 months after the completion of therapy. There was some recovery of spermatogenesis in twenty-nine patients (49%) but only twelve patients had absolute sperm counts of greater than 2×10^7 per ml. The time between the end of chemotherapy and when spermatogenesis was first seen to have returned, was a median of 17 months (range 11–68). Median follow-up of the patients who have remained azoospermic is 28 months (range 12–58).

Prior to chemotherapy, eighteen of the fifty-nine men who had sperm counts performed had fathered a total of thirty-six children. Since completion of chemotherapy eleven men have fathered twelve children. Two of these men who were reported as being oligospermic have fathered children within 1 year of their low sperm count. No congenital abnormalities have been detected among the children, but the wife of one patient had artificial insemination from a donor that was not her husband and has given birth to an anencephalic still born child.

Male hormone levels

Forty-six patients had FSH, LH and testosterone levels performed at least 1 year after completion of chemotherapy and on the same day that they had a sperm count performed. Testosterone levels were within the normal range in all but one patient who had a slightly low level. FSH and LH levels are shown in Table 1. Although a higher percentage of patients with sperm counts greater than 2×10^7 per ml have FSH and LH within the normal range than those with lower sperm counts, there was great variation.

Table 1. Absolute sperm count, and serum FSH and LH levels in forty-six patients at least 1 year after completion of chemotherapy

Sperm count	Serum FSH level Median	$\leqslant 7$ u/l	Serum LH level Median	$\leqslant 10$ u/l
Azoospermic	17 u/l	3/21	13 u/l	9/21
1×10^5 to 2×10^7 per ml	17 u/l	1/15	12 u/l	6/15
$> 2 \times 10^7$ per ml	14.6 u/l	3/10	7 u/l	7/10

Factors affecting recovery of spermatogenesis

Various factors were investigated to see whether they were associated with failure of recovery of spermatogenesis. Those factors shown by the Chi-square test to be significantly associated with lack of recovery are shown in Table 2. No patients who had received para-aortic radiotherapy in addition to chemotherapy recovered spermatogenesis. Only 41% of patients with bulky disease defined as greater than 5 cm nodal masses, greater than 2 cm lung metastases or brain or liver metastases had recovery. Chemotherapy lasting more than 6 months, which was presumably related to tumour bulk, was another adverse factor. There was no statistically significant association between failure of recovery of spermatogenesis and sperm count prior to chemotherapy ($P = 0.08$), age equal to or greater than 25 ($P = 0.13$), age equal to or greater than 30 ($P = 0.22$), and laparotomy ($P = 0.59$).

Table 2. Factors affecting recovery of spermatogenesis following chemotherapy

Factor	Recovery of spermatogenesis		Significance*
	Factor present/ no. of patients	Factor absent/ no. of patients	
Radiotherapy	0/11 (0%)	29/48 (60.4%)	
Bulky tumour† No radiotherapy	9/22 (40.9%)	20/26 (76.9%)	$P = 0.011$
Chemotherapy > 6 months No radiotherapy	9/21 (42.9%)	20/27 (74.1%)	$P = 0.029$
Any of above	12/38 (31.6%)		
None of above		17/21 (80.9%)	

*Chi-square test.
†See text.

Ovarian germ cell tumours

Between 1977 and 1985 thirty-one women successfully completed chemotherapy with the POMB/ACE regimen for ovarian germ cell tumours in this unit. Menstruation was not expected at the time of analysis after chemotherapy in fourteen of the women, because of extent of surgery in nine, young age in three, pelvic radiotherapy in one and 46XY karyotype in one. A further patient has been lost to follow-up.

All patients had amenorrhoea during chemotherapy but one patient restarted menstruation 2 months before the completion of chemotherapy. One 20-year-old girl has not yet restarted menstruation 7 months after completion of chemotherapy but her FSH and LH levels are within the normal range. All the remaining sixteen patients have restarted menstruation. Fourteen patients are currently menstruating regularly whilst two patients have been put on oral contraceptives to control irregular periods. The median period from completion of chemotherapy to start of regular menstruation was 4 months (−2 to 18 months). The median age at start of chemotherapy of those currently menstruating was 21 years (9–38 years).

Since the end of chemotherapy there have been seven pregnancies in five women resulting in three full-term normal deliveries, three miscarriages, one termination of pregnancy and one pregnancy is ongoing.

Discussion

It is encouraging that sixteen of seventeen women have had recovery of menstruation following chemotherapy and that five of these patients have already conceived following chemotherapy. The high success rate with chemotherapy in patients with ovarian dysgerminomas, malignant teratomas including endodermal sinus tumours (yolk sac tumours) coupled with the excellent chance of recovery of fertility after a median of 5 months of POMB/ACE chemotherapy suggests that this therapy should be given serious consideration as initial primary treatment for those patients. Radiotherapy and initial radical surgery should be avoided. Some women, however, will still become sterile because of the extent of their tumour and some may require aggressive surgery after chemotherapy to eradicate all their disease.

The study also shows some encouraging results regarding fertility after POMB/ACE chemotherapy for male germ cell tumours. Provided that patients are not given additional radiotherapy, do not have bulky disease and have treatment lasting less than 6 months, over 80% of them have recovery of spermatogenesis. Earlier diagnosis of metastatic disease will lead to fewer patients having bulky, advanced disease and therefore more patients requiring only a short duration of therapy after which they are likely to recover their fertility.

References

Drasga, R. E., Einhorn, L. H., Williams, S. D., Catel, D. N. & Stevens, E. E. (1983) Fertility after chemotherapy for testicular cancer. *Journal of Clinical Oncology*, **1**, 179–183.

Newlands, E. S., Bagshawe, K. D., Begent, R. H. J., Rustin, G. J. S., Crawford, S. M. & Holden, L. (1986) Current optimum management of anaplastic germ cell tumours of the testis and other sites. *British Journal of Urology*, **58**, 307–314.

Newlands, E. S., Begent, R. H. J., Rustin, G. J. S. & Bagshawe, K. D. (1982) A potential for cure in metastatic ovarian teratomas and dysgerminomas. *British Journal of Obstetrics and Gynaecology*, **89**, 555–560.

Rustin, G. J. S. (1983) Follow up, fertility and second tumours in germ cell tumours. *Clinics in Oncology* (ed. by K. D. Bagshawe, E. S. Newlands and R. H. J. Begent), pp. 267–279. Saunders, London.

Rustin, G. J. S., Booth, M., Dent, J., Salt, S., Rustin, E. & Bagshawe, K. D. (1984) Pregnancy after cytotoxic chemotherapy for gestational trophoblastic tumours. *British Medical Journal*, **1288**, 103–106.

Waxman, J. (1985) Cancer, chemotherapy and fertility. *British Medical Journal*, **290**, 1096–1097.

General discussion on fertility and testicular cancer

Chairman T. B. HARGREAVE

Hargreave In this discussion we shall consider fertility problems in association with testicular cancer and with testicular cancer treatment. It is important to distinguish whether fertility problems precede treatment or if they are the result of treatment. Infertility is a wide issue and we must look at possible ways of preventing its development as well as consideration of the possible effects of therapy on a man's fertility and indeed his subsequent offspring.

It is interesting to hear Dr Bosl's hormone data which seem to confirm my clinical impression that recovery after cancer chemotherapy may take up to 2 years. This is the time we often have to wait before making comment on the effects on a patient's fertility.

Skakkebæk Does anyone have evidence for improvement in fertility from the time of diagnosis till after treatment?

Bosl I have no specific data. In general terms I can say that 25–50% of our patients have had children before treatment, either before or after treatment, provided that a lymph node dissection had not been done. Six patients in our study did not have a lymph node dissection and three of these conceived children after therapy.

Berthelsen There are no data on fertility before and after treatment in terms of conception rates but we commonly see patients with better semen quality some years after treatment than before.

Hargreave It may surprise some people to learn that experience from my own infertility practice indicates that the statistical chance of achieving pregnancy does not deteriorate substantially until the motile sperm density falls below 0.5 million motile sperm/ml. This is a much lower figure than is generally accepted but does agree with Dr Rustin's observation that some of your patients fathered children even with an apparently low sperm count. Therefore the conventionally accepted criteria for normality in the general population do not reflect the true chances of pregnancy.

Rustin I agree, and I am not surprised. My two patients who fathered children within a few months of having sperm counts in the oligozoospermic range (both $<2\times10^6$ absolute count) are examples of this.

Safirstein Dr Bosl, are the effects of cisplatin expressed at the pituitary level or is it due to interruption of some feedback loop from the end organ to the pituitary?

Bosl We have performed provocative tests with gonadotrophin releasing hormone and demonstrated that the defect is at the gonadal (end organ) level. The pituitary responds usually to stimulation by releasing hormone resulting in a marked increase in LH levels.

Vogelzang Have you compared the toxicity of etoposide/cisplatin with VAB-6? Are they equitoxic *vis-à-vis* hormonal function?

Bosl We studied three patients and obtain equivocal results. One patient was above the mean, one was at the mean, and one was below the mean. This is very early data but we suspect that the effects of the different drug regimens will be exactly the same. More information will soon be available from a study of 10 patients receiving etoposide and cisplatin.

Friedman We must not get the impression that radiation damage to the germ cells is universal. In animals, the damage is dose dependent, and irradiation causes stem cell maturation arrest. Germ cells which have passed a certain point in spermatogenesis continue to develop into normal spermatozoa which are not significantly damaged but a hiatus develops so that the tubules contain only spermatogonia and sperm. Similar changes occur in many other tissues including the bone marrow and the effects at different sites are determined by the cell kinetics of the individual tissues. The atrophic tissue may then regenerate from the stem cell layer.

Dr Einhorn stated that the seminiferous epithelium is obliterated, as are the 'Skakkebæk' cells. I think this is incorrect. The 'Skakkebæk' cells along with germinoma/seminoma cells are exquisitely sensitive to irradiation even in small doses and these can be differentially destroyed leaving the spermatogonia alone (Friedman & Drutz, 1961, *Journal of Urology*, **85**, 609).

It should be noted that other antitumour agents have different effects on the testes.

Fried I agree that spermatogonia are among the most radiosensitive of all cells and sperm can mature after radiation-induced arrest of the spermatogonia. However, although the developing spermatozoa appear normal morphologically after irradiation, I must stress that these gametes may carry chromosomal abnormalities. Other antitumour agents may or may not act by the same mechanism.

Skakkebæk Dr Fried raised the very important point that many testicular tumour patients may have pre-existing congenital abnormalities such as the Sertoli-cell-only (SCO) syndrome in their testis. Dr Bethelsen and I (*Fertility and Sterility*, **39**, 68–75, 1983) showed a 20–25% incidence of congenital testicular defects (SCO, CIS, spermatogenic arrest) at the time of diagnosis of the original tumour. Therefore, if biopsy of the contralateral testis is going to be a routine procedure in different centres, we should look for nonmalignant changes in addition to CIS in order to substantiate, or otherwise, our findings.

Grigor Dr Fried, in your investigation, there is a high incidence of abnormal children (6/28) conceived by men *before* their testicular tumour. If a man has an abnormal child should he be considered at risk of developing a testicular tumour?

Fried This may be the case. However, our numbers are far too small to support or refute this hypothesis.

Schmoll This is a very important point you raised. Every study appears to report the abnormalities produced after treatment with radiotherapy or chemotherapy. We must now look at the incidence of abnormalities in children fathered before therapy, and future reports should compare the incidence before and after therapy rather than comparing offspring from treated men with the general population.

Fried We shall be very interested to see if our report will be confirmed by other investigators.

Hargreave Theoretically do you think that radiotherapy or chemotherapy is more likely to cause genetic damage which may affect children?

Berthelsen The dose of radiation reaching the remaining (shielded) testis is very small, in the region of 0.3–1.3 Gy. Thus there may indeed be a very small risk of permanent genetic damage although it will be extremely difficult to demonstrate.

I am more worried about chemotherapy because the dose which reaches the spermatogonia is much higher than with radiotherapy, and there is no way of protecting the gonad or germinal stem cells from chemotherapy.

Brada A technical point about radiotherapy to para-aortic and pelvic nodes for stage I seminoma. The dose of radiation received by the testis relates to the inferior border of the radiotherapy field. If the whole inguinal canal and ipsilateral scrotal sac are included – a policy in some centres – it becomes very difficult to shield the testis effectively.

Fried As long as the dose is kept constant and the remaining testis is well shielded, variation in the inferior border of the radiation field should not have a major effect on the dose received by the testis. The radiation reaching the remaining testis is mainly due to internal scatter rather than the penumbra of the rays.

Brada Senturia *et al.* (*Lancet*, **ii**, 766–769, 1985) reported on malformations in children fathered by 52 men treated for testicular tumours. There were four malformations detected in 30 children from men treated with chemotherapy which did not differ from the incidence of congenital abnormalities in a control group.

Fried This is further evidence that we can reassure anxious patients that they have no greater risk of having congenitally abnormal offspring than the general population, assuming they are able to fertilize their spouse successfully.

Hargreave It is a question how long follow-up studies should continue. Do we stop the follow-up period when a normal birth is recorded? Should we continue to follow these children throughout their lives even into adulthood to see if they are more likely to develop testicular tumours?

Dr Rustin, can you comment on the cause of the miscarriages in your two women who received POMB/ACE? Do you know the karyotype of the products of conception?

Rustin No. The products of conception were not karyotyped. Even if karyotypic abnormality had been detected, this would probably not be a significant finding as tissues from miscarriages are often abnormal; and also we do not know the actual natural miscarriage rate.

Hargreave What contraceptive advice do you give to your patients during and after chemotherapy?

Rustin Men should use contraceptives from 9 months after completion of chemotherapy if they do not want children and they should continue with contraceptives even if they are oligozoospermic. Azoospermic men should continue contraception until 3 years after chemotherapy because if no recovery is seen by then they are unlikely to recover spermatogenesis.

I advise my patients that they should not get their wives pregnant for at least 1 year after chemotherapy because we have worries that the sperm may be abnormal, although this is probably not the case.

Berthelsen We advise avoiding pregnancy for 2 years, not so much for the fear of having chromosomal abnormalities but more to ensure that the patients are cured of their disease before producing any more children. The patients should use contraceptives for at least 9 months after treatment. By then all irradiated post-spermatogonial cells ought to have been excreted.

Skakkebæk From a geneticist's point of view, what are the dangers of chromosomal abnormalities? How long should testicular tumour patients treated with radiation or cytotoxic drugs wait before trying to produce offspring in order to minimize the risk of genetic defects in their children?

Rustin Until we know the incidence of congenital abnormalities in this group we cannot make any comment. We have studied a large group of women treated for gestational choriocarcinoma who subsequently produced 212 full-term children, and the incidence of congenital abnormalities in these children was exactly the same as the national average. Other studies have shown that induced chromosomal changes in the chromatin of lymphocytes can persist for years after chemotherapy. Therefore, abnormalities are produced in some cells, but perhaps not in the germ cells.

Delozier-Blanchet As a clinical geneticist, I would suggest caution in concluding that the risk of genetic abnormalities in the offspring of treated testicular tumour patients is not increased. Although there is reason for optimism, information from hundreds of patients may be required to detect a small increase over the already high incidence (2–3%) of congenital malformation in the general population.

As radiotherapy and/or chemotherapy could have effects on the germ cells at both the chromosomal (breakage) and the gene (mutation) levels the case for careful pregnancy surveillance, including amniocentesis, can be made. Although we cannot exclude possible (albeit improbable) unrepaired gene mutation, we can exclude a chromosomal abnormality in the children of these patients by amniocentesis. The procedure is well established and of low risk: at the University Hospital in Geneva the incidence of miscarriage following amniocentesis is only about 1/250.

Although some oncologists may fear that the suggestion of prenatal diagnosis may cause unnecessary anxiety, we have found the opposite to be true. Cancer patients are generally quite concerned about the potential effects of their treatment on offspring, and are relieved by any means of surveillance which can be performed. In our genetic counselling service we offer amniocentesis as an option to the prospective parents; if the prenatal test is not desired, in selected cases we perform a cytogenetic study of the patient's lymphocytes to screen for genetic damage.

Rustin Surely there is no indication to do amniocentesis routinely on these patients. Our studies and other reports have not shown an increased incidence of congenital abnormalities in the children of these patients so I think amniocentesis not warranted.

Delozier-Blanchet On the question of performing amniocentesis, it actually depends on your philosophy about the test. In Switzerland, prenatal diagnosis is sometimes done purely for maternal anxiety, and is viewed as a safe procedure. We think that it is worthwhile in this group of cancer patients to detect possible chromosomal rearrangements.

Safirstein It is possible to separate sister chromatid exchanges from the ultimate cytotoxic effects of cisplatin. Therefore we do not appear to know what are the critical DNA–cisplatin interactions that are important in regard to ultimate genetic damage. This, coupled with what seems to be a very small increase in congenital defects, if any, makes one think that we are not justified in recommending mass amniocentesis screening of patients until we understand what DNA–cisplatin interactions are important.

Bosl There is much greater experience in patients with Hodgkin's disease in terms of both number of offspring and duration of follow-up. In this group of patients, there is no suspicion of increased incidence of developmental abnormalities in the offspring. The treatment of germ cell tumours is of shorter duration and uses less toxic drugs. Therefore, the offspring of germ cell tumour patients are unlikely to suffer a greater incidence of abnormalities.

Schmoll We should also look at possible long-term consequences of chromosomal defects by examining second generation children and not only the immediate offspring of treated patients. Do we have any information on second generation children in the large series of treated Hodgkin's disease patients?

Bosl The first generation children appear to be normal, but we have no information on second generation offspring.

Hargreave The message from this discussion is that there is no evidence of undue fetal abnormality associated with this group of patients, and that we must be careful not to panic our patients into unnecessary measures. For example, the indications for amniocentesis would seem to be those that normally prevail for the age of the woman and for the country concerned. We must remember that there is fetal loss, albeit small, from amniocentesis.

Treatment strategies of testicular cancer in the United States

L. H. EINHORN *Indiana University Medical Center, University Hospital, Indianapolis, Indiana, U.S.A.*

Summary

The treatment of testicular cancer has dramatically improved during the past decade. Combination chemotherapy with PVB was instituted at Indiana University in 1974. Subsequent studies demonstrated that: (1) post PVB, surgery can cure patients; (2) vinblastine dosage can be lowered from 0.4 to 0.3 mg/kg without sacrificing cure potential; (3) maintenance vinblastine is not necessary; (4) VP-16 can be substituted for vinblastine with equivalent cure rates and decreased neuromuscular toxicity.

Key words.   Testicular cancer, chemotherapy, cisplatin, vinblastine, bleomycin, etoposide, ifosfamide.

Platinum + vinblastine + bleomycin (PVB) studies

In August 1974 we began studies at Indiana University in disseminated testicular cancer with PVB chemotherapy (Einhorn & Donohue, 1977). The original PVB regimen is depicted in Table 1, and the therapeutic results are outlined in Table 2. Twenty-eight of forty-seven patients (60%) are currently alive with a minimal follow-up of 10 years.

The major serious toxicity was related to the high dose (0.4 mg/kg) vinblastine. Myalgias, constipation and paralytic ileus were all troublesome side effects, but severe granulocytopenia and potential sepsis was the most worrisome toxicity.

Thus, in 1976, we started a random prospective trial comparing our original PVB with the same regimen using a 25% dosage reduction (0.3 mg/kg) for vinblastine

Table 1. Original PVB regimen

Platinum 20 mg/m^2 × 5 i.v. every 3 weeks (four courses)	
Vinblastine 0.2 mg/kg i.v. day 1 and 2 every 3 weeks (four courses)	Induction
Bleomycin 30 unis i.v. push (starting on day 2) weekly × 12	
Maintenance vinblastine 0.3 mg/kg monthly × 21 (after induction therapy)	

Table 2. Results with PVB

No. of patients	47
Complete remission (CR)	33 (70%)
Disease-free after PVB + surgery	5 (11%)
5-year survivors	30 (64%)
No. presently alive	28 (60%)

Correspondence: Dr L. H. Einhorn, Indiana University Medical Center, University Hospital, Indianapolis, Indiana 46223, U.S.A.

during remission induction. It was felt that the reduced vinblastine dosage would reduce the haematological toxicity, but the more critical question was whether it could maintain the same therapeutic efficacy. A third arm adding doxorubicin to PVB was tested to see if the use of doxorubicin in combination with PVB would further improve the CR rate. The schema for this study is shown in Table 3.

Table 3. PVB study no. 2

Randomize
Platinum 20 mg/m^2 × 5 q 3 weeks × 4
Vinblastine 0.4 mg/kg q 3 weeks × 4
Bleomycin 30 units i.v. weekly × 12

Platinum 20 mg/m^2 × 5 q 3 weeks
Vinblastine 0.3 mg/kg q 3 weeks × 4
Bleomycin 30 units i.v. weekly × 12

Platinum 20 mg/m^2 × 5 q 3 weeks × 4
Vinblastine 0.2 mg/kg q 3 weeks × 4
Doxorubicin 50 mg/m^2 q 3 weeks × 4
Bleomycin 30 units i.v. weekly × 12

After 12 weeks of induction therapy, maintenance vinblastine (0.3 mg/kg monthly) given for a total of 2 years of chemotherapy.

Seventy-eight patients were entered on this study and all patients have been followed for a minimum of 7½ years. The 25% reduction in the vinblastine dosage resulted in the expected decrease in haematological and neuromuscular toxicity. The therapeutic results are shown in Table 4. There was no significant difference in any of the three induction arms. Fifty-seven of seventy-eight (73%) patients are currently alive and disease-free (NED). Based upon the results of this study, we abandoned our original PVB regimen in favour of the equally effective but less toxic regimen that utilized the reduced dosage (0.3 mg/kg) of vinblastine (Einhorn & Williams, 1980).

Table 4. Therapeutic results

	PVB (0.4 mg/kg)	PVB (0.3 mg/kg)	PVB + doxorubicin	Total
No. of patients	26	27	25	78
CR	18 (69%)	17 (63%)	18 (72%)	53 (68%)
NED* with surgery	5 (19%)	4 (15%)	2 (8%)	11 (14%)
Relapses	5 (19%)	2 (10%)	2 (8%)	10 (13%)
No. continuously NED*	18 (69%)	18 (67%)	17 (68%)	53 (68%)
No. presently NED*	20 (77%)	19 (70%)	18 (72%)	57 (73%)

* NED: no evidence of disease.

We began a third generation study in 1978, utilizing the resources of the Southeastern Cancer Study Group (SECSG). This study randomized patients achieving CR (or NED with PVB + resection of teratoma) to standard maintenance vinblastine (0.3 mg/kg monthly × 21) versus no maintenance therapy. This important study confirmed the fact that optimal cure rates in disseminated testicular cancer could be achieved with merely 12 weeks of PVB induction and that maintenance therapy was unnecessary (Einhorn et al., 1981b). One hundred and forty-seven patients from

Indiana University entered this SECSG protocol. With a minimal follow-up of 5 years, 117 (80%) patients are currently alive and disease-free.

Combination chemotherapy with PVB has been used at Indiana University since 1974. Overall, with follow-up of 5–10 years on these first three studies, 202 of 272 patients (74%) are currently alive and presumably cured of their disseminated testicular cancer. Furthermore, these results have been confirmed and published by numerous other investigators and cooperative groups around the world.

Salvage therapy

Although 80% of patients with disseminated testicular cancer will achieve a disease-free status with PVB (either with chemotherapy alone or surgical resection of residual disease), there still remains a patient population eligible for salvage therapy. There are still 20% of the patients who have unresectable partial remission (or no response at all to PVB) and another 10% who will relapse from a PVB-induced CR.

It is our philosophy to resect surgically residual disease after four courses of induction therapy if the serum markers (hCG and AFP) are normal and if it is anatomically feasible to extirpate persistent disease. If a patient has an unresectable PR and has normal serum markers, after four courses of cisplatin combination chemotherapy, he is observed monthly (on no chemotherapy) until he develops serological or radiographic evidence of progressive disease. This practice is followed because some patients with an 'unresectable PR' have no remaining carcinoma, i.e. they have persistent necrotic fibrous tissue with or without teratoma. In fact, some of these patients will become radiographic CR with the passage of time as their necrotic fibrous deposits eventually spontaneously dissipate.

The two-drug combination of cisplatin + VP-16 has been found to be highly synergistic in preclinical studies (Schabel et al., 1979). Single agent VP-16 has been found to be an active, albeit noncurative, drug in refractory testicular cancer. The initial results of our salvage chemotherapy regimen, which began in 1978, were published by Williams et al. (1980). These results have been confirmed by numerous other single institutions as well as the SECSG (Hainsworth et al., 1985). Overall, approximately 25% of PVB failures can be salvaged and potentially cured with cisplatin + VP-16 combination chemotherapy. This represents the first curative salvage regimen for an adult solid tumour.

Another active drug in refractory disease is ifosfamide (Wheeler et al., 1986). VP-16 and ifosfamide are the only single agents capable of achieving a greater than 20% objective response rate in patients who progress during cisplatin combination chemotherapy. We have evaluated the combination of VP-16 + ifosfamide + cisplatin as third line chemotherapy in refractory testicular cancer and have produced a significant number of durable complete remissions (Loehrer, Einhorn & Williams, 1986). Our treatment strategy is to combine cisplatin (unless the patient progressed during previous cisplatin combination chemotherapy) with other active agents not previously utilized in the individual patient. We now currently utilize cisplatin + ifosfamide + either VP-16 or vinblastine (depending upon prior chemotherapy) as initial salvage chemotherapy.

PVB versus platinum + VP-16 + bleomycin (PVP$_{16}$B)

From 1981 to 1984 the SECSG has evaluated PVB versus PVP$_{16}$B as initial induction chemotherapy for disseminated testicular cancer. The VP-16 dosage was 100 mg/m^2 × 5 every 3 weeks for four courses and was combined with the usual dosages of cisplatin + bleomycin. The therapeutic results were similar, with 72% NED with PVB and 79% NED with PVP$_{16}$B (p = NS). However, the reduction in myalgias and peripheral neuropathies with PVP$_{16}$B was highly statistically significant (Williams et al., 1985). Therefore, in 1984, based upon these results, PVP$_{16}$B became our standard induction regimen for disseminated testicular cancer.

New studies

It has been clear for many years that the most important prognostic factor related to a favourable outcome of chemotherapy in disseminated testicular cancer was the volume of metastatic disease. Several staging systems are already available; however, most of them were at least partially developed prior to the advent of successful cisplatin combination chemotherapy. Therefore we have developed a new staging system placing patients with disseminated tumour into three categories: minimal, moderate, or advanced disease, based upon disease extent (Table 5). One hundred and eighty-one patients were retrospectively classified by this scheme (PVB with or without maintenance vinblastine) and additional patients were prospectively stratified on our recently completed SECSG protocol (PVB versus PVP$_{16}$B). Overall, 99%, 91% and 57% of patients in these three categories achieved a favourable response to chemotherapy (CR or NED with chemotherapy plus surgical resection of teratoma) (Birch et al., 1986).

Our present studies utilize this new staging system. For minimal and moderate disease, it would be statistically impossible to demonstrate therapeutic superiority for a new regimen. However, once again, we can demonstrate equivalent results with decreased toxicity and cost, as we did when we reduced vinblastine to 0.3 mg/kg, eliminated maintenance vinblastine, and substituted VP-16 for vinblastine. In this

Table 5. Staging system

A. Minimal
  1. Elevated markers only
  2. Cervical ± retroperitoneal nodes
  3. Unresectable, nonpalpable retroperitoneal disease
  4. Minimal pulmonary metastases: less than five per lung field and largest less than 2 cm (± nonpalpable abdominal disease ± cervical nodes)

B. Moderate
  1. Palpable abdominal mass with no supradiaphragmatic disease
  2. Moderate pulmonary metastases: five to ten per lung field with largest less than 3 cm; or, solitary pulmonary mass of any size; or, mediastinal lymphadenopathy less than 50% intrathoracic diameter

C. Advanced
  1. Advanced pulmonary metastasis: primary mediastinal germ cell tumour; or, greater than ten pulmonary metastases per lung field; or, multiple pulmonary metastases with largest metastasis greater than 3 cm
  2. Palpable abdominal mass + pulmonary metastases
  3. Hepatic, osseous, or CNS metastases

new study we are evaluating the standard four courses (12 weeks) of $PVP_{16}B$ and comparing it in a random prospective study to three courses (9 weeks) of $PVP_{16}B$.

In advanced disease, only about half of the patients are curable with standard chemotherapy, and, therefore, we can ask a therapeutic question. Ozols (1987) have demonstrated safety and efficacy for double dose cisplatin. We are now evaluating standard $PVP_{16}B$ versus double dose cisplatin ($40 \text{ mg/m}^2 \times 5$) + VP-16 + bleomycin in advanced disseminated testicular cancer.

References

Birch, R., Williams, S. D., Cone, A. et al. (1986) Prognostic factors for favorable outcome in disseminated germ cell tumors. *Journal of Clinical Oncology*, **4**, 400–407.

Einhorn, L. H. & Donohue, J. P. (1977) Cis-diamminedichloroplatinum, vinblastine, and bleomycin combination chemotherapy in disseminated testicular cancer. *Annals of Internal Medicine*, **87**, 293–298.

Einhorn, L. H. & Williams, S. D. (1980) Chemotherapy of disseminated testicular cancer. *Cancer*, **46**, 1339–1344.

Einhorn, L. H., Williams, S. D., Mandelbaum, I. & Donohue, J. (1981a) Surgical resection in disseminated testicular cancer following chemotherapeutic cytoreduction. *Cancer*, **48**, 904–908.

Einhorn, L. H., Williams, S. D., Troner, M. et al. (1981b) The role of maintenance therapy in disseminated testicular cancer. *New England Journal of Medicine*, **305**, 727–731.

Hainsworth, J. D., Williams, S. D., Einhorn, L. H., Birch, R. & Greco, F. A. (1985) Successful treatment of resistant germinal neoplasms with VP-16 and cisplatin: Results of a Southeastern Cancer Study Group Trial. *Journal of Clinical Oncology*, **3**, 666–671.

Lange, P. H., McIntire, K. R., Waldmann, T. et al. (1976) Serum alphafeto-protein and human chorionic gonadotropin in the diagnosis and management of nonseminomatous germ cell testicular cancer. *New England Journal of Medicine*, **295**, 1237–1240.

Loehrer, P. J., Einhorn, L. H. & Williams, S. D. (1986) Salvage therapy for refractory germ cell tumors with VP-16 plus ifosfamide plus cisplatin. *Journal of Clinical Oncology* (in press).

Mackay, E. N. & Sellers, A. H. (1966) A statistical review of malignant testicular tumors based on the experience of the Ontario Cancer Foundation Clinics, 1938–1961. *Canadian Medical Association Journal*, **94**, 889–899.

Ozols, R. F. (1987) Treatment of poor prognosis germ cell tumours with high dose cisplatin regimens. *International Journal of Andrology*, **10**, 291–300.

Schabel, F. M., Trader, M. W., Lester, W. R. et al. (1979) Cis-dichlorodiammineplatinum (II): Combination chemotherapy and cross resistance studies with tumors of mice. *Cancer Treatment Reports*, **63**, 1459–1473.

Wheeler, B. M., Loehrer, P. J., Williams, S. D. & Einhorn, L. H. (1986) Ifosfamide in refractory male germ cell tumors. *Journal of Clinical Oncology*, **4**, 28–34.

Williams, S. D., Einhorn, L. H., Greco, F. A. et al. (1980) VP-16-213 salvage therapy for refractory germinal neoplasms. *Cancer*, **46**, 2154–2158.

Williams, S. D., Einhorn, L. H., Greco, F. A., Birch, R. & Irwin, R. (1985) Disseminated germ cell tumors: a comparison of cisplatin plus bleomycin plus either vinblastine or VP-16. *Proceedings of American Society of Clinical Oncology*, **4**, 102.

Discussion

Grigor Could you summarize the improved prognosis for nonseminomatous germ cell tumours over the last decade?

Einhorn As you can see from the table (p. 404), there has been a dramatic world-wide improvement in survival since 1974 with an overall survival now of 95% compared to 50%. This has been the greatest success story in the treatment of all cancers over this period.

Treatment strategies of testicular cancer in Europe

G. STOTER *Department of Oncology, Rotterdam Cancer Institute*

Key words. Seminoma, nonseminoma, radiotherapy, chemotherapy, RPLND.

Introduction

Since 1974 curative cisplatin containing chemotherapy has been available for the treatment of disseminated testicular cancer, yielding a 70% long-term disease-free survival. For patients with low volume metastatic disease the complete remission (CR) rates are 90–100%, whereas for patients with high volume metastases the CR rates vary from 30% to 60%.

STAGE I

Nonseminoma

Clinical stage I is defined as tumour confined to the testis. With modern staging techniques including the use of CT-scans of chest and abdomen, bipedal lymph-angiography, and the determination of serum tumour markers such as β-hCG, AFP and LDH, it is estimated that patients with a diagnosis of stage I disease have a 20% chance of harbouring microscopic retroperitoneal lymph node metastases, rendering the overall chance of progression of disease to an average of 20–30%.

In a U.S. intergroup study (Weiss *et al.*, 1986) 267 patients who underwent bilateral retroperitoneal lymph node dissection (RPLND) appeared to have pathological stage I disease, defined as there being no microscopic metastases in the removed specimen. Twenty-five (11%) developed progression of disease, exclusively outside the retroperitoneum, showing that this form of local treatment is effective in preventing the development of retroperitoneal metastases, whereas the progression rate of above 10% is due to haematogenous metastases, already present at the time of surgery. These results are in accordance with older data from Skinner and Donohue.

In the Royal Marsden Hospital (Peckham *et al.*, 1979) 85 patients with clinical stage I disease were treated with radiotherapy to the retroperitoneal lymph nodes following orchidectomy. Thirteen patients (15%) developed progression of disease, predominantly outside the retroperitoneum, indicating that radiotherapy may have some effect on micrometastases in the retroperitoneum, whereas by its nature it does not influence the progression of systemic disease.

Although the mortality of lymph node dissection and radiotherapy is negligible, the morbidity cannot be ignored with anejaculation and infertility occurring in

Correspondence: Dr G. Stoter, Department of Oncology, Rotterdam Cancer Institute, Groene Hilledijk 301, 3075 EA Rotterdam, The Netherlands.

most patients following bilateral RPLND, and gastrointestinal side effects, subcutaneous sclerosis, and retroperitoneal fibrosis after radiotherapy.

It is clear that RPLND and radiotherapy are overtreatment for approximately 70% of the patients in clinical stage I, when modern staging has been performed accurately, while both treatment forms cannot prevent the progression of systemic disease in 10–15% of the patients, who in retrospect already had haematogenous metastases. These facts, combined with the side effects involved with RPLND and radiotherapy constitute the rationale for a surveillance policy following orchidectomy in patients in clinical stage I, with chemotherapy in reserve for those patients who develop progression of disease.

The Danish Testicular Carcinoma Study Group (DATECA Study Group) (Schultz et al., 1985) have performed a randomized study of retroperitoneal radiotherapy versus surveillance. From 1981 to 1983, seventy-six patients were randomized to irradiation and eighty-one patients to surveillance by an intensive follow-up programme with chest X-rays, abdominal CT-scans, and determinations of serum tumour markers for a period of 2 years after orchidectomy.

Ten (13%) patients on the radiotherapy arm and twenty-three (28%) patients on the surveillance arm developed progressive disease ($P < 0.05$). Median time to progression in the irradiated group was $4\frac{1}{2}$ months (range 2–16 months) and 4 months (range 1–34 months) in the surveillance group. In the irradiated group all relapses occurred outside the retroperitoneum, whereas in the surveillance group thirteen (57%) of the relapses were exclusively observed in the retroperitoneum. All thirty-three relapsing patients achieved no-evidence-of-disease (NED) status with induction chemotherapy consisting of cisplatin, vinblastine and bleomycin (PVB). By 1985, two patients have died from nonmalignant causes. There have been no deaths from malignant disease. The results of this study have led the DATECA Study Group to recommend the surveillance procedure as the standard approach in view of the small therapeutic advantage of radiotherapy and the enhanced toxicity when chemotherapy has to be given to relapsing patients, in addition to the unequivocal demonstration that irradiation is superfluous in 70–80% of the patients.

At the Royal Marsden Hospital (Peckham, 1985) between 1979 and 1984, 133 patients have been registered in a surveillance study following orchidectomy. The results have been reported for 105 patients with a minimum follow-up of 1 year. The protocol consisted of monthly visits in the first year, 2-monthly for the second year and 3-monthly for the third year. CT-scans of the abdomen were performed every 2 months only in the first year. Twenty-eight (27%) patients developed progressive disease. 35% of the relapsing patients had their metastases exclusively in the retroperitoneum. The median time to progression was 5 months (range 2–31 months) with twenty-four (86%) relapses occurring in the first year. One patient relapsed in the third year. By 1985 all patients were alive and 27/28 were free of disease. Based on the results of this study and the Danish one, the Medical Research Council of the United Kingdom recommend the surveillance programme for patients with clinical stage I, provided that patient and physicians strictly adhere to the requirements of such a protocol.

At the National Cancer Institute in Milan (Pizzocaro et al., 1986) between 1981 and 1983, fifty-nine patients were entered on a surveillance protocol. The results have been reported after a minimum follow-up period of 18 months. Eighteen (31%) patients developed progression of disease; fifteen (83%) within the first year, two in the second year and one in the third year. The median time to progression was 6 months (range 2–36 months). Retroperitoneal lymph node metastases as the only site of relapse appeared in eight (44%) patients. Four (22%) of eighteen patients had retroperitoneal masses > 5 cm. Serum tumour markers were elevated in 67% of the relapses. Seventeen (94%) of eighteen patients achieved CR following induction chemotherapy or surgery (two patients with lymph nodes < 6 cm). One patient refused therapy and died. Fifty-eight (98%) of fifty-nine patients had NED at the time of analysis (30 June 1985).

These investigators feel that the surveillance procedure is a difficult time and money consuming procedure, in which patients are in particular exposed to the risk of retroperitoneal metastases which may not be detected until they have become bulky. Therefore they recommend a unilateral RPLND as the standard approach for all patients without intraoperative evidence of (micro)metastases. They have performed this type of surgery in sixty-one patients and have not observed retroperitoneal relapses, whereas ejaculation was preserved in 87% of the cases.

The view of the Milan Cancer Institute is supported by investigators from the Norwegian Radium Hospital (Fosså & Ous, 1985), who performed unilateral RPLND in seventy-five pathological stage I patients. Three patients developed progressive disease (one lung, two markers). Seventy-two patients (96%) remain disease-free after a median follow-up of 2 years. Of note, none of thirty-three patients with right-sided dissection and thirteen (33%) of forty with left-sided dissection had anejaculation.

A multicentre German testicular cancer study group (Bonn Testicular Cancer Study Group) (Weissbach et al., 1984) have performed unilateral RPLND in fifty-five patients, four (9%) of whom relapsed, a similar rate as compared to fourteen (13%) relapses in 132 patients who had been treated with bilateral dissection. Presently, a randomized multicentre German study of unilateral versus bilateral RPLND is under way.

For those who do not participate, the Bonn Group recommend a unilateral dissection as the standard approach, although they admit that the surveillance procedure may also be attractive in clinical stage I patients with good prognosis characteristics.

In 1986 the EORTC Genitourinary Tract Cancer Research Group (EORTC GU Group) has initiated a registration study for patients with clinical stage I to be closely surveilled. The reasons for such a study are (1) to prevent laxity with regard to follow-up examinations, and (2) to pool large numbers of patients to enable a reliable analysis of prognostic characteristics which predict a high probability of progression of disease. Putative factors of prognostic significance are histology, pT (post-surgical assessment of extent of tumour) category, invasion of lymphatic and blood vessels, tumour marker staining in the orchidectomy specimen, pre-orchidectomy serum concentration of markers, and scrotal violation. So far, the literature suggests that malignant teratoma, undifferentiated (MTU), pT3–4, and vascular invasion may be factors of poor prognosis, correlated with an increased risk of progression of disease.

In conclusion, in Europe, there is a trend in favour of the surveillance procedure in patients with clinical stage I, provided that doctor and patient comply to the strict requirements of follow-up for a period of 3 years. The main goal of ongoing studies is to identify factors of poor prognosis which predict a high probability of progression of disease. If such a subset of patients can be identified, they are probably candidates for a short term of induction chemotherapy (two cycles) adjuvant to orchidectomy.

Seminoma

A surveillance programme is more difficult to accomplish for seminoma than for nonseminoma patients, because of the lack of serum tumour markers such as β-hCG and AFP (although LDH and placental alkaline phosphatase (PlAP) may be of some help) in addition to the fact that the patients are at risk of relapse for a longer period of time, up to 5 years. Until now, only the Royal Marsden Hospital investigators have embarked on such a study (Peckham, 1985). Elsewhere in Europe, radiotherapy to the para-aortic and ipsilateral para-iliac lymph nodes ('dog-leg' field) is considered standard treatment. Mediastinal and supraclavicular irradiation for clinical stage I have been abandoned.

STAGE II

Nonseminoma

Clinical stage II is defined as metastatic disease to the retroperitoneal lymph nodes. The most important stratification within this stage is between high volume metastases (HVM) and low volume metastases (LVM). Definitions differ between surgico-pathological and clinical staging systems as well as between investigators with regard to their opinion on what is LVM or HVM. For example, some call retroperitoneal lymph node metastases > 5 cm high volume, whereas others think that the cut-off point is 10 cm.

There is consensus throughout the world that unresectable stage II tumours should be treated with induction chemotherapy and debulking surgery in case of residual tumour in marker-negative patients.

The therapeutic approach to resectable stage II is open for discussion. The U.S.A. Intergroup is performing a study of bilateral RPLND with a randomization for adjuvant chemotherapy with two cycles of PVB or VAB-6 (cyclophosphamide, vinblastine, bleomycin, cisplatin, actinomycin) versus no further treatment (Williams *et al.*, 1986). Forty-eight (49%) of ninety-eight patients on the observation arm relapsed: two died despite adequate chemotherapy, one committed suicide and one died after refusal of chemotherapy. Six (6%) of patients on the adjuvant chemotherapy arm relapsed: five before the start of chemotherapy. One patient died despite salvage chemotherapy. Since the survival results in both arms are similar, the results of this study can be used to argue in favour of each treatment approach.

Traditionally, RPLND has not been favoured in Europe, with the exception of a few institutes. In most countries, radiotherapy has been omitted even for early stage II and most patients will receive induction chemotherapy in all substages of stage II. RPLND is occasionally performed in the few patients with retroperitoneal lymph node metastases < 2 cm in diameter. If RPLND is attempted in stage II with lymph node metastases > 2 cm, adjuvant chemotherapy is usually administered.

At the National Cancer Institute in Milan (Pizzocaro & Monfardini, 1984) RPLND is attempted in all stage II patients. In twenty-six patients with lymph node metastases ≤ 5 cm without macroscopic extranodal extension, the progression rate was 35%, and eight of nine patients could be cured with chemotherapy. However, seven patients with more extensive retroperitoneal metastases all relapsed after RPLND. These data have led the Milan investigators to withhold adjuvant chemotherapy after RPLND, with the exception of the latter category of patients who are treated with four cycles of PVB after surgery.

In conclusion, patients with stage II will be treated with induction chemotherapy in most European institutes. The EORTC protocols for induction chemotherapy of disseminated disease accept all subcategories of stage II.

Seminoma
Patients with stage II are usually treated with radiotherapy to the retroperitoneal region, with the exception of bulky disease. At the Royal Marsden Hospital (Ball, Bassett & Peckham, 1982), twenty-three patients with retroperitoneal lymph nodes > 5 cm in diameter had a 5-year disease-free survival following radiotherapy of less than 60%. This has led the investigators to recommend radiotherapy for stage I and II A and B (lymph nodes smaller than 2 cm and 5 cm, respectively) and to give induction chemotherapy for higher stages.

ADVANCED DISEASE

Nonseminoma
The three most widely used induction chemotherapy regimens are BEP (bleomycin, etoposide, cisplatin), PVB and VAB-6. With these regimens 70% long-term disease-free survival is obtained. However, the results in patients with bulky disease (HVM) are worse than in patients with small metastases (LVM). In the EORTC studies HVM is defined as lymph node metastases > 5 cm in diameter, or lung metastases > 2 cm. The CR rate following four cycles of PVB induction chemotherapy was 87% for LVM as compared to 60% for HVM, whereas the difference in 3-year survival was 15% to the disadvantage of HVM (Stoter *et al.*, 1986a,b). Also, patients with high serum concentrations of tumour markers have a worse prognosis. In the EORTC experience in two subsequent protocols using PVB or BEP or an alternating regimen of PVB and BEP, patients with β-hCG levels above 10,000 ng/ml consistently have a CR rate below 25%. Most investigators agree that the most important prognostic factors are the volume of metastatic disease and the concentration of serum markers (Stoter *et al.*, 1987). On the basis of these prognostic variables, patients can be divided into good risk and bad risk categories. The main goal of research is to decrease the intensity and toxicity of

chemotherapy in good risk patients and to intensify the treatment in bad risk patients. The toxic death rate with standard regimens varies from 3% to 5% (Stoter et al., 1986a,b; Williams et al., 1985).

The EORTC (Stoter et al., 1986a,b) has confirmed the Indiana University data that the lower dose of vinblastine of 0.3 mg/kg/cycle is as effective as the higher dose. Meanwhile, the Milan investigators have demonstrated that an even lower dose of 0.2 mg/kg/cycle is effective in good risk patients (Pizzocaro et al., 1986). The deletion of bleomycin does not jeopardize the therapeutic results as has been shown by the Australasian Germ Cell Neoplasm Trial Group (Levi et al., 1986), and the Memorial Sloan-Kettering Cancer Center investigators (Bosl, Bajorin & Leitner, 1986). The preliminary results of an ongoing EORTC trial appear to confirm these data.

In patients with a poor prognosis the treatment is being intensified. Most studies are either still ongoing or have only been published in abstract form. At NCI, the preliminary results of a randomized comparison of standard PVB with PVeBV, including cisplatin 40 mg/m^2 i.v. days 1–5 and VP-16 100 mg/m^2 i.v. days 1–5, suggest improved results with the latter combination (Ozols et al., 1984). In a BEP study at the Finsen Institute (Daugaard & Rørth, 1986) cisplatin 40 mg/m^2 i.v. days 1–5, VP-16 200 mg/m^2 i.v. days 1–5 and bleomycin 15 mg/m^2 i.v. weekly was administered to twenty-two previously untreated patients with poor prognosis characteristics. Nineteen (86%) patients achieved CR, seventeen (77%) remain disease-free after 1+ to 19+ months. Bone-marrow toxicity, ototoxicity and nephrotoxicity was severe, including three (14%) toxic deaths. At Hannover University (Schmoll et al., 1986) similar results (70% NED) were demonstrated with a medium high dose BEP regimen, including cisplatin 35 mg/m^2 i.v. days 1–5 and VP-16 120 mg/m^2 i.v. days 1–5. Remarkably, the Milan investigators (Pizzocaro et al., 1985) have achieved identical results (83% NED) in a comparable group of patients with standard BEP: bleomycin 30 mg i.v. weekly, VP-16 100 mg/m^2 i.v. days 1–5 and cisplatin 20 mg/m^2 i.v. days 1–5.

Investigators at Memorial Sloan-Kettering Cancer Center (Leitner et al., 1985) have failed to demonstrate a benefit from alternating treatment with VAB-6 (no VP-16) and EP (VP-16 + cisplatin). A retrospective comparison with VAB-6 alone showed an identical 45% CR rate in both studies. The EORTC (Stoter et al., 1986a,b) has performed a randomized comparison of four cycles of BEP versus an alternating regimen of PVB and BEP for a total of four cycles. No superiority of PVB/BEP could be demonstrated.

Only recently, studies with bone marrow ablative high dose chemotherapy have started (Pico et al., 1985). The preliminary results in heavily pretreated patients with refractory disease justify further clinical research in this direction.

In conclusion, the approach to the treatment of LVM disease is shorter induction treatment with fewer drugs and lesser amounts of drugs and the replacement of drugs by less toxic agents. In contrast, the tendency in HVM is more intensive treatment. However, the studies reported so far are either negative or inconclusive.

Conclusion

Nonseminoma

The European approach to stage I will probably grow into the direction of surveillance programmes in the framework of registration studies to enable the recognition of a possible subset of patients with a high probability of progressive disease, for whom it may be more optimal to give a short term of induction chemotherapy after orchidectomy.

The European strategy to stage II is generally induction chemotherapy with debulking surgery for patients with residual tumour, with the possible exception of patients with small retroperitoneal lymph node metastases < 2 cm, who may be candidates for (unilateral) RPLND.

In patients with disseminated disease, much emphasis is placed on the analysis of prognostic variables to select prospectively patients who are good risk (less aggressive treatment) and bad risk (more intensive treatment). If poor risk patients can be identified with a sufficient degree of specificity (i.e. patient will not achieve CR), it is ethically justified to expose them to intensive experimental therapy, including first-line ablative chemotherapy with autologous bone marrow transplantation. Since testicular cancer is a rare disease and poor risk patients form the minority of them, it is important to standardize classification systems of histology and extent of disease, and to have uniformity in assays for marker determination. This will allow multi-institutional prospectively randomized studies; the only way to prove whether or not these patients will benefit from intensified therapy. The available results from recent phase II studies are at best inconclusive.

Seminoma

It is unclear whether stage I patients will be suitable candidates for surveillance after orchidectomy because of the lack of reliable tumour markers and a prolonged period (up to 5 years) in which the patients are at risk of progression of disease, whereas 30 Gy of radiotherapy to the retroperitoneal lymph nodes produces a nearly 100% cure rate.

There is much disagreement in Europe with respect to stage II patients. There seems to be a tendency towards chemotherapy for patients with retroperitoneal lymph node metastases > 5 cm. Seminoma appears to be at least as sensitive to cisplatin-based chemotherapy as nonseminoma. It is likely that in Europe in the near future radiotherapy will be given only to patients with stage I and stage II with lymph nodes ≤ 5 cm, whereas all other stages will be treated with chemotherapy. The role of radiotherapy and surgery after chemotherapy is unclear.

Acknowledgement

The author is indebted to Mrs A. Sugiarsi for typing the manuscript.

References

Ball, B., Barrett, A. & Peckham (1982) The management of metastatic seminoma testis. *Cancer*, **50**, 2289–2294.

Bosl, G. J., Bajorin, D. & Leitner, S. (1986) A randomized trial of etoposide (E) + cisplatin (P) and VAB-6 in the treatment of "good risk" patients with germ cell tumors. *Proceedings of the American Society for Clinical Oncology*, **5**, 104.

Daugaard, G. & Rørth, M. (1986) High-dose cisplatin and VP-16 with bleomycin in the management of advanced metastatic germ cell tumors. *European Journal of Cancer and Clinical Oncology*, **22**, 477–485.

Fosså, S. D. & Ous, S. (1985) In: *Testicular Cancer* (ed. by S. Khoury and R. Küss), p. 319. Alan R. Liss, New York.

Leitner, S. P., Israel, A. M., Bosl, G. L. & Schneider, R. J. (1985) Treatment of poor prognosis germ cell tumors with alternating cycles of VP-16/cisplatin and VAB-6: an update. *Proceedings of the American Society for Clinical Oncology*, **4**, 104.

Levi, J., Raghavan, D., Harvey, V., Thomson, D., Gill, G., Byrne, M., Burns, I. & Woods, R. (1986) Deletion of bleomycin from therapy for good prognosis advanced testicular cancer: a prospective randomized study. *Proceedings of the American Society for Clinical Oncology*, **5**, 97.

Ozols, R. F., Ihde, B., Jacob, J., Steiss, R., Veach, S. R., Wesley, M. & Young, R. C. (1984) Randomized trial of PVeBV (high dose cisplatin, vinblastin, bleomycin, VP-16) versus PVeB in poor prognosis non-seminomatous testicular cancer. *Proceedings of the American Society for Clinical Oncology*, **3**, 155.

Peckham, M. J. (1985) Surveillance following orchidectomy for clinical stage I testicular germ-cell malignancy. *Acta Urologica Belgica*, **53**, 155–164.

Peckham, M. J., McElwain, T. J., Barrett, A. & Hendry, W. F. (1979) The combined management of malignant teratoma of the testis. *Lancet*, **ii**, 267–270.

Pico, J. L., Droz, J. P., Goyette, A., Beaujean, E., Kamonier, D., Laplaige, P., Baume, D., Amiel, J. L. & Hayat, M. (1985) High dose chemotherapy followed by autologous bone marrow transplantation for poor prognosis non-seminomatous germ cell tumors. *Proceedings of the American Society for Clinical Oncology*, **4**, 108.

Pizzocaro, G. & Monfardini, S. (1984) No adjuvant chemotherapy in selected patients with pathologic stage II non-seminomatous germ cell tumors of the testis. *Journal of Urology*, **131**, 677–680.

Pizzocaro, G., Salvioni, R. & Piva, L. (1986) Successful treatment of good risk metastatic testicular cancer with cisplatin, bleomycin and 0.2 mg/kg vinblastine. *Proceedings of the American Society for Clinical Oncology*, **5**, 97.

Pizzocaro, G., Zanoni, F., Milani, A., Salvioni, R., Piva, L., Pilotti, S., Bombardieri, E., Tesoro-Tess, J. D. & Musumeci, R. (1986) Orchidectomy alone in clinical stage I non-seminomatous testis cancer: a critical appraisal. *Journal of Clinical Oncology*, **4**, 35–40.

Pizzocaro, G., Zanoni, F., Salvioni, R., Piva, L. & Milani, A. (1985) High complete remission rate with cisplatin, etoposide, bleomycin (BEP) and surgery in poor prognosis germ cell tumors of the testis. *Proceedings of the American Society for Clinical Oncology*, **4**, 110.

Schmoll, H. J., Arnold, A., Bergmann, L., Illiger, J., Preiss, J., Pfreundschuh, M. & Fink, U. (1986) Effective chemotherapy in testicular cancer with bulky disease: platinum ultra high dose/VP-16/bleomycin. *Proceedings of the American Society for Clinical Oncology*, **5**, 102.

Schultz, H. P., Rørth, M., von der Maase, H., Sandberg, E., Pedersen, M. & the Dateca Study Group (1985) Results from recent clinical trials in non-seminomatous testicular tumours. *Acta Urologica Belgica*, **53**, 234–242.

Stoter, G., Kaye, S., Sleijfer, D., Ten Bokkel Huinink, W., Jones, W., Van Oosterom, A., Splinter, T., Pinedo, H., Sylvester, R. & Keizer, J. (1986a) Preliminary results of BEP (bleomycin, etoposide, cisplatin) versus an alternating regimen of BEP and PVB (cisplatin, vinblastine, bleomycin) in high volume metastatic (HVM) testicular non-seminomas. An EORTC study. *Proceedings of the American Society for Clinical Oncology*, **5**, 106.

Stoter, G., Sleijfer, D. Th., Ten Bokkel Huinink, W. W., Kaye, S. B., Jones, W. G., Van Oosterom, A. T., Vendrik, C. P. J., Spaander, S., de Pauw, M. & Sylvester, R. (1986b) High dose versus low dose vinblastine in cisplatin-vinblastine-bleomycin (PVB) combination chemotherapy of non-seminomatous testicular cancer: a randomized study of the EORTC Genito-Urinary Tract Cancer Cooperative Group. *Journal of Clinical Oncology* (in press).

Stoter, G., Sylvester, R., Sleijfer, D. Th., Ten Bokkel Huinink, W. W., Kaye, S. B., Jones, W. G., Van Oosterom, A. T., Vendrik, C. P. J., Spaander, P. & de Pauw, M. (1987) Multivariate analysis of prognostic variables in patients with disseminated non-seminomatous testicular cancer: results from an EORTC multi-institutional phase III study. *International Journal of Andrology*, **10**, 239–246.

Weiss, R. B., Stablein, D. M., Muggia, F. M., Einhorn, L. H., Stephens, R. L., Spaulding, J. T. & De Wijs, W. D. for the Testicular Cancer Intergroup Study (1986) Toxicity of chemotherapy as adjuvant or salvage treatment in early stage non-seminomatous testicular cancer (NSTC). *Proceedings of the American Society for Clinical Oncology*, **5**, 99.

Weisbach, L., Boedefeld, E. A., Oberdörster, W. & Vahlensieck, W. (1984) Therapy in stage I non-seminomatous testicular tumor. A critical review of current strategies. *European Journal of Urology*, **10**, 1–9.

Wiliams, S., Einhorn, L., Greco, A., Birch, R. & Irwin, L. (1985) Disseminated germ cell tumors: a comparison of cisplatin plus bleomycin plus either vinblastine (PVB) or VP-16 (BEP). *Proceedings of the American Society for Clinical Oncology*, **4**, 100.

Williams, S., Muggia, F., Einhorn, L., Hahn, R., Donohue, J., Brunner, K., Stablein, D., De Wijs, W., Crawford, D. & Spaulding, J. for the Testicular Cancer Intergroup Study (1986) Resected stage II testicular cancer: immediate adjuvant chemotherapy versus observation. *Proceedings of the American Society for Clinical Oncology*, **5**, 98.

Discussion

Rørth With modern therapy how does the prognosis of seminoma compare with nonseminomatous germ cell tumours, and what improvements have occurred over the last decade?

Stoter Today, stage for stage seminoma and nonseminoma carry a similar prognosis. Advanced seminoma is uncommon and does not usually respond to radiotherapy. The prognosis of advanced seminoma is much better when chemotherapy is used as first line therapy.

Tumour stage	5 year survival rate (%)		
	1973*		1986
	Seminoma	Nonseminoma	Seminoma/nonseminoma
I	90–95	90	~100
II	70	50	98
III	5–10	5–10	~80

* *From*: Main J. G. & Sulak, M. H. (1973) Radiation therapy in malignant testis tumors. *Cancer*, **32**, 1212–1216.

Biology of germ cell tumours: concluding remarks

M. NIEMI *Department of Anatomy, University of Turku, Turku, Finland*

The present 'state of the art' of testicular cancer is somewhat paradoxical. On the one hand, the disease can be detected early with a great degree of accuracy, and effectively treated. In fact the most remarkable change since the first Workshop on Testicular Cancer (1980) has been the very substantial increase in the number of patients who can be completely cured (95%). On the other hand, our knowledge of the aetiology of testicular cancer and of the early steps in carcinogenesis and differentiation of the primordial germ cells, is still extremely poor. Virtually no significant progress in these fields has been made during the past 6 year period.

Therefore, one noticed with satisfaction during the present workshop that there are now several laboratories which have made efforts to apply modern techniques of genetics, cell culture and histo- and cytochemistry to elucidate the biological nature of normal and malignant germ cells. Although many of the new techniques are promising and one may look forward with some enthusiasm, it became clear during the debate in the workshop that classical histological techniques, when adequately applied and interpreted, still have an important role in testicular pathology. Dr Holstein's experience with well fixed (glutaraldehyde for a short time) testicular tissue and semithin (1 µm) sections demonstrates that the quality of testicular histology can be markedly improved with relatively simple measures. If these techniques can be widely accepted and properly used we will certainly be able to gather in the future comparable information on a wide collection of normal and malignant human tissues. More detailed information is certainly needed about the morphology of the embryonic germ cells as well as about abnormal but benign changes in mature type A spermatogonia and primary spermatocytes.

In the 1980 workshop the concept of carcinoma-in-situ (CIS) germ cells was still fresh and caused only 'considerable interest'. The concept has been well established during the present workshop and there have been no doubts that it is a pre-invasive state, which ultimately leads to invasive cancer, although the 'incubation' period may be several years.

Whether the carcinoma-in-situ germ cells arise through a malignant transformation from spermatogonia or whether they exist in the susceptible testis from early days of embryonic life is still a matter of debate. It was therefore of interest that the 'father' of the CIS concept, Dr Skakkebæk, took a strong stand in favour of the latter explanation. If this can be proven to be the case, then another hypothesis of Dr Skakkebæk will have strong support, namely that the CIS gonocytes may regress to totipotent embryonic cells and hence give rise to all kinds of testicular germ cell tumours except spermatocytic seminoma.

Although there were some differing opinions in the workshop about adequate or appropriate nomenclature, this type of debate was not at all as exhaustive as it often is when the pathologists alone are debating their classifications. Nevertheless, evidence was brought about to show that the term 'seminoma' ('semen tumour') is indeed a misnomer and should be replaced by 'gonocytoma'. Consequently carcinoma-in-situ should be renamed 'gonocytoma-in-situ'. Independently of whether this change in terminology can be effected (could a working group be assembled?), it became clear that cases where the malignant germ cells have occupied the whole tubule, although not invaded out of them, should be called 'intratubular seminomas' (gonocytomas) and not carcinomas-in-situ.

One of the most significant new innovations since the first workshop has been the introduction of placental alkaline phosphatase (PlAP) as a marker of malignant transformation of the germ cells. In many of the photomicrographs shown during the workshop, and notably in those presented by Dr Hustin, it became obvious that we have in PlAP a very useful marker for the identification of CIS cells. The staining method will certainly find much use in, for example, detecting malignant germ cells in the spermatic cord and in the regional lymph nodes.

Of a great fundamental importance may be Dr Hustin's observation that PlAP is present in the embryonic germ cells only at stages preceding the formation of the first sex cords in the testicular anlage. Whether the stem cell for CIS cells is ultimately a transformed primordial germ cell instead of a gonocyte remains to be shown.

Recent immunological studies have indicated that the haematopoietic system, the nervous system and the gonads may share some antigenic properties. The migration of the stem cells of these systems in the early embryos is therefore getting renewed interest and we listened with enthusiasm to the description by Dr Friedman about the function and route of the primordial germ cells into extragonadal tissues.

New useful markers for normal and malignant germ cells are to be expected in due course, but the intermediate filament proteins seem already to be available as tools for characterization of testicular tumours. They may also give evidence as to the nature of the ultimate stem cell of the testicular CIS cells.

The workshop was held at a time which could perhaps be called a period of gene engineering. So much hope and enthusiasm is directed to the use of various molecular manipulations at the cellular level that it was only natural that genes and the oncogenes in particular were a main topic in the workshop. The future seems very exciting indeed: in the germinal tumours not only the transcripts of many genes but also their ultimate protein products can be identified, which certainly brings the classification of the tumours to a molecular level, and also may open new avenues for understanding the carcinogenesis of testicular tumours.

The biology of any human cancer form is difficult to study because of the scarcity of the material and the interference by various pre-operative treatment procedures. Therefore tissue brought into *in vitro* culture is extremely valuable and during the workshop we learned about several human testicular tumour cell lines which are available and useful, for example, in studies where the effect of new chemotherapeutic agents are going to be tested. Cultured cell lines can be transferred into nude mice to induce solid tumours, which might be even more sensible targets for cytotoxic trials. Tumour cell lines apparently are useful also for giving evidence of the hormone production of the cancer cells and may in due course lead to the finding of new markers for monitoring the development of human tumours *in-situ*.

As in other cancer forms the cell surface molecules of the normal and malignant germ cells are of utmost importance for the understanding of the appearance and development of the malignant transformation. The use of specific monoclonal antibodies for mapping the molecules on the outer surface of the cell membrane seems to be very promising. The glycolipid antigens identified by Dr Andrews on human embryonal carcinoma cells serve as a model along which further studies on the differentiation of the germ cells should be designed.

Another new technique which has already proved useful for producing significant new results is flow cytometry. The fact that normal paraffin-embedded sections can be enzymatically dispersed for analysis opens wide perspectives for the use of this sophisticated technology for cancer studies. As Dr Sledge showed, a flow cytometric analysis of tumour tissue may give information about prognosis and choice of treatment of the patients.

Clinical aspects of carcinoma-in-situ (CIS): concluding remarks

T. B. HARGREAVE *Department of Surgery/Urology, Western General Hospital, Edinburgh, Scotland*

The morning of the second day of the meeting was devoted to clinical aspects of carcinoma-in-situ (CIS) and the Danish experience was presented. There is now no doubt that this lesion exists but we must be cautious before extrapolating the Danish findings to other countries because the total experience is still limited to small numbers of patients and there could possibly be local environmental factors.

It is clear, however, that when carcinoma-in-situ is diagnosed there is a high chance of progression to testicular tumour (seminoma and nonseminoma) and furthermore preliminary results presented by Dr von der Maase suggest that this progression can be prevented by low dose radiotherapy (20 Gy to the involved testis). This report of radiotherapy treatment should make us think again about programmes to detect CIS because we now have a more acceptable method of treatment. Almost certainly there has been a reluctance to search for CIS for the following reasons: firstly, because treatment up till now has been castration and this is hard for patients to accept and difficult for doctors to recommend; secondly, because testicular biopsy may leave small scars which are later felt as nodules making follow-up clinical examination difficult to interpret; and thirdly, because of a lack of awareness amongst clinicians of CIS.

Following the report of radiotherapy treatment for CIS and the lack of side effects, it should now be easier to set up further investigative programmes in Denmark and other countries to define the true role of CIS. Some aspects of the problem that need further work are:

Who to screen. The Danish experience is that CIS may be detected in the contralateral testis in 5.7% of patients with unilateral testicular malignancy and biopsy of the contralateral testis would seem indicated. We do not know if CIS is effectively treated by platinum-based combination chemotherapy although it is very likely that it is. If so, biopsy may only be necessary in those patients who are unliklely to require chemotherapy. Thus, contralateral biopsy could be taken at the same time as the orchidectomy if the surgeon believes the testicular tumour to be localized (negative chest X-ray and negative abdominal ultrasound before the original orchidectomy). This policy would result in some unnecessary biopsies because later CT scans would reveal abdominal nodes but has the advantage that both biopsy and orchidectomy could be performed under the same anaesthetic. The Danish experience is that carcinoma-in-situ is found in a high percentage of patients with gonadal dysgenesis, androgen insensitivity and 45,X0/46,XY karyotype, and there can now be no doubt that bilateral testicular biopsy is indicated for these patients. More difficult to define is the role of biopsy in patients with a history of testicular maldescent or infertility, or both. Studies are needed to evaluate whether the apparent increased risk associated with infertility (1.1% of unselected Danish infertility testicular biopsies) is accounted for by testicular maldescent or whether other subgroups can be defined. Poor sperm analysis, low testicular volume (<10 ml), history of a testis shrinking and then expanding, and testicular pain may all be additional indicators of CIS in infertility and maldescent patients. Furthermore there is a need to distinguish testicular maldescent into those testes which have passed through the external inguinal ring and lie in the superficial inguinal pouch from other maldescended testes (in the inguinal canal or intra-abdominal).

When to screen. There was some evidence that CIS may be present at an early age (2 months in a baby with gonadal dysgenesis and 10 years in a boy with maldescent). If this is true, screening of any at-risk population should be attempted before the age at which testicular tumours appear (<15 years). Further information is needed about the occurrence of CIS in boys and male babies. This also raises the question of whether CIS is a precursor lesion for all testicular tumours and not an acquired lesion.

How to screen. Testicular biopsy remains the only method of screening but less invasive methods would be desirable. Currently used serum markers are negative in patients with CIS and cannot be used. Ultrasound and nuclear magnetic resonance may be useful, but further information is needed. Testicular biopsy is not without problems and in particular further evaluation of sampling error is needed. It must also be remembered that when investigating infertile patients other information may be needed – for example, information about the appearance of the testis, rete testis, epididymis and vas deferens, and in these cases small stab biopsies or Trucut needle biopsies are not adequate. In previously unoperated cases, testicular biopsy should include any small areas of scar tissue as carcinoma-in-situ is more likely to be found in these areas, but if a previous testicular biopsy has been performed then the scar from that previous biopsy should be avoided otherwise the pathologist may not be able to comment about whether any residual CIS remains or not.

Testicular cancer and fertility. Now that up to 95% of men with testicular cancer can be offered curative therapy, there is increased interest in post-treatment fertility. Data presented by Drs Berthelsen and Rustin suggest that up to 20% of men may have subfertility before any treatment and this must be taken into account before infertility is attributed to the treatment. Chemotherapy is damaging, however, and evidence from hormonal studies is consistent with damage to the gonad and preservation of normal pituitary function, as would be expected. More contentious is the possibility of genetic abnormality in any children fathered after chemotherapy. It is worth noting from Dr Fried's presentation that there may be abnormalities in children conceived before chemotherapy and therefore we must be very careful before ascribing any genetic risk to cancer chemotherapy. Currently there is no evidence of any increase in the incidence of fetal abnormality in children fathered after treatment of testicular cancer, although very large numbers would be needed to detect a small risk.

Treatment of germ cell tumours: concluding remarks

N. J. VOGELZANG *Section of Hematology/Oncology, University of Chicago Medical Center, Chicago, Illinois, USA*

Several dogmas in the treatment of testicular cancer were challenged and others were confirmed at the Copenhagen Workshop on testicular cancer.

In clinical stage I nonseminoma Peckham *et al.*, Rørth *et al.* and Oliver confirmed a 30% relapse rate with two-thirds of the patients having retroperitoneal disease at relapse when observation alone was offered. Apparently 97–100% of patients will be salvaged yet concern persists regarding the widespread use of surveillance approach because of the following factors:
1 Late relapses (>3 years);
2 Prolonged reliance upon a high level of patient compliance;
3 High cost and variable reliability of noninvasive assessments of the retroperitoneum;
4 Marker negative relapses;
5 Complications associated with the retroperitoneal relapse (i.e. need for resection of postchemotherapy teratoma);
6 Relative ease and safety of a unilateral or bilateral retroperitoneal lymph node dissection when performed by experienced urologists.
Follow-up reports on all surveillance studies will be vital.

In clinical stage I seminoma a 12% relapse rate (to date) with observation only may increase because of the prolonged time to relapse. The difficulty in assessing relapse by a marker-negative tumour in the retroperitoneum has been demonstrated.

The options open for treatment of clinical stage II tumours will continue to be a cause for concern and discussion. Dr Pizzocaro provided a timely warning that masses less than 3 cm visualized by CT scan or lymphangiogram should *not* be assumed to be metastases as 15–30% of such patients will not have pathological confirmation of metastases. The Testicular Cancer Intergroup Study results with two cycles of adjuvant PVB or VAB have been confirmed by Hartlapp *et al.* The relapse rate for pathological stage IIA may be lower than that for stage IIB disease. Observation following surgery continues to be warranted in these patients.

Stage III patients have an excellent prognosis with high dose cisplatin-based chemotherapy, i.e. ≥ 100 mg/m^2/course. However, much dispute remains as to which patients (if any) will die of their disease. The dispute is fuelled by several major factors:
1 Stage migration;
2 Physician experience and the 'learning curve';
3 The increased use of etoposide and ifosfamide as salvage and as initial therapy;

4 A more frequent and effective use of postchemotherapy surgery;
5 Variability in data base collection and reporting (i.e. hCG reports in mIU/ml, lack of LDH data, exclusion from the data base of certain clinical subgroups of patients, etc.).

There exist at least four to six formulas which can be easily used to estimate probability of complete remission. Given the precision and reproducibility of marker assays, formulas which utilize the continuum of marker values are preferred. The prognosis of marker-negative disease also appears to be related to a continuum of disease bulk and a usable formula should so reflect that fact. Future multivariate analyses of defined patient populations continue to be needed. Use of the existing formulations is strongly encouraged.

Drs Ozols, Schmoll and Daugaard reported apparent improvement in poor prognosis patients using ultra-high-dose platinum-based regimens — at the cost of substantial toxicity. Opposing opinions were expressed by Drs Pizzocaro and Einhorn. Precise comparisons of various 'poor risk' groups are impossible due to the bewildering diversity of selection factors. All future reports of poor risk patients must use the published prognostic formulations.

Late toxicity of treatment with cisplatin-based chemotherapy or radiotherapy continues to be a concern. The cisplatin-treated kidney and inner ear show long-term changes. Vascular toxicity remains fortunately a rare event. Fertility studies show recovery with time after both chemotherapy and irradiation.

Research in progress will elucidate the role of etoposide/cisplatin as compared to VAB-6 in good risk patients, the necessity of three or four cycles of cisplatin-based chemotherapy in good risk patients, the value of ultra-high dose platinum, VP-16 and bleomycin as compared to standard doses of the drugs in poor risk patients, ifosfamide's role in initial treatment of good and poor risk patients and the value of carboplatin-based therapy as compared to cisplatin-based therapy in poor risk patients. Lastly, the value of cisplatin alone compared to cisplatin-based chemotherapy in good risk patients will also be examined.

Author index

Abildgaard N.   203
Abildgaard U.   347
Amtorp O.   347
Andrews P.W.   95
Arnold H.   311
Atlas S.A.   353

Bagger-Sjöbäck D.   359
Bagshawe K.D.   301, 389
Bajorin D.   285
Bajorunas D.   381
Becker H.   1
Begent R.H.J.   301, 389
Bergmann L.   311
Berthelsen J.G.   19, 173, 203, 371
Boiesen P.   181
Bonfert B.   311
Bosl G.J.   285, 353, 381
Brada M.   247
Bruun E.   187, 199
Bussar-Maatz R.   277

Casper J.   105, 139
Casileth B.   385
Collette J.   29
Crawford S.M.   301

Daugaard G.   319, 347
De Pauw M.   239
DeLozier-Blanchet C.D.   69
Debruyne F.M.J.   51
Dikman S.   325
Dölken G.   311

Eble J.N.   115
Einhorn L.H.   115, 399
Engel E.   69
Engström B.   359
Engström W.   79
Evan G.   57

Feitz W.F.J.   51
Fenderson B.   95
Fink U.   311
Fonatsch C.   105
Franchimont P.   29
Fried P.   385
Friedman N.B.   43
Frimodt-Møller C.   187, 199

Geller N.L.   285
Giwercman A.   19, 173, 187, 191, 199, 209
Guttenplan J.   325

Hakamori S.-i.   95
Hansen H.H.   319
Hansen S.O.   203
Hargreave T.B.   221, 393, 421
Harstrick A.   139
Hartlapp J.H.   277
Hartmann M.   1
Hecht Th.   311
Hecker H.   311
Henriksen O.   191
Hirsch A.   359
Ho A.D.   311
Hoffmann L.   311
Holden L.   301
Holstein A.F.   1
Holstein-Rathlou N.H.   347
Hopkins B.   79
Hustin J.   29

Illiger J.   311

Jackobsen G.K.   121
Jensen H.   203
Jensen K.E.   191
Johansen B.   203
Jones W.G.   239

Kaulen H.   311
Kaye S.B.   239
Kennedy B.J.   363
Kjær L.   191

Laurell G.   359
Lehmann D.   163
Leitner S.P.   353
Lenz S.   187, 199
Leyssac P.P.   347

Malmi R.   157
Manegold C.   311
Mayr A.   311
Moel D.   325
Munck-Hansen J.   203
Müller Hj.   163
Müller J.   19, 147, 173, 209

Newlands E.S.   301, 389
Nielsen E.S.   255
Niemi M.   37, 169, 417

Oliver R.T.D.   85, 263
Østerlind A.   203
Ozols R.F.   291

425

Author index

Parkinson M.C. 147
Peckham M.J. 247
Pedersen K.V. 181
Pedersen M. 255
Pektasides D. 389
Pfreundschuh M. 311
Pizzocaro G. 269
Preibisz J.J. 353
Preiss J. 311
Pöllänen P. 37

Rabes H.M. 127
Ramaekers F.C.S. 51
Rasmussen L.H. 203
Rørth M. 255, 319
Roth B.J. 115
Rustin G.J.S. 301, 389

Safirstein R. 325
Samuels B.L. 363
Scheiner E. 353
Schmoll H.-J. 105, 139, 311
Schnaidt U. 105
Schofield P. 79
Schubert I. 311
Schultz H. 255
Schütte B. 1
Sealey J.E. 353
Sehested M. 121

Sikora K. 57
Skakkebæk N.E. 19, 147, 173, 187, 191, 199, 209
Sledge G.W. 115
Sleijfer D. Th. 239
Söderström K.-O. 157
Spaander P. 239
Steinfeld A. 385
Steinfeld R. 385
Stoter G. 239, 407
Sylvester R. 239

Ten Bokkel Huinink W.W. 239
Thomsen C. 191

Van Oosterom A.T. 239
Vaugnat P. 69
Vendrik C.P.J. 239
Vogelzang N.J. 225, 363, 423
Von der Maase H. 173, 209, 255

Walt H. 69
Watson J. 57
Weiss J. 311
Weissbach L. 277
Winston J. 325
Wuhrman B.P. 115

Zetterlund C.G. 181

Subject index

Advanced disease, treatment 311
AFP
  poor prognosis patients 225
  production in testicular tumour cell lines 105
Aldosterone levels in patients treated with chemotherapy 353
Alkaline phosphatase, embryonal carcinoma cells 95
Androgen insensitivity syndrome, CIS 176, 209
Aneuploidy, testicular cancer 57
Antisperm antibodies, CIS 163
Autoimmunity, testicular cancer 163

Bilateral testicular cancer
  age at diagnosis 203
  histology 203
  time lag between tumours 203
Biopsy, testicular
  complications 199
  screening for CIS 199, 173
Birth defects after radiation therapy 385
Bleomycin, lung toxicity 311
Bone metastases in patients with testicular cancer 225
Brain metastases, treatment 301

Carbohydrate antigens, SSEA-3, SSEA-4 95
Carcinoma-in-situ *see* CIS
Cell growth, oncogenetic control 57
Cell lines
  testicular cancer 95, 105, 139
    hormone production 105
Chemotherapy
  and CIS 209
  and fertility 391
Chromosomal changes
  after radio- and chemotherapy 391
  testicular cancer cells 69, 105
CIS cells
  androgen insensitivity syndrome 173
  antisperm antibodies 163
  chemotherapy 209
  contralateral testis, incidence of 173
  detected by magnetic resonance imaging 173, 191
  detected by ultrasound 173, 187
  glycoconjugates 157
  glycogen 19
  glycoproteins 163
  gonadal dysgenesis 173
  gonadoblastoma 19
  IgG 163
  incidence 173, 181, 209
  infertility 173
  invasive cancer 19
  irradiation therapy 209
  lectin binding 157, 163
  morphology
    in relation to gonocytes 19
    in relation to seminoma cells 19
  orchidectomy 95
  screening 173, 199
  somatosexual ambiguity 173
  spontaneous course 209
  staining for PlAP 19, 29
  testicular feminization syndrome 291
  undescended testis 173, 181
Cisplatin
  and ifosfamide salvage therapy 399
  and vinblastine salvage therapy 399
  and VP-16 salvage therapy 399
  antitumour activity in xenografts 29
  cardiovascular toxicity 353
  effect on glomerular filtration rate 325, 347
  effect on LH, FSH and testosterone 381
  effect on serum phosphorus 353
  haemodynamic effect 325, 347
  high dose regimens 291, 311, 319
  hypomagnesaemia induction 325, 353
  mechanism of cytotoxicity 325
  nephrotoxicity 325, 347
  nephrotoxicity effect of frusemide 325
  nephrotoxicity effect of hypertonic solutions 325
  ototoxicity 359
  polyuria induction 325, 347
  renal excretion 325
  renal metabolism 325
  renal uptake 325
  toxicity of high dose 311
Cisplatin analogue, antitumour activity in xenografts 139
Concanavalin A 157
  binding to CIS cells 157, 163
Conception rates, before and after antineoplastic treatment 371
Contralateral testicle, incidence of testicular cancer 203
Cryopreservation of semen in patients with testicular cancer 371
Cryptorchid testis, staining for PlAP 29
Cryptorchidism
  carcinoma-in-situ detected by ultrasound 187
  incidence of CIS 173, 181

Subject index

Cytogenetics, testicular cancer 69
Cytokeratin
  normal testicular tissue 51
  testicular cancer tissue 51, 95

Desmin, testicular tissue 51
DNA content
  advanced germ cell tumours, prognostic value 115
  spermatocytic seminoma cells 147

Embryonal carcinoma
  biochemical cell properties 95
  cell lines
    human 95
    murine 95
  differentiation of cells in culture 95
Embryonal germ cells, morphology 1
Extragonadal germ cell tumours, proposed aetiology 43

Familial occurrence, testicular cancer 85
Feminization, testicular and CIS 173, 209
Fertility
  after chemotherapy for testicular cancer 371, 389
  after lymphadenectomy for testicular cancer 371
  after radiotherapy for testicular cancer 371
  before testicular cancer 371
Fetal germ cells, morphology 1
Fibronectin, embryonal carcinoma cells 95
Flow cytometry, DNA content in testicular cancer 115
FSH patients treated with chemotherapy 381

Genetic implications, radio- and chemotherapy 371, 385
Germ cells
  adult, staining for PlAP 29
  embryonal, staining for PlAP 29
  fetal, staining for PlAP 29
  glycoconjugates 157
  infantile, staining for PlAP 29
  lectin-binding sites 157
  morphological characterization 1
  normal ultrastructure 1
  primordial 43
Glycoconjugates
  CIS cells 157
  germ cells 157
  seminoma cells 157
Glycogen
  CIS cells 19
  germ cells 1, 19
Glycolipids, embryonal carcinoma cells 95
Glycoproteins, CIS cells 163
Glycosyltransferase, embryonal carcinoma cells 95
Gonadal dysgenesis and CIS 173
Gonadotrophins
  development of testicular cancer 19
  levels, patients treated with chemotherapy 381
Gonocyte morphology in relation to CIS cells 19
Gonocytoma (see also Seminoma) 19
Gonocytoma-in-situ (see also CIS) 19
Growth regulatory genes, malignant testicular tumour cells 79

hCG
  poor prognosis patients 225
  production, testicular tumour cell lines 105
High dose chemotherapy 291, 311, 319
HLA antigens
  familial germ cell tumour 85
  normal testicular tissue 37
  testicular cancer 85
HMG-CoA reductase gene, testicular cancer 79
HPA 157
Hypogonadism after chemotherapy 381
Hypomagnesaemia patients treated with cisplatin 325, 353

Ifosfamide salvage therapy 399
IGF II gene, testicular cancer 79
IgG, CIS cells 163
Immunological environment, normal testis 37
Incidence
  bilateral testicular cancer 203
  CIS 173, 181, 209
Infertility and CIS 173
Insulin gene, testicular cancer 79
Interferon, effect on embryonal carcinoma cells in culture 95
Intermediate filament protein
  normal testicular tissue 51
  testicular cancer 51
Irradiation therapy of CIS 209
Isochromosome 12p, testicular cancer 69

LDH, poor prognosis patients 225
LDL-receptor gene, testicular cancer 79
Lectin-binding sites in normal and malignant germ cells 157
Leydig cell, function after irradiation of the testis 209
LH patients treated with chemotherapy 381
Liver metastases, patients with testicular cancer 225
LSA 157
Lung metastases, patients with testicular cancer 225
Lymphadenectomy, stage IIA and IIB nonseminoma 269
Lymphocytes, normal testicular tissue 37

Macrophages, normal testicular tissue 37
Magnetic resonance imaging
  CIS 173, 191
  normal testis 191
maldescent, incidence of CIS 173, 181
MHC antigens, embryonal carcinoma 95
Morphology
  CIS cells 1, 19

Subject index 429

germ cells 1, 19
gonocytes 19
nonseminoma cells 1, 19
normal testicular tissue 1
seminoma cells 1, 19
Multivariate analysis 225, 239

Nephrotoxicity, cisplatin-based chemotherapy 325, 347, 353
Nonseminoma
lymphadenectomy in stage IIA and IIB 269
prognostic variables 239, 301
proliferation pattern 127
proliferation rate 127
relapse rate, stage I 247
stage II prognosis 277
staging 407
surveillance stage I 255
treatment of poor prognosis patients 291, 311, 319
treatment stage I 407
treatment stage II 277, 407
Nude mice, testicular cancer cells 105

Oestrogen, tumour marker 105
Oncogenes
c-myc 57
testicular cancer 57, 69
Oncoprotein level in relation to prognosis of testicular cancer 57
normal testicular tissue 57
p62-c-myc 57
testicular cancer 57
Ototoxicity induced by cisplatin 359

Pituitary–testicular axis, testicular cancer patients 381
Placental alkaline phosphatase *see* PlAP
Placental-like alkaline phosphatase *see* PlAP
PlAP
CIS cells 19, 29
cryptorchid testis 29
developing testis 29
immunohistochemical demonstration 19, 29
normal testicular tissue 29
serum concentration in seminoma patients 263
testicular cancer cells 29
Ploidy status, testicular cancer 57, 69, 115
PNA 157
Poor prognosis
identification of patients 225
treatment 291, 301, 319
Prognosis and oncoprotein level 57
Prognostic factors
disseminated testicular cancer 225, 239, 319
stage I testicular cancer 247
Prognostic variables, testicular cancer patients 285
Proliferation rate, testicular cancer 127

Radiation treatment, effect on offspring 385
Radiotherapy
and fertility 371
stage I nonseminoma 255
RCA I 157
Relapse rate
stage I nonseminoma 247
stage I seminoma 247
Renin levels in patients treated with cisplatin-based chemotherapy 353
Risk group, for CIS 173, 181, 209
Risk group assignment, patients with testicular cancer 285

SBA 157
Screening for CIS
methods 173
testicular biopsy 199
Seminoma
oncoproteins 363
proliferation pattern 127
relapse rate stage I 247
staging 407
surveillance of stage I patients 263
syncytiotrophoblast-like cells 121
treatment 407
Seminoma cells
glycoconjugates 157
lectin binding 157
morphology in relation to CIS cells 19
Seminoma, spermatocytic
histology of adjacent tissue 147
nuclear DNA distribution 147
pathogenesis 147
Somatosexual ambiguity and CIS 173
Spermatocytic seminoma *see* Seminoma, spermatocytic 19
Spermatocytoma *see* seminoma, spermatocytic 19
Spermatogenesis, patients with testicular cancer 371
Staging, testicular cancer 407
Steroid hormones
development of testicular cancer 19
production in testicular cancer cell lines 105
Surgery, stage IIA and IIB nonseminoma 269
Surveillance, stage I testicular cancer 247, 263
Syncytiotrophoblast-like cells, ultrastructure 121

Teratoma oncoprotein 57
Testosterone levels in patients treated with chemotherapy 381
Tumour markers
poor risk patients 285
production in testicular cancer cell lines 105

UEA I 157
Ultrasound detection of CIS 187, 209
Undescended testis, incidence of CIS 181

Vascular toxicity induced by combination chemotherapy 363

Vimentin
  normal testicular tissue 51
  testicular cancer tissue 51
VP-16
  high dose in bulky disease patient 311, 319
  high dose toxicity 311, 319
  salvage therapy 399

WGA 157

Xenografts, testicular cancer 139